57121

S0-BIQ-751

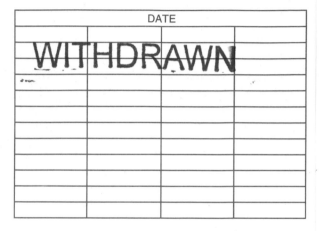

DATE		
WITHDRAWN		

BAKER & TAYLOR

Explaining epidemics and other studies in the history of medicine

This book brings together for the first time many of Professor Rosenberg's most important essays. The first two parts, which focus on ideas and institutions, are meant to underline interactions between these realms. The essays treat topics such as therapeutics and its relationship to social change in the nineteenth century; the practice of medicine in New York in the 1860s; and the rise and fall of the dispensary. The third part of the book focuses on the attempt to use history as a resource for discussion of a contemporary medical world that often seems out of control and in a semipermanent crisis – economic, organizational, and humane. The essays discuss themes that have become visible to the public: deinstitutionalization of the mentally ill and the status of psychiatry; the hospital as a social and economic problem; and the social negotiations surrounding AIDS.

Other books by Charles E. Rosenberg

The Cholera Years: The United States in 1832, 1849, and 1866 (1962; revised edition 1987)

The Trial of the Assassin Guiteau: Psychiatry and Law in the Gilded Age (1968)

No Other Gods: On Science and American Social Thought (1976)

The Care of Strangers: The Rise of America's Hospital System (1987)

Explaining epidemics and other studies in the history of medicine

CHARLES E. ROSENBERG

University of Pennsylvania

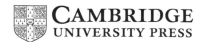

CAMBRIDGE UNIVERSITY PRESS

Published by the Press Syndicate of the University of Cambridge
The Pitt Building, Trumpington Street, Cambridge CB2 1RP
40 West 20th Street, New York, NY 10011–4211, USA
10 Stamford Road, Oakleigh, Victoria 3166, Australia

First published 1992

Printed in the United States of America

Library of Congress Cataloging-in-Publication Data

Rosenberg, Charles E.
  Explaining epidemics and other studies in the history of medicine /
  Charles E. Rosenberg.
      p.   cm.
  Includes index.
  Consists largely of Prof. Rosenberg's essays reprinted from various
sources.
  ISBN 0-521-39340-X (hardback). – ISBN 0-521-39569-0 (pbk.)
    1. Medicine – History – 19th century.   2. Epidemiology –
History – 19th century.   I. Title.
    [DNLM: 1. Delivery of Health Care – history – collected works.
2. Disease Outbreaks – history – collected works.   3. Socioeconomic
Factors – collected works.   WZ 40 R813e]
R149.R67   1992
610'.9'034 – dc20
DNLM/DLC
for Library of Congress   91-46538
                                                                          CIP

A catalog record for this book is available from the British Library.

ISBN 0-521-39340-X hardback
ISBN 0-521-39569-0 paperback

FOR
JESSICA

Contents

III The past in the present: Using medical history

Acknowledgments

I should like to thank the following publishers and journals for permission to reprint material: the Johns Hopkins University Press and the *Bulletin of the History of Medicine* for permission to reprint Chapters 2, 4, 7 and 10, which appeared in the *Bulletin* 57 (1983), 22–42; 63 (1989), 185–197; 41 (1967), 223–253; and 64 (1990), 163–186; the University of Pennsylvania Press for permission to reprint Chapter 1, which appeared in Morris J. Vogel and Charles E. Rosenberg, eds., *The Therapeutic Revolution. Essays in the Social History of American Medicine* (Philadelphia: University of Pennsylvania Press, 1979), pp. 3–25; the *Journal of the History of Medicine* for permission to reprint Chapter 8, which appeared in 29 (1974), 32–54; the University Press of Virginia for permission to reprint Chapter 11, which appeared in George Kriegman et al., eds., *American Psychiatry: Past, Present, and Future* (Charlottesville: University Press of Virginia, 1975), pp. 135–148; Watson Publishing International for permission to reprint Chapter 5, which appeared in Charles E. Rosenberg, ed., *Healing and History: Essays for George Rosen* (New York: Science History Publications, 1979), pp. 116–136; Rutgers University Press for permission to reprint Chapter 15, which appears (with some minor changes) as the introduction to Charles E. Rosenberg and Janet Golden, eds., *Framing Disease: Studies in Cultural History* (New Brunswick, N.J.: Rutgers University Press, 1992); *Daedalus*, Journal of the American Academy of Arts and Science, for permission to reprint Chapter 13, which appeared in 118/2 (1989), 1–17; the Milbank Memorial Fund, publisher of the *Milbank Quarterly*, for permission to reprint Chapters 9, 12, and portions of 15, which appeared in 60 (1982), 108–154; 64 (1986, supplement 1), 34–55; and 67 (1989, supplement 1), 1–15; *Comparative Studies in Society and History* for permission to reprint Chapter 6, which appeared in 8 (1966), 135–162; the College of Physicians of Philadelphia for permission to reprint Chapter 16, which appeared in their *Transactions & Studies* 12 (1990), 127–150; and the University of Tennessee Press for permission to reprint Chapter 3, which appeared in *Gunn's Domestic Medicine* by John C. Gunn (Knoxville:

University of Tennessee Press, 1986), pp. v–xxi. The general Introduction, Chapter 14, and headnotes for each chapter appear for the first time.

It would be difficult to thank everyone who has helped one way or another in the writing of these essays; mv obligations cover decades of editorial help, critical reading, and knowledgeable insights from teachers, students, colleagues, friends, and family. I would, however, like to acknowledge briefly the help I received from Shari Rudavsky and Susan Scholten in the preparation of this lengthy manuscript.

C.E.R.

Introduction: Why care about the history of medicine?

Medicine has always had its historians; but until recently it was a history written by and for practitioners. Until the early nineteenth century, in fact, history and practice could hardly be distinguished. Galen and Hippocrates could be and were used to bolster arguments about the nature of fever or the logic of a particular therapeutic choice. A learned physician read Latin and Greek, not simply to mystify the laity but to work with those master texts that still figured meaningfully in his intellectual life.

By the late nineteenth century, of course, the writings of classical and Hellenistic antiquity were no longer alive in the thought and practice of even educated practitioners. History had become quite clearly history – something in the past. This is not to suggest that interest in the medicine of previous eras disappeared. It remained and was to become gradually – if even today incompletely – an academic field. But the history of medicine was still populated almost entirely by scholars trained in medical schools, the great majority of whom made their living as physicians. They were fascinated with the past (or some aspect of it), especially a past that could be construed as progressing upward toward an enlightened and ethical present. The intellectual significance of particular individuals and events was seen, for example, in terms of their relationship to the development of a contemporary understanding of the body and not to the particular historical context in which those individuals worked and thought. Thus William Harvey was to be understood as a founder of modern experimental physiology and not as a man of the seventeenth century, a Royalist and neo-Platonist.

An interest in medicine's history served also in the late nineteenth and early twentieth centuries as one badge of allegiance to the profession's humane and humanistic craft tradition, to the vision of the profession as art, not science. Scholarship in the history of medicine could attest to a gentleman's learning and experience, attributes different from and in some ways superior to the mechanical skills and one-dimensional certainties of the laboratory. The origins of medical history as an institutionalized academic field lie in the twentieth century and took place on the Continent;

I

but the leaders of this incipient professionalization were still products of
the profession's humanist tradition – physicians trained in an era in which a
well-educated practitioner might still be presumed to have a familiarity
with classical languages and literature, philosophy, ethics, and general
history.[1]

Medicine remained a marginal subject matter among academic practitioners of the new "scientific" history – holders of the doctorate who began
to dominate the teaching and writing of history in the late nineteenth
and twentieth centuries. Fitful calls for a "new history" incorporating
and integrating social, cultural, and economic aspects of life were voiced
periodically but remained episodic and isolated; academic history continued to be dominated by the traditional spheres of politics and policy, war
and diplomacy. In university departments of classics, oriental language, and
modern literature, a handful of scholars pursued medical subjects but often
in terms of limited textual problems.

Meanwhile the world of medicine guarded its history with a kind of
essentialist zeal; no one without medical training, the unspoken argument
followed, could really understand the nuances and content of the field.
It was not simply a question of esoteric technical knowledge, but of
experience – of empathy, ethics, and a cognitive understanding that could
only grow out of clinical experience. This exclusive claim was aided by
a mixture of caution and skepticism that discouraged most nonmedical
scholars from treading in what seemed so specialized an area; medicine
remained marginal as a subject matter to academic history's established
canon of significance. Until the 1960s, the history of medicine was fundamentally a professional history, written by and largely for physicians.[2]

This was certainly the impression I gathered as a beginner in the field in
the early 1960s.[3] I can recall distinctly a good many illustrative conversations. Ludwig Edelstein, the distinguished classicist and authority on
Hippocratic medicine, was one of the teachers who influenced me most;
and I recall his explaining how he had waged a decades-long – and

---

1 We do not have a comprehensive modern history of the history of medicine. For a
   significant personal view, see Owsei Temkin, *The Double Face of Janus and other Essays
   in the History of Medicine* (Baltimore: Johns Hopkins University Press, 1977), especially
   the autobiographical title essay (pp. 3–37).
2 This is not to deny the existence of an enthusiastic audience for accessible
   presentations of medical history; the popular successes of Paul de Kruif and Hans
   Zinsser nicely illustrate this potential. Nor is it to deny the significant efforts of a
   handful of professional historians, such as Richard H. Shryock in the United States.
3 I have sketched some impressions of this period elsewhere, in the form of an afterword
   to a new (1987) edition to my first book, *The Cholera Years. The United States in 1832,
   1849 and 1866* (Chicago: University of Chicago Press, 1962, new ed. 1987).

generally defensive – battle for the right and necessity of non–medically certified scholars to practice medical history. I remember as well parallel conversations in the spring of 1961 with Owsei Temkin, then director of the Institute for the History of Medicine at the Johns Hopkins University School of Medicine, where I held a postdoctoral fellowship. Temkin convinced me that he too felt that key aspects of medicine's history would remain inaccessible to holders of the Ph.D. – no matter how keen their interest or appropriate their specifically historical training. And this despite his impressive ability to place medical thought and practice in a broad cultural context.

Things have changed enormously in the three decades since those conversations took place. Developments in academic history and the social sciences – and in society generally – have changed the intellectual visibility of medical history and recast the status of its increasingly numerous practitioners. First, clinical medicine has become increasingly discouraging to the humanities-minded. Premedical studies – despite gestures toward diversity in curriculum – have remained consistently and necessarily oriented toward the technical and the scientific. And contemporary medical education, with its enormously increasing burden of information for undergraduates, followed by the physically, emotionally, and intellectually demanding years in internship, residency, and specialized fellowship, leave little room for the kind of broad humanistic education that an older generation of medical historians, many of them European-trained, took for granted. And much of the scholarship in the field has until the recent past been the avocational product of practicing physicians. But such historian-clinicians seem not to be reproducing themselves in our late twentieth-century schools of medicine – European as well as British and American – even if those schools have betrayed twinges of guilt about their often narrowly technical orientation.

At the same time, and somewhat ironically, the American audience for descriptions, prescriptions, and analyses of medicine has increased both within and without the professional world. A generation of critics has focused on the way in which the system has responded poorly to the human needs of those it treats with such technical competence. A parallel and even more vigorous critique – and thus audience constituency – has developed around the economic and institutional problems of American medicine. How can we pay for the medicine we have come to believe we want? And what are the human costs that go along with our intrusive, acute-care-oriented health care system? Both genuine concern and a preemptive prudence have motivated a good many medical school administrators to experiment with offerings in "medical humanities" and – even more frequent – medical ethics. History has a logical, but still largely potential, role in such programs.

Yet medicine, and the body – over which the profession has historically been granted cultural authority – have never enjoyed more prominence in the world of academic scholarship. Professors of English and of sociology, for example, like historians, have developed an interest in past systems of medicine and past styles of constructing the body and its functions. Paralleling this interest in the body as raw material for the imprinting of cultural messages has been an even more widespread growth in the history of medicine as social function. The social and institutional aspects of medicine and their relationship to underlying cultural values and social structural realities have become fashionable subjects for historical research. Social history and demography have turned their attention to the everyday life of men and women: how long they live, how they think about their bodies, about life and death, health and disease, childbearing and child rearing. In all of these areas, medical texts and medical authority not only played a legitimating role, but often provide the only surviving historical record. Even if they do not think of themselves as *medical* historians, scholars are often dependent on medical sources for the data that allow them to begin to reconstruct these aspects of life.

But this vigorous interest in medicine's social and cultural past is in some fundamental ways divorced from the much older intraprofessional tradition in medical history and from its progress-oriented, intellectualistic canon. Our newer practitioners of the social history of medicine are as likely to be interested in the patient's experience as in the physician's, or in medicine as marketplace phenomenon, and in the way in which constructions of the body serve as a language for representing and legitimating gender and class relationships; they are much less likely to be interested in Louis Pasteur or William Harvey, the origins of cell theory, or immunology. There has in fact developed a kind of oppositional clustering of interests and skills – with the intellectual history of medicine still being dominated by physicians and by historians credentialed in a relatively new subdiscipline, the history of science. (The technical history of the several specialties remains in particular the province of practitioners.)

The past generation has also seen a parallel and complexly related shift in the way we approach medicine's internal intellectual development and the history of care. There has been a growing awareness of the problematic quality of the relationship between bedside care and the formal rationalization of that therapeutic interaction. Medicine is behavior as well as cognition; it is the everyday life of village apothecaries as well as the lectures and experiments of professors. In addition, historians, social scientists, and some philosophers have moved toward an increasingly sophisticated contextualism, a willingness to place ideas in specific historical settings.[4] A variety of scholars have begun to think of science as well as medicine as a set of generation- and place-specific practices, and not accumulations of knowledge advancing ineluctably – if sometimes erratically – toward a deeper understanding of nature. This concern with practice and with the imperfect, with the way in which communities of the learned negotiate what they choose to accept as truth, has, since the work of Thomas Kuhn and others in the 1960s, become an important theme in the sociology of knowledge and the history of science. It is an epistemology that has implied a program of historical sociology – for would-be students of every period from classical antiquity to the present. And it has added an important dimension to the collective, if disparate, effort that constitutes the history of medicine at the end of the twentieth century. In fact, explosive fragmentation now characterizes the field as much as any other single tendency, except perhaps the waning dominance of the physician-historian.

It is unfortunate in a way because the most fundamental theme – and attraction – of the history of medicine is its potentially integrative quality. What originally attracted me to the field is medicine's necessary integration of theory and practice, of life and death, of family and institutional life, of the historical and the timeless. Medicine has its origins in the social response to unchanging realities: pain, death, childbirth, trauma and disease, the working out of the life cycle in men and women. The fear, pain, and isolation of these events have not changed in some ways – just as the human body remains constrained by innate biological limits. Change in medical ideas and medical practice has always to be judged against this baseline. There has always been something special about medicine, a sacred dimension based on the physician's relationship to life, death, and pain – and on the consequent social acceptance of his or her touching of bodies and minds. There has never been a time that physicians did not employ some framework within which these events and relationships could be explained and rationalized.

This implies a second aspect of medical history as research field. It necessarily breaks down the boundaries between applied and pure; the clinical interaction brings together the social context in which the patient is treated – whether family bedroom or teaching hospital – with the intellectual assumptions that guide the interaction. Historians of the past two centuries must be particularly sensitive to the institutional structures that contain and constrain the clinical encounter.

Some years ago I was charged with the writing of a general essay on the

4 Only a handful of historians of medicine and science can be described as relativists in the technical, philosophical sense. A great many have become contextualists to some degree or another; but this is a very different question.

institutionalization of knowledge in the United States; and in doing so I
tried to communicate my vision of the interactive and interdependent
nature of that relationship. I finally struck upon the metaphor of ecology,
titling the essay "Towards an Ecology of Knowledge."[5] It was a metaphor
and a way of thinking that came naturally to a student of medicine. For
medical knowledge and practice are always integrated in what can be
thought of as ecological – that is, interdependent, dynamic, and interactive
– terms. Ideas always have a structural role: in earlier centuries it could be
in creating a common frame of reference in which the physician could
rationalize and reassure.[6] In the twentieth century it implies the relationship between the internal logic and development of ideas about the natural
world and the social forms in which that knowledge is used, validated,
and reproduced. Conventional divisions between intellectual, social, and
institutional approaches cannot be justified in theory – even if they still
describe the limitations of much contemporary historical work.

The following essays reflect this general point of view in a number of
ways. The first two parts, which focus on ideas and institutions, are meant
to underline interactions between these realms. They reflect as well, in
their chronological development, something of the past quarter-century's
changing intellectual climate in academic history as experienced by one
practitioner. The last part, "The past in the present," reflects my desire to
make some sense out of a medical world that often seems out of control
and in semipermanent crisis – economic, organizational, and humane.
There has never been a larger potential audience for a discussion of the
fundamental bases of contemporary medicine. This final group of essays
constitutes an effort to use history as a resource in that discourse, to define
limits and provide an historical context for a debate that is often marked by
narrow, erratically informed, and self-serving polemic. The essays pursue
themes that have become visible to the public, such as deinstitutionalization
of the mentally ill and the status of psychiatry, the hospital as social and
economic problem, and the social negotiations surrounding AIDS, and
they attempt to speak to professional and nonacademic audiences at the
same time. It is my hope, however, that all of these chapters, those written
for historians as well as general readers, will be accessible to anyone with
an interest in one of humankind's oldest professions.

5 "Towards an Ecology of Knowledge: On Discipline, Context and History," in
   Alexandra Oleson and John Voss, eds., *The Organization of Knowledge in Modern
   America* (Baltimore: Johns Hopkins University Press, 1979), pp. 440–455. See also my
   "Woods and Trees? Ideas and Actors in the History of Science," *Isis* 74 (1988),
   356–367.
6 At the same time, possession of an esoteric body of learning could legitimate the
   physician's social identity and specify a relationship between that professional identity
   and a more general class identity.

PART I

Ideas as actors

1

The therapeutic revolution: Medicine, meaning, and social change in nineteenth-century America

&ev. Therapeutics has always been central to medical practice, but not to the practice of the profession's historians. My first teacher, Erwin H. Ackerknecht, once wryly cited by way of explanation the German saying that one should not mention rope in the house of the hanged; little glory was to be harvested from the annals of pre-twentieth-century therapeutics. It was more an occasion of embarrassment than of pride, largely ignored by historians except as a source of anecdote and as counterpoint to the laudable accumulation of effective knowledge in more recent generations.

I too could make little sense of traditional therapeutics when I first began to study medical history. Those of my teachers and contemporaries willing to take the older healing tradition seriously saw the physician's role as essentially consolatory and psychological; past therapeutic practices could then be construed as a mixture of ritual and placebo. Little serious attention was paid to the actual drugs and procedures that made up the content of practice – the cathartics, emetics, diuretics, bleeding, and the like – and to the way in which they were understood by patients, families, and practitioners.

Only gradually did the system begin to seem coherent – to seem in fact to be a *system* of social relations and shared conceptual frameworks. The ideas of both physician and patient had to be taken seriously, even if they seemed arbitrary and irrational in twentieth-century terms, in terms that is of measurable physiological efficacy. Ideas have to be seen as actors in the endlessly repetitive drama of the sickroom – but so do drugs and procedures. Therapeutics was a complex and interactive system, centering on the doctor–patient interaction but incorporating the specific physiological activity of drugs, social relationships at the bedside, and the expectations of participants as well as views concerning the nature of the human body and the physiological basis of health and disease. This essay was written originally for a bicentennial symposium on the history of

9

medicine in America. By 1976 it seemed unthinkable that a retrospective evaluation of American medicine should ignore therapeutics; it is and was the center of medical care, of the physician's role, and of the legitimacy that surrounds it. ✌️

Medical therapeutics changed remarkably little in the two millennia preceding 1800; by the end of the century, traditional therapeutics had altered fundamentally. This development is a significant event not only in the history of medicine, but in social history as well. Yet historians have not only failed to delineate this change in detail; they have hardly begun to place it in a framework of explanation which would relate it to all those other changes which shaped the twentieth-century Western world.

Medical historians have always found therapeutics an awkward piece of business. On the whole, they have responded by ignoring it.[1] Most historians who have addressed traditional therapeutics have approached it as a source of anecdote, or as a murky bog of routinism from which a comforting path led upward to an ultimately enlightened and scientifically based therapeutics. Isolated incidents such as the introduction of quinine or digitalis seemed only to emphasize the darkness of the traditional practice in which they appeared. Among twentieth-century students of medical history, the generally unquestioned criterion for understanding pre-nineteenth-century therapeutics has been physiological, not historical: Did a particular practice act in a way that twentieth-century understanding would regard as efficacious? Did it work?

Yet therapeutics is after all a good deal more than a series of pharmacological or surgical experiments. It involves emotions and personal relationships and incorporates all of those cultural factors which determine belief, identity, and status. The meaning of traditional therapeutics must be sought within a particular cultural context; and this is a task more closely akin to that of the cultural anthropologist than the physiologist. Individuals become sick, demand care and reassurance, and are treated by designated

---

1 For examples of works which try to place traditional therapeutics in a more general framework, see: Erwin H. Ackerknecht, "Aspects of the History of Therapeutics," *Bulletin of the History of Medicine* 36 (1962): 389–419; Ackerknecht, *Therapie von den Primitiven bis zum 20. Jahrhundert* (Stuttgart: Ferdinand Enke, 1970); and Owsei Temkin, "Therapeutic Trends and the Treatment of Syphilis before 1900," *Bulletin of the History of Medicine* 29 (1955): 309–316.

I should like to acknowledge the advice and encouragement given to me over many years by my teachers, the late Erwin H. Ackerknecht and Ludwig Edelstein. Drew Gilpin Faust, Saul Jarcho, Owsei Temkin, and Anthony F. C. Wallace read the manuscript carefully and made a number of important suggestions. A somewhat different version of this paper appeared in *Perspectives in Biology and Medicine* 20 (1977): 485–506.

healers. Both physician and patient must share a common framework of explanation. To understand therapeutics in the opening decades of the nineteenth century, its would-be historian must see that it relates, on the one hand, to a cognitive system of explanation, and, on the other, to a patterned interaction between doctor and patient, one which evolved over centuries into a conventionalized social ritual.

Instead, however, past therapeutics has most frequently been studied by scholars obsessed with change as progress and concerned with defining such change as an essentially intellectual process. Historians have come to accept a view of nineteenth-century therapeutics which incorporates such priorities. The revolution in practice which took place during the century, the conventional argument follows, reflected the gradual triumph of a critical spirit over ancient obscurantism. The increasingly aggressive empiricism of the early nineteenth century pointed toward the need for evaluating every aspect of clinical practice; nothing was to be accepted on faith, and only those therapeutic modalities which proved themselves in controlled clinical trials were to remain in the physician's arsenal. Spurred by such arguments, increasing numbers of physicians grew skeptical of their ability to alter the course of particular ills and by mid-century – this interpretation continues – traditional medical practice had become far milder and less intrusive than it had been at the beginning of the century. Physicians had come to place ever-increasing faith in the healing power of nature and the natural tendency toward recovery which seemed to characterize most ills.

This view of change in nineteenth-century therapeutics constitutes accepted wisdom, though it has been modified in recent years. An increasingly influential emphasis sees therapeutics as part of a more general pattern of economically motivated behavior which helped to rationalize the regular physician's place in a crowded marketplace of would-be healers.[2] Thus the competition offered by sectarians to regular medicine in the middle third of the century was at least as significant in altering traditional therapeutics as a high-culture-based intellectual critique; the sugar pills of homeopathic physicians or the baths and diets of hydropaths might possibly do little good, but they could hardly be represented as harmful or dangerous in themselves. The often draconic treatments of regular physicians – the bleeding, the severe purges and emetics – constituted a real handicap in competing for a limited number of paying patients and were accordingly modified to fit economic realities. Indeed, something approaching an inter-

2 For an example of this position, see William Rothstein, *American Physicians in the Nineteenth Century: From Sects to Science* (Baltimore: Johns Hopkins University Press, 1972).

pretive consensus might be said to prevail in historical works of recent vintage, a somewhat eclectic but not illogical position which views change in nineteenth-century therapeutics as proceeding both from a high-culture-based shift in ideas and the sordid realities of a precarious marketplace.

Obviously, both emphases reflect a measure of reality. But insofar as they do, they serve essentially to identify sources of instability in an ancient system of ideas and relationships. For neither deals with traditional therapeutics as a meaningful question in itself. As such, therapeutic practices must be seen as a central component in a particular medical system, a system characterized by remarkable tenacity over time.[3] The system must, that is, have worked, even if not in a sense immediately intelligible to a mid-twentieth-century pharmacologist or clinician. It is my hope in the following pages to suggest, first, the place of therapeutics in the configuration of ideas and relationships which constituted medicine at the beginning of the nineteenth century, and then the texture of the change which helped to create a very different system of therapeutics by the end of the century.

The key to understanding therapeutics at the beginning of the nineteenth century lies in seeing it as part of a system of belief and behavior participated in by physician and layman alike. Central to the logic of this social subsystem was a deeply assumed metaphor – a particular way of looking at the body and of explaining both health and disease. The body was seen, metaphorically, as a system of dynamic interactions with its environment. Health or disease resulted from a cumulative interaction between constitutional endowment and environmental circumstance. One could not well live without food and air and water; one had to live in a particular climate, subject one's body to a particular style of life and work. Each of these factors implied a necessary and continuing physiological adjustment. The body was always in a state of becoming – and thus always in jeopardy.

Two subsidiary assumptions organized the shape of this lifelong interaction. First, every part of the body was related inevitably and inextricably with every other. A distracted mind could curdle the stomach, a dyspeptic stomach could agitate the mind. Local lesions might reflect imbalances of nutrients in the blood; systemic ills might be caused by fulminating local lesions. Thus the theoretical debates which have bemused historians of medicine over local as opposed to systemic models of disease causation,

3 Within the meaning of the term *therapeutics*, I include any measures utilized by physician or layperson in hopes of ameliorating or curing the felt symptoms of illness. In the great majority of instances this implied the administration of some drug, but it might include bleeding or alterations in diet or other aspects of lifestyle. This essay avoids the question of surgery and its relationship to the cognitive system which explained nonsurgical therapeutic practices.

solidistic versus humoral emphases, models based on tension or laxity of muscle fibers or blood vessels – all of these models served the same explanatory function relative to therapeutics; all related local to systemic ills; they described all aspects of the body as interrelated; they tended to present health or disease as general states of the total organism. Second, the body was seen as a system of intake and outgo – a system which had necessarily to remain in balance if the individual were to remain healthy. Thus the conventional emphasis on diet and excretion, perspiration, and ventilation. Equilibrium was synonymous with health, disequilibrium with illness.

In addition to the exigencies of everyday life which might destabilize that equilibrium which constituted health, the body had also to pass through several developmental crises inherent in the design of the human organism. Menstruation and menopause in women, teething and puberty in both sexes – all represented points of potential danger, moments of struc-tured instability as the body established a new internal equilibrium.[4] Seasonal changes in climate constituted another kind of recurring cyclical change which might imply danger to health and require possible medical intervention – thus the ancient practice of administering cathartics in spring and fall to help the body adjust to the changed seasons. The body could be seen, that is – as in some ways it had been since classical antiquity – as a kind of stewpot, or chemico-vital reaction, proceeding calmly only if all its elements remained appropriately balanced. Randomness was minimized, but at a substantial cost in anxiety; the body was a city under constant threat of siege, and it is not surprising that early nineteenth-century Americans consumed enormous quantities of medicines as they sought to regulate assimilation and excretion.

The idea of specific disease entities played a relatively small role in such a system. Where empirical observation pointed unavoidably toward the existence of a particular disease state, physicians still sought to preserve their accustomed therapeutic role. The physician's most potent weapon was his ability to "regulate the secretions" – to extract blood, to promote the perspiration, urination, or defecation, which attested to his having helped the body to regain its customary equilibrium. Even when a disease seemed not only to have a characteristic course but (as in the case of smallpox) a specific causative "virus," the hypothetical pathology and indicated therapeutics were seen within the same explanatory framework.[5]

---

4 For a more detailed discussion of one such cyclical crisis, see Carroll Smith-Rosenberg, "Puberty to Menopause: The Cycle of Femininity in Nineteenth-Century America," *Feminist Studies* 1 (1973): 58–72.
5 In some ways, it should be emphasized, constitutional ills fit more easily into this model than the acute infectious – and especially epidemic – ills. Cancer or tu-

The success of inoculation and later vaccination in preventing smallpox could not challenge this deeply internalized system of explanation. When late eighteenth- and early nineteenth-century physicians inoculated or vaccinated, they ordinarily accompanied the procedure with an elaborate regimen of cathartics, diet, and rest. Though such elaborate medical accompaniments to vaccination might appear, from one perspective, as a calculated effort to increase the physician's fees, these preparations might better be seen as a means of assimilating an anomalous procedure into the physician's accustomed picture of health and disease.

The pedigree of these ideas can be traced to the rationalistic speculations of classical antiquity. They could hardly be superseded, for no information more accurate or schema more socially useful existed to call them into question. Most importantly, the system provided a rationalistic framework in which the physician could at once reassure the patient and legitimate his own ministrations. It is no accident that the term "empiric" was pejorative until the mid-nineteenth century, a reference to the blind cut-and-try practices which regular physicians liked to think characterized their quackish competitors. The physician's own self-image and his social plausibility depended on the creation of a shared faith – a conspiracy to believe – in his ability to understand and rationally manipulate the elements in this speculative system. This cognitive framework and the central body metaphor about which it was articulated provided a place for his prognostic as well as his therapeutic skills; prognosis, diagnosis, and therapeutics had all to find a consistent mode of explanation.

The physician in 1800 had no diagnostic tools beyond his senses and it is hardly surprising that he would find congenial a framework of explanation which emphasized the importance of intake and outgo, of the significance of perspiration, of pulse, of urination and menstruation, of defecation, of the surface eruptions which might accompany fevers or other internal ills. These were phenomena which he as physician, the patient, and the patient's family could see, evaluate, and scrutinize for clues to the sick person's fate. These biological and social realities had several implications for therapeutics. Drugs had to be seen as adjusting the body's internal equilibrium; in addition, the drug's action had, if possible, to alter these visible products of the body's otherwise inscrutable internal state. Logically enough, drugs were not ordinarily viewed as specifics for particular disease entities; materia medica texts were often arranged not by drug or disease,

berculosis, for example, could naturally be seen as resulting from long-term problems of assimilation. Acute and especially epidemic diseases seemed more sharply defined in time and, ordinarily, in their courses; nevertheless, the pathological mechanisms which caused the symptoms that constituted the disease were still represented in terms similar to those we have described.

but in categories reflecting the drug's physiological effects: diuretics, cathartics, narcotics, emetics, diaphoretics. Quinine, for example, was ordinarily categorized as a tonic and prescribed for numerous conditions other than malaria.[6] Even when it was employed in "intermittent fever," quinine was almost invariably prescribed in conjunction with a cathartic; as in the case of vaccination, a drug with a disease-specific efficacy ill-suited to the assumptions of the physician's underlying cognitive framework was assimilated to it. (Significantly, the advocacy of a specific drug in treating a specific ill was ordinarily viewed by regular physicians as a symptom of quackery.)

The effectiveness of the system hinged to a significant extent on the fact that all the weapons in the physician's normal armamentarium worked – "worked," that is, by providing visible and predictable physiological effects: purges purged, emetics induced vomiting, opium soothed pain and moderated diarrhea. Bleeding, too, seemed obviously to alter the body's internal balance, as evidenced both by a changed pulse and the very quantity of blood drawn.[7] Blisters and other purposefully induced local irritations certainly produced visible effects – and presumably internal consequences corresponding to their pain and location and to the nature and extent of the matter discharged.[8] Not only did a drug's activity indicate to both physician and patient the nature of its efficacy (and the physician's competence) but it provided a prognostic tool, as well; for the patient's response to a drug could indicate much about his condition, while the product elicited – urine, feces, blood, perspiration – could be examined so as to shed light on the body's internal state. Thus, for example, a patient could report to her physician that

6 Digitalis was, similarly, categorized as a diuretic and prescribed in many cases in which the edema which indicated its employment was unrelated to a cardiac pathology.

7 The rapid fluid loss in severe bloodletting or purging might indeed lower temperature, while extremely copious bloodletting quieted agitation, as well!

8 The vogue of blisters, plasters, and other purposeful excoriations or irritations of the skin was related as well to the prevailing assumption concerning the interdependence of every part of the body and the necessary balancing of forces believed to determine health or disease. Thus, for example, the popularity of "counterirritation" in the form of skin lesions induced by the physician through chemical or mechanical means was based on the assumption that the excoriation of one area and consequent suppuration could "attract" the morbid excitement from another site to the newly excoriated one, while the exudate was significant in possibly allowing the body an opportunity to rid itself of morbid matter, of righting the disease-producing internal imbalance. Such a path to healing could follow natural as well as artificial lesions. "Every physician of experience," one contended as late as 1862, "can recall cases of internal affections, which, after the use of a great variety of medicines, have been unexpectedly relieved by an eruption on the skin; or of ailments of years' continuance, which have been permanently cured by the formation of a large abcess." J. D. Spooner, *The Different Modes of Treating Disease: or the Different Action of Medicine on the System in an Abnormal State* (Boston: David Clapp, 1862), p. 17.

the buf on my blood was of a blewish Cast and at the edge of the buf it
appeared to be curded something like milk and cyder curd after
standing an hour or two the water that came on the top was of a
yellowish cast.[9]

The patient's condition could thus be monitored each day as the doctor
sought to guide its course to renewed health.

The body seemed, moreover, to rid itself of disease in ways parallel to
those encouraged or elicited by drug action. The profuse sweat, diarrhea,
or skin lesions often accompanying fevers, for example, seemed all way
stations on a necessary course of natural recovery. The remedies he employed, the physician could assure his patients, only acted in imitation of
nature:

> Blood-letting and blisters find their archtypes in spontaneous
> haemmorrhage and those sero-plastic exudations that occur in some
> stage of almost every acute inflammation; emetics, cathartics, diuretics,
> diaphoretics, etc. etc. have each and all of them effects in every way
> similar to those arising spontaneously in disease.[10]

Medicine could provoke or facilitate, but not alter, the fundamental patterns of recovery inherent in the design of the human organism.

This same explanatory framework illuminates as well the extraordinary
vogue of mercury in early nineteenth-century therapeutics. If employed for
a sufficient length of time and in sufficient quantity, mercury induced a
series of progressively severe and cumulative physiological effects: first,
diarrhea, and ultimately, full-blown symptoms of mercury poisoning. The
copious involuntary salivation characteristic of this toxic state was seen as
proof that the drug was exerting an "alterative" effect – that is, altering the
fundamental balance of forces and substances which constituted the body's
ultimate reality. Though other drugs, most prominently arsenic, antimony,
and iodine, were believed able to exert such an "alterative" effect, mercury
seemed particularly useful because of the seemingly unequivocal relationship between varying dosage levels and its consequent action (and the
convenient fact that it could be administered either orally or as a salve).[11]

---

9 Mary Ballard to Charles Brown, May 12, 1814. Charles Brown Papers, College of
William and Mary, Williamsburg, Va.
10 E. B. Haskins, *Therapeutic Cultivation: Its Errors and its Reformation; An Address delivered
the Tennessee Medical Society, April 7, 1857* (Nashville: Cameron & Fall, 1857), p. 22.
11 Bleeding in a single large quantity was also seen as exerting such an alterative effect
(and thus might be indicated where a number of smaller bleedings would have the
opposite and undesirable effect). The term *alterative* was, in addition, most frequently
associated with the treatment of longstanding constitutional ills, in the words of one
physician, "subverting any vitiated habit of body or morbid diathesis existing." Samuel
Hobson, *An Essay on the History, Preparation and Therapeutic Uses of Iodine* (Philadelphia:
The Author, 1830) p. 22n.

Moderate doses appeared to aid the body in its normal healing pattern, while in larger doses, mercury could be seen as a forceful intervention in pathological states which had a doubtful prognosis. Mercury was, in this sense, the physician's most flexible, and, at the same time, most powerful weapon for treating ailments in which active intervention might mean the difference between life and death. In such cases he needed a drug with which he might alter a course toward death – one stronger than those with which he routinely modified the secretions and excretions in less severe ailments.

Both physician and educated layman shared a similar view of the manner in which the body functioned, and the nature of available therapeutic modalities reinforced that view. The secretions could be regulated, a plethoric state of the blood abated, the stomach emptied of a content potentially dangerous. Recovery must, of course, have often coincided with the administration of a particular drug and thus provided an inevitable post hoc endorsement of its effectiveness. A physician could typically describe a case of pleurisy as having been "suddenly relieved by profuse perspiration" elicited by the camphor he had prescribed.[12] Fevers seemed, in fact, often to be healed by the purging effects of mercury or antimony. Drugs reassured insofar as they acted, and their efficacy was inevitably under-written by the natural tendency toward recovery which characterized most ills. Therapeutics thus played a central role within the system of interaction between doctor and patient. On the cognitive level, therapeutics confirmed the physician's ability to understand and intervene in the ongoing physio-logical processes which defined health and disease; on the emotional level, the very severity of drug action assured the patient and his family that something was indeed being done.

In the medical idiom of 1800, "exhibiting" a drug was synonymous with administering it (and the administration of drugs so routine that "prescrib-ing for" was synonymous with seeing a patient). The use of the term *exhibit* was hardly accidental. For the therapeutic interaction we have sought to describe was a fundamental cultural ritual, in a literal sense – a ritual in which the legitimating element was, in part at least, a shared commitment to a rationalistic model of pathology and therapeutic action. Therapeutics served as a pivotal link in a stylized interaction between doctor and patient, encompassing organically (the pun is unfortunate but apposite) the cog-nitive and the emotional within a framework of rationalistic explanation.[13]

12 Benjamin H. Coates, Practice Book, entry for February 25, 1836. Historical Society of Pennsylvania, Philadelphia.
13 For a parallel discussion of medical explanation in relation to cosmology and symbolic form, see: Victor Turner, *The Forest of Symbols: Aspects of Ndembu Ritual* (Ithaca, N.Y.: Cornell University Press, 1967); Mary Douglas, *Purity and Danger: An Analysis of Concepts of Pollution and Taboo* (London: Routledge and Kegan Paul, 1966); and Douglas, *Natural Symbols, Exploration in Cosmology* (New York: Pantheon, 1970).

To "exhibit" a drug was to act out a sacramental role in a liturgy of healing. The analogy to religious ritual is not exact, but it is certainly more than metaphorical. A sacrament, after all, is conventionally defined as an external, visible symbol of an invisible, internal state. Insofar as a particular drug caused a perceptible physiological effect, it produced phenomena which all – the physician, the patient, and the patient's family – could witness (again, the double meaning, with its theological overtones, is instructive) and in which all could participate.

This was a liturgy calculated for the sickroom, of course, not for church. And indeed, the efficacy and tenacity of this system must be understood in relation to its social setting. Most such therapeutic tableaux took place in the patient's home, and thus the healing ritual could mobilize all those community and emotional forces which anthropologists have seen as fundamental, in their observations of medical practice in traditional, non-Western societies. Healing, in early nineteenth-century America, was in the great majority of cases physically and emotionally embedded in a precise, emotionally resonant context. The cognitive aspects of this system of explanation, as well, were appropriate to the world-view of such a community. The model of the body, and of health and disease, which we have described was all-inclusive, antireductionist, and capable of incorporating every aspect of man's life in explaining his physical condition. Just as man's body interacted continuously with his environment, so did his mind with his body, his morals with his health. The realm of causation in medicine was not distinguishable from the realm of meaning in society generally.

There was no inconsistency between this world of rationalistic explanation and traditional spiritual values. Few Americans in the first third of the nineteenth century felt any conflict between these realms of reassurance. If drugs failed, this expressed merely the ultimate power of God, and constituted no reason to question the truth of either system of belief. Let me quote the words of a pious mid-century physician who sought in his diary to come to terms with the dismaying and unexpected death of a child he had been treating. "The child seemed perfectly well," the troubled physician explained,

> till it was attacked at the tea table. Remedies, altho' slow in their action, acted well, but were powerless to avert the arm of death. The decrees of Providence . . . cannot be set aside. Man is mortal, & tho' remedies often seem to act promptly and effectually to the saving of life – they often fail in an accountable manner! 'So teach me to number my days that I may apply my heart unto wisdom'.[14]

14 Diary of Samuel W. Butler, July 25, 1852, Historical Collections, College of Physicians of Philadelphia, Philadelphia.

The Lord might give and the Lord take away – but until He did, the physician dared not remain passive in the face of those dismaying signs of sickness which caused his patient anxiety and pain.

The physician's art, in the opening decades of the nineteenth century, centered on his ability to employ an appropriate drug or combination of drugs and bleeding to produce a particular physiological effect. This explains the apparent anomaly of physicians employing different drugs to treat the same condition; each drug, the argument followed, was equally legitimate so long as it produced the desired physiological effect. The selection of a proper drug or drugs was no mean skill, authorities ex-plained, for each patient possessed a unique physiological identity, and the experienced physician had to evaluate a bewildering variety of factors, ranging from climatic conditions to age and sex, in the compounding of any particular prescription. A physician who knew a family's constitutional idiosyncrasies was necessarily a better practitioner for that family than one who enjoyed no such insight – or even one who hailed from a different climate, for it was assumed that both the action of drugs and reaction of patients varied with season and geography.[15] The physician had to be aware, as well, that the same drug in different dosages might produce different effects. Fifteen grams of ipecac, a young Southern medical student cautioned himself, acted as an emetic, five induced sweating, while smaller doses could serve as a useful tonic.[16]

The same rationalistic mechanisms which explained recovery explained failure as well. One could not predict recovery in every case; even the most competent physician could only do that which the limited resources of medicine allowed – and the natural course of some ills was toward death. The treatment indicated for tuberculosis, as an ancient adage put it, was opium and lies. Cancer too was normally incurable; some states of dis-equilibrium could not be righted.

Early nineteenth-century American physicians unquestionably believed in the therapeutics they practiced. Physicians routinely prescribed severe cathartics and bleeding for themselves and for their wives and children. A New England physician settling in Camden, South Carolina, for example, depended for health in this treacherous climate upon his accustomed cathartic pills. "Took two of the pills last night," he recorded in his diary,

15 As Benjamin Rush could explain to an English correspondent, for example, "The extremes of heat and cold, by producing greater extremes of violence in our fevers than in yours, call for more depletion, and from more outlets, than the fevers of Great Britain." Rush to John Coakley Lettsom, May 13, 1804, L. H. Butterfield, ed., *Letters of Benjamin Rush*, 2 vols. (Princeton, N.J.: American Philosophical Society, 1951), vol. 2, p. 881.

16 Anonymous notebook, Materia Medica Lectures of John P. Emmett, University of Virginia, 1834–1836, Perkins Library, Duke University, Durham, N.C.

"they have kept me busy thro' the day and I now feel like getting clear of my headache."[17] Even when physicians felt some anxiety in particular cases, they could take assurance from the knowledge that they were following a mode of practice endorsed by rational understanding and centuries of clinical experience. A young New York City physician in 1795, for example, felt such doubts after having bled and purged a critically ill patient:

> I began to fear that I had carried the debilitating plan too far. By degrees I became reassured; & when I reflected on his youth, constitution, his uniform temperance, on the one hand; & on the fidelity which I had adhered to those modes of practice recommended by the most celebrated physicians, on the other, I felt a conviction that accident alone, could wrest him from me.[18]

Such conviction was a necessary element in medical practice; without belief the system could hardly have functioned.

Individuals from almost every level in society accepted, in one fashion or another, the basic outlines of the world-view which we have described. Evidence of such belief among the less articulate is not abundant, but it does exist. Patients, for example, understood that a sudden interruption of perspiration might cause a cold or even pneumonia, and that such critical periods as teething, puberty, and menopause were particularly dangerous. The metabolic gyroscope which controlled the balance of forces within the body was delicate indeed, and might easily be thrown off balance. Thus it was natural for servants and laborers reporting the symptoms of their fevers to an almshouse physician to ascribe their illnesses to a sudden stoppage of the perspiration.[19] It was equally natural for young ladies complaining of amenorrhea to ascribe it to a sudden chill. The sudden interruption of any natural evacuation would presumably jeopardize the end implicit in that function; if the body did not need to perspire in certain circumstances, or

---

17 The "busy" referred to the "operation" of the drug and not to the physician's schedule! See Diary of William Blanding, July 4, 1807, South Caroliniana Library, University of South Carolina, Columbia, S.C. As usual Benjamin Rush was particularly enthusiastic. "Ten of my family have been confined with remitting fevers," he wrote to John Redman Coxe on October 5, 1795. "Twenty-four bleedings in one month have cured us all. I submitted to two of them in one day. Our infant of 6 weeks old was likewise bled twice, and thereby rescued from the grave." *Letters*, vol. 2, p. 763.

18 Entry for September 18, 1795. *The Diary of Elihu Hubbard Smith (1771–1798)* (Philadelphia: American Philosophical Society, 1973), p. 59.

19 Such comments were made to examining physicians, for example, by laborer James McSherry, thirty-nine, and houseworker Sarah Mullin, nineteen, at the Philadelphia Almshouse, Hospital Casebook, 1824–1827, Records of the Board of Guardians of the Poor, Philadelphia City Archives.

discharge menstrual blood at intervals, it would not be doing so.[20] These were mechanisms through which the body maintained its health-defining equilibrium – and could thus be interrupted only at great peril.

Such considerations dictated modes of treatment as well as views of disease causation. If, for example, the normal course of a disease to recovery involved the formation of a skin lesion, the physician must not intervene too aggressively and interrupt the process through which the body sought to rid itself of offending matter. Thus a student could record his professor's warning against the premature "exhibition" of tonics in a continued fever; such stimulants were "highly prejudicial they lock in the disease instead of liberating it from the system. After evacuations have been premised," the young man continued, "then the tonic medicine may be employed."[21] Yet physicians assumed that fevers normally accompanied by skin lesions could not "find resolution" without an appropriately bountiful crop of such blisters; and if they seemed dilatory in erupting, the physician might appropriately turn to blisters and counterirritation in an effort to encourage them. To "drive them inward," on the other hand, was to invite far graver illness. In such ailments it was the physician's task to prescribe mild cathartics in an effort to aid the body in its efforts to expel the morbid material. Mercury, for example, might be desirable in small doses but perilous in "alterative" ones.

In any case, it was the physician's primary responsibility to "regulate or restore" the normal secretions whenever interrupted. Chronic constipation, diarrhea, and irregular menstruation similarly called for active steps on the physician's part. In constipation, mild cathartics were routine; in amenorrhea, drugs to restore the flow (emmenagogues) were indicated. (The use of emmenagogues could represent an ethical dilemma to physicians who feared being imposed upon by seemingly innocent young ladies who sought abortifacients under the guise of a desire to restore the normal

20 The logic of the system is usefully illustrated by the assumption that suppressed menstruation would cause a plethora, or superabundance, of blood. During pregnancy, it was believed that the blood was utilized by the developing embryo; during lactation, by the body's need to produce milk for the nursling. If the mother became ill and the infant stopped nursing, a student in David Hosack's lectures noted during the winter of 1822–1823, the lancet might be needed to "take off" the "plethora induced by the stoppage of the monthly discharge." J. Barratt, Medical Notebook, Lecture 49th, South Caroliniana Library, University of South Carolina, Columbia, S.C. "A partial suppression of the menses," a house-pupil at the Philadelphia Almshouse noted in 1825, "is sometimes the cause of Plethora. Give first an emetic of ipecac and then a laxative." Unpaged medical notebook in the Nathan Hatfield Papers, Historical Collections, College of Physicians of Philadelphia.

21 Abraham Bitner, "Notes taken from the Philadelphia Almshouse, Nvr. 1824," p. 3. Historical Collections, College of Physicians of Philadelphia.

menstrual cycle interrupted by some cause other than pregnancy.)[22]

The widespread faith in emetics, cathartics, diuretics, and bleeding is evidenced as well by their prominent place in folk medicine. Domestic and irregular practice, that is, like regular medicine, was shaped about the eliciting of predictable physiological responses; home remedies mirrored the heroic therapeutics practiced by regular physicians. In the fall of 1826, for example, when a Philadelphia tallow chandler fell ill, he complained of chills, pains in the head and back, weakness in the joints, and nausea. Then, before seeing a regular physician, he

> was bled till symptoms of fainting came on. Took an emetic, which operated well. For several days after, kept his bowels moved with Sulph. Soda, Senna tea &c. He then employed a Physician who prescribed another Emetic, which operated violently and whose action was kept up by drinking bitter tea.[23]

Only after two more days did he appear at the Almshouse Hospital. Physicians skeptical of traditional therapeutics complained repeatedly of lay expectations which worked against change; medical men might well be subject to criticism if they should, for example, fail to bleed in the early stages of pneumonia. Parents often demanded that physicians incise the inflamed gums of their teething infants so as to provoke a "resolution" of this developmental crisis. Laypersons could, indeed, be even more importunate in their demands for an aggressive therapy than the physicians attending them thought appropriate. The indications for bleeding were carefully demarcated in formal medical thought, for example, yet laypersons often demanded it even when the state of the pulse and general condition of the patient contraindicated loss of blood. Some patients demanded, as well as expected, the administration of severe cathartics or emetics; they suspected peril in too languid a therapeutic regimen.

Botanic alternatives to regular medicine in the first third of the century were also predicated upon the routine use of severe cathartics and emetics, of vegetable origin. (In the practice of Thomsonian physicians, the most prominent organized botanic sect, such drugs were supplemented by sweat baths designed, in theory, to adjust the body's internal heat through the eliciting of copious perspiration.)[24] Botanic physicians shared many of the

22 Pious physicians sometimes found it difficult to balance their professional desire to restore a normal menstrual flow against a fear of being placed in the position of inducing abortion. For an example, see Diary of R. P. Little, November 28, 1842, Trent Collection, Duke University Medical Library. Durham, N.C.

23 Case of George Devert, November 15, 1826, Hospital Casebook, 1824–1827, Philadelphia City Archives.

24 The most detailed account of the Thomsonian movement is still that by Alex Berman, "The Impact of the Nineteenth-Century Botanico-Medical Movement in American

social problems faced by their regular competitors; they dealt with the same emotional realities implicit in the doctor–patient relationship, and in doing so appealed to a similar framework of physiological assumption.

Nevertheless, there were differences of approach among physicians and in the minds of a good many laypersons who questioned both the routinism and the frequent severity of traditional therapeutics. (The criticisms which greeted the atypically severe bleeding and purging advocated by Benjamin Rush are familiar to any student of the period.) America, in 1800, was in many ways already a modern society, diverse in religion, in class, and in ethnic background. It would be naive to contend that the unity of vision which, presumably, united most traditional non-Western cultures in their orientation toward particular medical systems could apply to this diverse and labile culture. Yet, as we have argued, there are surprisingly large areas of agreement. Even those Americans skeptical of therapeutic excess and inconsistency (and, in some cases, more generally of the physician's authority) did not question the fundamental structure of the body metaphor which I have described, however much they may have doubted the possible efficacy of medical intervention in sickness.[25]

In describing American medical therapeutics in the first quarter of the nineteenth century we have been examining a system already marked by signs of instability. Fundamental to this instability was rationalism itself. A key legitimating aspect of the traditional view of the body was its rationalistic form (even if we regard that rationalism as egregiously speculative); yet by 1800, this structure of explanation was tied irrevocably to the institutions and findings of world science. And as this world changed and provided data and procedures increasingly relevant to the world of clinical medicine, it gradually undercut the harmony between world-view and personal interaction which had characterized therapeutics at the opening of the century.

By the 1830s, criticism of traditional therapeutics had become a cliché in sophisticated medical circles; physicians of any pretension spoke of

Pharmacy and Medicine," (Ph.D. diss., University of Wisconsin, 1954); Berman, "The Thomsonian Movement and its Relation to American Pharmacy and Medicine," *Bulletin of the History of Medicine* 25 (1951): 519–538.

25 The absolute rejection of traditional therapeutics enunciated by mid-century hydropaths and other evangelically oriented critics of medicine did not involve a rejection of the central body metaphor, but rather an absolute rejection of "artificial" drugs and bleeding. They did not question, but, on the contrary, emphasized the traditional view of the body; it served, indeed, as the logical basis for their dismissal of conventional therapeutics. They emphasized instead the body's capacity to heal itself when aided by appropriate regimen alone. The physician's therapeutic intrusions into that system seemed literally blasphemous.

self-limited diseases, of skepticism in regard to the physician's ability to intervene and change the course of most diseases, of respect for the healing powers of nature. This point of view emphasized the self-limiting nature of most ailments and the physician's duty simply to aid the process of natural recovery through appropriate and minimally heroic means. "It would be better," as Oliver Wendell Holmes put it in his usual acerbic fashion, "if the patient were allowed a certain discount from his bill for every dose he took, just as children are compensated by their parents for swallowing hideous medicinal mixtures."[26] Rest, a strengthening diet, and a mild cathartic were all the aid nature required in most ills. In those ailments whose natural tendency was toward death, the physician had to acknowledge his powerlessness and simply try to minimize pain and anxiety. This noninterventionist position was accompanied by increasing acceptance of the parallel view that most diseases could be seen as distinct clinical entities, each with a characteristic cause, course, and symptomatology.

These positions are accepted by most historians as reflecting the fundamental outline for the debate over therapeutics in the middle third of the nineteenth century. And, as a matter of fact, it does describe one significant aspect of change – the influence of high-culture ideas and of a small opinion-forming elite in gradually modifying the world-view of a much larger group of practitioners and, ultimately, of laypersons. But when we try to evaluate the impact of such therapeutic admonitions on the actual practice of actual physicians, realities become a good deal more complex. Medical practice was conducted at a number of levels – intellectual, economic, and regional – but demonstrated in each the extraordinary tenacity of traditional views.

American physicians were tied to the everyday requirements of the doctor–patient relationship and thus, even among the teaching elite, no mid-century American practitioner rejected conventional therapeutics with a ruthless consistency. The self-confident empiricism which denied the efficacy of any therapeutic measure not proven efficacious in clinical trials seemed an ideological excess suited to a handful of European academics, not to the realities of practice. It is no accident that the radically skeptical position was christened "therapeutic nihilism" by its critics. Nihilism, with its echoes of disbelief and destructive change, of "total rejection of current religious beliefs and morals" (to borrow a defining phrase from the *Oxford English Dictionary*) was not chosen as a term of casual abuse, but represented precisely the gravity of the challenge to a traditional world-view

26 Oliver Wendell Holmes, *Valedictory Address, Delivered to the Medical Graduates of Harvard University, at the Annual Commencement, ... March 10, 1858* (Boston: David Clapp, 1858), p. 5.

implied by a relentless empiricism, and the materialism which seemed so often to accompany it.

There were enduring virtues in the old ways. "There is," as one leader in the profession explained, "a vantage ground between the two extremes, neither verging towards meddlesome interference on the one hand, nor imbecile neglect on the other."[27] The physician had to contend, moreover, with patient expectations: "The public," as another prominent clinician put it, "expect something more of physicians than the power of distinguishing diseases and of predicting their issue. They look to them for the relief of their sufferings, and the cure or removal of their complaints."[28]

The physician had to create an emotionally, as well as intellectually, meaningful therapeutic regimen; throughout the middle third of the nineteenth century this meant the administration of drugs capable of eliciting a perceptible physiological response. No mid-century physician doubted the efficacy of placebos (as little as he doubted that the effectiveness of a drug could depend on his own manner and attitude), but in a grave illness the physician's own awareness of their inertness made it impossible for him to rely on sugar or bread pills and the healing power of nature. One medical man, for example, after conceding the uselessness of every available therapeutic means in cholera, still contended that "a noble profession whose aims and purpose are the preservation of human life should not be content with anything short of the adoption of remedial measures for so fatal a disease, which promise positive and beneficent results in every individual case."[29] Hospital case records indicate that even elite physicians maintained a more than lingering faith in cathartic drugs throughout the middle third of the century. (And in hospital practice economic considerations could have played no role in the doctor's willingness to prescribe.)

Physicians shaped a number of intellectual compromises in order to maintain such continuity with traditional therapeutic practice. First, despite the growing plausibility of views emphasizing disease specificity, most physicians still maintained an emphasis on their traditional ability to modify symptoms. The older assumption that drugs acted in a way consistent with the body's innate pattern of recovery was easily shifted toward new emphases; the physician's responsibility now centered on recognizing the natural course of his patient's ailment and supporting the body in its path to renewed health with an appropriate combination of drugs and regimen. Even the course of a self-limited disease might be shortened, its painful

27 T. Gaillard Thomas, *Introductory Address Delivered at the College of Physicians and Surgeons, New York, October 17th, 1864* (New York: 1864), p. 31.
28 Jacob Bigelow, *Brief Expositions of Rational Medicine, to which is Prefixed the Paradise of Doctors* ... (Boston: Phillips, Sampson and Co., 1858), p. iv.
29 A. P. Merrill, *Medical Record* 1 (1866): 275.

symptoms mitigated. The secretions had still to be regulated, diet specified and modified, perhaps a plethora of blood lessened by cupping or leeching. Even in ills whose natural course led to death, the physician might still avail himself of therapeutic means to ease the grim journey. Finally, no one doubted, there were ailments in which the physician's intervention could make the difference between life and death. Scurvy, for example, was often cited as a disease "that taints the whole system, [yet] yields to a mere change in diet."[30] The surgeon still had to set bones, remove foreign bodies, drain abscesses.

Second, even an explicit affirmation of the natural tendency to recovery, in most ills, did not obviate the place of traditional views of the body in explaining that recovery. Physicians, for example, spoke habitually of "vital power" and the need to support that vitality if the natural healing tendency were to manifest itself. The body could, that is, still be seen in traditional holistic terms, vital power constituting the sum of all its internal realities and, by implication, a reflection of the body's necessary transactions with its environment. The use of the term *vital power* suggests, moreover, how deeply committed the medical profession still was to communication of meaning through metaphor – in this case, a metaphor incorporating a shorthand version of the age-old view of the body we have outlined, yet appearing in the necessary guise of scientific truth.

The decades between 1850 and 1870 did see an increased emphasis on diet and regimen among regular physicians, most strikingly a vogue for the use of alcoholic beverages as stimulants. It is hardly surprising that one reaction to the varied criticisms of traditional therapeutics was a consequent acceptance of a "strengthening and stimulating" emphasis in practice; the new emphasis not only responded to criticisms by sectarian healers of "depleting" measures such as bleeding and purging, but preserved an active role for the physician within the same framework of attitudes toward the body which had always helped order the doctor–patient relationship.

Practice changed a good deal less than the rhetoric surrounding it would suggest. "Nature," a South Carolina medical man explained to a patient troubled by a "derangement of the Abdominal organs" in 1850, "must restore their natural condition by gradually building them up anew, & time is necessary for the accomplishment of this." But drug treatment was appropriate as well, the physician continued.

> The Medicinal treatment is to aid nature, by correcting irregularities
> and meeting untoward symptoms as they may occur. . . . The Medicinal

---

30 C. W. Parsons, *An Essay on the Question, Vis Medicatrix Naturae, How far is it to be relied on in the Treatment of Diseases?* Fiske Fund Prize Dissertation No. 11 (Boston: Printed for the Rhode Island Medical Society, 1849), p. 7.

treatment consisted of an Alterative course of Tonics, chiefly Metallic, not Mercurial – so combined with Laxatives as to regulate the Secretions of the Digestive organs.[31]

Less aggressive than it might have been a generation earlier, such a course of treatment still allowed the physician an active role.

The inertia of traditional practice was powerful indeed; older modes of therapeutics did not die, but, as we have suggested, were employed less routinely, and drugs were used in generally smaller doses. Dosage levels decreased markedly in the second third of the century, and bleeding, especially, sank into disuse. The resident physician at the Philadelphia Dispensary could, for example, report in 1862 that of a total of 9,502 treated that year, "general blood-letting has been resorted to in one instance only, . . . cupping twelve times and leeching thrice."[32] Residents at Bellevue in New York and Massachusetts General Hospital in Boston had reported the previous year that bloodletting was "almost obsolete."[33] Mercury, on the other hand, still figured in the practice of most physicians; even infants and small children endured the discomfort of mercury poisoning until well after the Civil War. Purges were still administered routinely in spring and fall to facilitate the body's adjustment to the changing seasons. The blisters and excoriated running sores so familiar to physicians and patients at the beginning of the century were gradually replaced by mustard plasters or turpentine applications, but the ancient concept of counterirritation still rationalized their use. Even bleeding still lingered, though increasingly in the practice of older men, and in less cosmopolitan areas. To divest themselves of such reliable means of regulating the body's internal equilibrium was, as older physicians contended, to succumb to an intellectual fad with no justification other than a morally irresponsible, if intellectually modish, emphasis on the healing powers of nature. It seemed to many physicians almost criminal to ignore their responsibility to regulate the secretions, even in ailments whose natural course was toward either death or recovery. Thus the continued vogue of cathartics and diuretics (though emetics, like bleeding, faded in popularity as the century progressed).

The debate over therapeutics was characterized more by moderation than by a full-fledged commitment either to the old or to the new and radically skeptical. Few physicians occupied either of these extreme posi-

---

31 Edmund Ravenel to unknown correspondent, draft, [November 1850], Ford-Ravenel Collection, South Carolina Historical Society, Charleston.
32 Report of the Resident Physicians, Philadelphia Dispensary, *Rules of . . . with the Annual Report for 1862* (Philadelphia: J. Crummill, 1863), pp. 12–13.
33 Oliver Wendell Holmes, *Medical Essays* (Boston: Houghton Mifflin, 1911), p. 258. Cited from an essay published originally in 1861.

tions. In the intellectual realm as well as in that of practice, clinicians sought, in a number of ways, to insure the greatest possible degree of continuity with older ideas. When smaller doses seemed as efficacious as those heroic prescriptions they had employed in their youth, it could be explained as a consequence of change in the prevailing pattern of disease incidence and perhaps even in the constitution of Americans.[34] More fundamentally, most physicians still found it difficult to accept the reductionist implications of the view that disease ordinarily manifested itself in the form of discrete clinical entities, with unique causes, courses, and pathologies. Physicians still spoke of epidemic influences, of diarrheas shifting into cholera, or minor fevers efflorescing into typhoid or yellow fever, if improperly managed.[35] The system was rich in confirmatory evidence; did not cases of "incipient" yellow fever and cholera recover, if treated in a timely fashion? Traditionalists still found it natural to speak of general constitutional states – sthenic or asthenic – as underlying the symptomatology of particular ills or the response of the body to particular drugs. Drugs, on the other hand, were still assumed to reflect the influence of climate in their action. Man was still an organism reacting unceasingly, and at countless levels, with its environment.

Perhaps most significantly, even those who were most radical in their criticisms of traditional routinism and severity of dosage still emphasized that the physician's therapeutic effectiveness depended, to a good extent, on his familiarity with the patient's constitutional idiosyncrasies. "No two patients have the same constitutional or mental proclivities," the *Boston Medical and Surgical Journal* editorialized in 1833: "No two instances of typhoid fever or of any other disease, are precisely alike. No 'rule of thumb,' no recourse to a formula-book, will avail for the treatment of the typical diseases."[36]

Indeed, it was not until the very end of the nineteenth century that an outspoken and thoroughgoing therapeutic skepticism came actually to be pronounced from some of the country's most prestigious medical chairs. "In some future day," as one authority put it,

34 See, for example, Samuel Henry Dickson, "Therapeutics," *Richmond Medical Journal* 3 (1867); 12; Jared Kirtland, *An Introductory Lecture, on the Coinciding Tendencies of Medicines* (Cleveland: M. C. Younglove, 1848), p. 7.

35 A New Orleans physician could, for example, write in 1849 that "we have some cases of *Yellow Fever* – that is, they are yellow fever at the death, though but few look like it at the *beginning*. It is the mildest type of Intermittent and Remittent fever, of which 99 in the 100 cases can be cured if taken in time & properly treated; but *neglected* or *maltreated* [they shift into classic yellow fever]." E. D. Fenner to James Y. Bassett, September 18, 1849, Bassett Papers, Southern Historical Collection, University of North Carolina, Chapel Hill, N.C.

36 "Routine Practice," *Boston Medical and Surgical Journal* 108 (January 11, 1883): 43.

it is certain that drugs and chemicals will form no part of a scientific therapy. This is sure to be the case, for truth is finally certain to prevail. . . . The principal influence or relation of materia medica to the cure of bodily disease lies in the fact that drugs supply material upon which to rest the mind while other agencies are at work in eliminating disease from the system, and to the drug is frequently given the credit. . . . Sugar of milk tablets of various colors and different flavors constitute a materia medica in practice that needs for temporary use only, morphin, codein, cocain, aconite and a laxative to make it complete.[37]

A dozen drugs, a Johns Hopkins clinician argued, "suffice for the pharmaco-therapeutic armamentarium of some of the most eminent physicians on this continent."[38] Not surprisingly, the sometimes aggressive depreciation of therapeutic routinism by such leaders in the profession as William Osler or Richard Cabot still provoked aggressive counterattack. "Expectant treatment," Abraham Jacobi contended bitterly in 1908, "is too often a combination of indolence and ignorance. . . . Expectant treatment is no treatment. It is the sin of omission, which not infrequently rises to the dignity of a crime."[39] Not all medical men were willing or able to accept the newer kind of reassurance which characterized the world of scientific medicine.

Indeed, many nineteenth-century American physicians were keenly aware of the potential inconsistency between the demands of science and those of clinical practice – and, by implication, humanity. This perceived conflict had a pedigree extending backward at least to the presidency of Andrew Jackson, and it is hardly a moot question today. The debate over therapeutics naturally reflected this conflict of values. "The French have departed too much from the method of Sydenham & Hippocrates to make themselves good practitioners," an indignant New York physician complained in 1836. "They are tearing down the temple of medicine to lay its foundations anew. . . . They lose more in Therapeutics than they gain by morbid anatomy – They are explaining how men die but not how to cure them."[40] To some American medical teachers, the newly critical demands

37 Elmer Lee, "How Far does a Scientific Therapy depend upon the Materia Medica in the Cure of Disease," *Journal of the American Medical Association* 31 (1898): 827.
38 Lewllys F. Barker, "On the Present Status of Therapy and its Future," *Johns Hopkins Hospital Bulletin* 11 (1900): 153. Critics of his skeptical position, the often acid William Osler put it, "did not appreciate the difference between the giving of medicines and the treatment of disease." Osler, *The Treatment of Disease. The Address in Medicine Before the Ontario Medical Association, Toronto, June 3, 1909* (London: Oxford, 1909), p. 13.
39 Abraham Jacobi, "Nihilism and Drugs," *New York State Journal of Medicine* 8 (1908): 57–65.
40 Alexander H. Stevens to James Jackson, April 14, 1836, James Jackson Papers, Francis Countway Library of Medicine, Boston.

of the Paris Clinical School and its emphasis on reevaluating traditional therapeutics in the light of "numerical" standards seemed almost antisocial, a reversion to a sterile and demeaning empiricism.

> The practice of medicine according to this view, is entirely empirical, it is shorn of all rational induction, and takes a position among the lower grades of experimental observations, and fragmentary facts.[41]

The polarization of values implied by such observations grew only more intense in the second half of the century, as traditionally oriented physicians expressed their resentment of a fashionable worship of things German, and what they felt to be a disdain for clinical acumen. The appeal of the laboratory and its transcendent claims seemed to many clinicians a dangerous will-o'-the-wisp. Even S. Weir Mitchell, onetime experimental physiologist, could charge that "out of the false pride of the laboratory and the scorn with which the accurate man of science looks down upon medical indefiniteness, has arisen the worse evil of therapeutic nihilism."[42] The danger, as another prominent chairholder put it, was that young men, "allured by the glitter of scientific work, will neglect the important and really more difficult attainments of true professional studies."[43] To some extent, of course, this was a conflict between the elite and the less favored; but it was, as well, a clash of temperament and world-view within America's medical elite. Willingness to accept the emotional and epistemological transcendence of science, even at the expense of traditional clinical standards, provided an emotional fault line which marked the profession throughout the last two-thirds of the century and paralleled the kind of change and conflict implied by modernization in other areas of society.

In the second half of the twentieth century, the relationship between doctor and patient is much altered; its context has in the great majority of cases shifted from the home to the physician's office or some institutional setting. The healer is in many cases unknown, or known only casually, to the patient. Even the place of drug therapeutics has changed, changed not only in the sense that the efficacy of most drugs is beginning to be understood, but in the social ambience which surrounds their use. The patient still maintains a faith in the physician's prescription (often, indeed, demands such a prescription) but it is a rather different kind of faith than that which

41 L. M. Lawson, *Western Lancet* 9 (1849): 196.
42 S. W. Mitchell, *The Annual Oration before the Medical and Chirugical Faculty of Maryland, 1877* (Baltimore: Inness and Col, 1877), p. 5.
43 Roberts Bartholow, *The Present State of Therapeutics: A Lecture Introductory to the Fifty-sixth Annual Course in Jefferson Medical College... October 1, 1879* (Philadelphia: J. B. Lippincott, 1879), p. 21.

shaped the interaction of physician, patient, and therapeutics at the beginning of the nineteenth century.

Clearly the physician and the great majority of his patients no longer
share a similar view of the body and the mechanisms which determine
health and disease. Differing views of the body and the physician's ability
to intervene in its mysterious opacity divide groups and individuals, rather
than unifying, as the widely disseminated metaphorical view of body function had still done in 1800. Physician and patient are no longer bound
together by the physiological activity of the drugs administered. In a sense,
almost *all* drugs now act as placebos, for with the exception of certain
classes of drugs such as diuretics, the patient experiences no perceptible
physiological effect. He does ordinarily have faith in the efficacy of a
particular therapy, but it is a faith based not on a shared nexus of belief and
participation in the kind of experience we have described, but rather in the
physician and his imputed status, and, indirectly, in that of science itself.
Obviously, one can draw facile parallels to many other areas in which
an older community of world-view and personal relationship has been
replaced by a more fragmented and status-oriented reality. Such observations have become commonplace as we try to ascertain the shape of a
gradually emerging modernity in the nineteenth-century West.

It is less easy to evaluate the moral implications of such change, and its
existential meaning for the participants in the healing ritual. Our generation is tempted by an easy romanticization of community lost; it would be
tempting, that is, to bewail the destruction of a traditional medicine, of a
nexus of shared belief and assured relationship. Clearly we have lost
something; or, to be more accurate, something has changed. But it would
be arrogant indeed to dismiss the objective virtues of modern medicine
with the charge that it is somehow less meaningful emotionally than it
was in 1800. For after all, if we have created new dimensions of misery
through technology, we have allayed others. To the historian familiar with
nineteenth-century medicine and conditions of life, it would be naive
indeed to dismiss the compensatory virtues of twentieth-century medicine
– its humane failings notwithstanding.

2

Medical text and social context: Explaining William Buchan's Domestic Medicine

ᔥ One can make a strong case for William Buchan's *Domestic Medicine* being the most widely read – nonreligious – book in English during the half century following its Edinburgh publication in 1769. Certainly it was the most frequently reprinted medical treatise in Britain and the United States. Its pages illustrate with particular clarity the shared knowledge and assumptions that bound professionals and lay people together in a community of ideas and healing practice. Buchan concedes the reality of lay practice and the widespread distribution of medical knowledge, yet seeks to define a special role for the credentialed physician.

I had long felt a bookshop browser's interest in Buchan's treatise; it was the only pre-1850 medical text that one was almost certain to find in the "old medical"section of any used or rare bookshop. But when I began my academic work in the early 1960s, it had not seemed an appropriately dignified subject for research. After writing the previous chapter on traditional therapeutics in the mid-1970s, however, I began to think more systematically about the day-to-day aspects of Anglo-American medical care and Buchan seemed an obvious place to start. A growing interest among professional historians in popular ideas and world-views also made the Edinburgh physician's effort to improve "domestic medicine" a potential tool for use in evaluating the relationships among high, low, and middle orders. Material that had seemed marginal – quaint and anecdotal – when I began graduate school in the late 1950s had gradually become acceptable, even exciting to a growing number of professional historians. By the early 1980s, when this essay was written, popular health and healing and ideas about the body seemed well on the way to fashionable status – as approaches that called themselves "cultural history" and "cultural studies" moved from the periphery to the center of academic concern. ᔥ

In the last decade, historians have shown a growing interest in medical care. One consequence has been the awkward realization that the larger part of such care provided to the sick has always been offered by individuals who did not consider themselves and were not considered by their contemporaries to be physicians. This implies a practical challenge to the would-be medical historian, for lay practitioners rarely kept systematic records. Diary entries and references in private correspondence have survived in scores of manuscript repositories; but voluminous collections of personal papers are not easily sampled by the historian searching specifically for descriptions of domestic practice. Thus prospective chroniclers of popular medicine are particularly dependent on the advice books and manuals which often guided and rationalized household doctoring. Even within this genre there is a significant gap between behavior and prescription; the appearance of an argument or recipe on a printed page does not mean the idea was understood (at least in the form in which it was presented) or that the recipe was in fact administered.

A few books, however, enjoyed such an extraordinary vogue that the historian of medical practice must assume that their very popularity tells us something significant about the medical system that produced them. No single health guide before the twentieth century enjoyed a greater popularity than William Buchan's *Domestic Medicine*. Between the 1769 publication of its first edition in Edinburgh and the appearance of its last English-language version just over a century later in Philadelphia, Buchan's *Domestic Medicine* appeared in at least 142 separate editions.[1] Still ubiquitous in secondhand bookstores, copies of Buchan are as remarkable for their uniformly shabby condition as for their omnipresence: covers

---

1 The first edition was published by Balfour, Auld, and Smellie in 1769, the last in Philadelphia by Claxton in 1871. A London edition was announced in 1769 but seems never to have actually appeared. (The announcement appeared among advertisements at the rear of S. A. Tissot's *Essay on Diseases of Sedentary and Literary Persons* [London: J. Nourse, E. and C. Dilly, 1769].) The figure of 142 includes only English-language editions and excludes multiple issues of the same edition. It has been compiled from entries in the *National Union Catalogue*, New York Public Library Catalogue, British Museum Catalogue, Wellcome Institute Catalogue, R. H. Shoemaker's *A Checklist of American Imprints for 1820–1829* (New York: Scarecrow Press, 1964–1971), and Robert Austin's *Early American Medical Imprints . . . 1668–1820* (Washington, D.C.: National Library of Medicine, 1961) with John Blake's unpublished supplement. I have used copies of Buchan in the Countway Library, National Library of Medicine, College of Physicians of Philadelphia, Library Company of Philadelphia, and my own collection. I should like to thank Richard J. Wolfe, Curator of the Rare Book Department at the Countway Library, and John Blake, Chief of the History of Medicine Division of the National Library of Medicine, for allowing me to make copies of their catalogue cards for William Buchan. In the absence of a union catalogue for the United Kingdom, it is certain that I have failed to locate editions held by local and regional libraries in Britain.

loose, signatures shaky, handwritten recipes and newspaper clippings adorning endpapers. In this case at least, the historian can be confident that he or she is dealing with a text that was widely and carefully read. Certainly, the dozens of publishers who chose to print and reprint Buchan's hardy perennial were aware of their several generations' intellectual inclinations; they had no wish to create opinion, but to reflect it. Their self-serving economic choices confirm the relevance of this book to at least four generations of British and American domestic physicians.

The most striking aspect of Buchan's *Domestic Medicine* is its novel format. The making of health books was an ancient art – but Buchan's treatise marked something of a departure; it had only one obvious prede-cessor, S. A. Tissot's *Avis au peuple sur sa santé*, which appeared in 1761 in Lausanne and was soon translated into English.[2] Until the mid-eighteenth century, books on health for laypeople fell into two broad categories. First, there were books on regimen and long life, clearly if implicitly written for the educated and leisured. Such texts were as much moral philosophy as medical treatise; they emphasized regimen and offered prospective advice on the preservation of health. "Let us," as one put it,

> by virtuous course of life, and by the practice of such rules as the experience of ages has established, endeavour to preserve health of body and soundness of mind, until we arrive at the boundaries which providence (unless we are our own enemies) seems to have nearly marked out for our respective constitutions.[3]

These guides to right living provided little in the way of description of specific diseases and equally little by way of therapeutics. George Cheyne's *An Essay of Health and Long Life* and Luigi Cornaro's *Discourses on a Sober and Temperate Life* were probably the most widely read exemplars of this genre in the half-century before Buchan.[4] A second category of health

---

2 *A Short Title Catalogue of Eighteenth Century Printed Books in the National Library of Medicine*, compiled by John Blake (Bethesda, Md.: U.S. Department of Health, Education, and Welfare, 1979), notes a dozen English-language editions between 1765 and 1778. Only four of these editions appeared after 1769; see p. 451. Insofar as the early success of Tissot in Great Britain indicated the existence of an appropriate audience, Buchan's ability to supersede it in the marketplace implies that the *Domestic Medicine* was far more effective in meeting the needs of that market.

3 James MacKenzie, *The History of Health, and the Art of Preserving it...*, 2d ed. (Edinburgh: William Gordon, 1759), p. 436.

4 George Cheyne, *An Essay of Health and Long Life* (London: George Strahan, 1725). See also Cheyne's *An Essay on Regimen... Serving to Illustrate the Principles and Theory of Philosophical Medicin* [sic], *And Point Out Some of its Moral Consequences* (London: C. Rivington, 1740). Cornaro's seventeenth-century text was printed in various forms and under several titles throughout the eighteenth century. I have used the Glasgow edition of 1770: *Discourses on a Sober and Temperate Life* (Glasgow: Robert Ure, 1770). These

manual was more pragmatic, consisting essentially of recipes or lists of medicaments and their applications in the home treatment of perceived illness. John Wesley's *Primitive Physick*, John Theobald's *Every Man His Own Physician*, and Nicholas Culpeper's *English Physician* were perhaps the best known of such works in mid-eighteenth-century Britain.[5] Cheyne and Cornaro were books to read and contemplate; Wesley and Culpeper, books to use in kitchen or sickroom. Buchan's *Domestic Medicine* broke away from these genre conventions; it was both a book to read and a book to use.

Approximately the first third of Buchan's original edition was a general treatise on health and the means necessary for its preservation; the remainder of the book was organized around particular ills (many, but not all, corresponding to entities recognizable to the twentieth-century physician).[6] A description of the disease and its symptoms is followed by a discussion of causes, appropriate regimen, and treatment. Recipes for drug mixtures, poultices, and the like were run into the text, an arrangement altered in the second edition three years later; this London revision of 1772 provided a separate index of remedies and moved a good many of those provided in 1769 out of the text and into footnotes. The third edition published two

texts centered on regimen and individual control of the so-called non-naturals – diet, evacuation and retention, air, exercise, sleep, and the "passions." William Coleman has recently emphasized the consistency between these traditional doctrines and "Enlightenment rationalism," in "Health and Hygiene in the *Encyclopédie*: A Medical Doctrine for the Bourgeoisie," *J. Hist. Med.* 29 (1974): 399–421, at p. 399. See also Peter H. Niebyl, "The Non-naturals," *Bull. Hist. Med.* 44 (1970): 372–377; L. J. Rather, "The 'Six Things Non-Natural': A Note on the Origins and Fate of a Doctrine and a Phrase," *Clio Medica* 3 (1968): 337–347. On Cheyne, see Lester S. King, "George Cheyne, Mirror of Eighteenth-Century Medicine," *Bull. Hist. Med.* 48 (1974): 517–539. There were occasional attempts to present the admonitions of proper regimen in inexpensive, "tract" form, but these were atypical. See, for example, *Directions and Observations Relative to Food, Exercise and Sleep* (London: S. Bladon, 1772).

5 Wesley's *Primitive Physick* was first published in 1747; it has been conveniently reprinted with an introduction by A. Wesley Hill (London: Epworth Press, c. 1960). See also: A. Wesley Hill, *John Wesley Among the Physicians: A Study of 18th-Century Medicine* (London: Epworth Press, 1958). Theobald's little manual appeared first in 1764 – when it was issued in four separate printings. The full title is instructive: *Every Man his Own Physician. Being a complete Collection of efficacious and Approved Remedies, for every Disease incident to the Human Body. With Plain Instructions for their Common Use. Necessary to be had in all families, particularly those residing in the country. The Fourth Edition, Improved* (London: W. Griffin, R. Withy, and G. Kearsly, 1754). The price was eighteen pence. Culpeper's herbal and astrological *English Physitian: or an astrologo-physical discourse of the vulgar herbs of this Nation* appeared first in 1652 and was reprinted many times in the following two centuries.

6 Smallpox, epilepsy, measles, and consumption, for example, correspond in general to twentieth-century nosological entities; other sections such as those on "costiveness," "headache," "suppression of urine," and "excessive vomiting" describe symptoms rather than diseases. Buchan also organized sections around diseases of women, diseases of children, and surgery.

years later added a separate dispensatory in the form of an appendix.[7] Buchan's treatise was evolving steadily into a manual for home use.

But for whose use? Who constituted the audience for this enormously successful book? Buchan, like Tissot, offered his domestic guide for the ostensible needs of a rural elite whose presumed noblesse would lead them to minister to the ills of neighbors and dependents unable to find or employ a physician; landowners, clergymen, even schoolteachers might be expected to help in treating nearby "rusticks." One-half of mankind, Buchan emphasized, would never have the means to consult a trained physician; nor would they provide the audience for his *Domestic Medicine*.[8] Buchan was simply reaffirming the assumptions of his Swiss forerunner; Tissot did not intend – despite its title – that his *Advice to the People*

> would become a Piece of Furniture, as it were, in the House of every Peasant. Nineteen out of twenty will probably never know of its Existence. Many may be unable to read, and still more unable to understand it, plain and simple as it is. I have principally calculated it for the Perusal of intelligent and charitable Persons who live in the Country; and who seem to have, as it were, a Call from Providence, to assist their less intelligent poor Neighbors with their Advice.[9]

Like Tissot, Buchan also hoped that his manual would help the respectable to protect the lower orders from the dangerous impositions of quacks – and the consequences of their own superstitious beliefs.

Yet such statements of purpose seem more a preemptive defense against the potential antagonism of regular physicians than an accurate description

---

7 The second (1772) edition, "with considerable additions," was published in London by W. Strahan and T. Cadell and in Edinburgh by A. Kincaid, W. Creech, and J. Balfour. The third (1774) edition, also "with considerable additions," was published by Strahan and Cadell in London and J. Balfour and W. Creech in Edinburgh. The dispensatory occupies an appendix, pp. 685–749. Tissot's *Advice* had provided a numbered table of remedies and references by number throughout the text to the several remedies. A helpful modern evaluation of Buchan and his *Domestic Medicine* is to be found in C. J. Lawrence, "William Buchan: Medicine Laid Open," *Med. Hist.* 19 (1975): 20–35. There is some evidence that publisher and popularizer William Smellie may have been editor or part-author of Buchan's book. See Lawrence, "Buchan," pp. 21–22. The evidence for a definitive attribution of the roles of Buchan and Smellie does not seem to exist and I have chosen in the following pages to treat "William Buchan" as the single author of what is an internally consistent text and concentrate on that text. There does not seem to be any evidence that later (1772 and following) editions were not actually revised by Buchan. A letter from Buchan to his publisher William Strahan (dated December 21, 1771) strongly supports this view. Misc. Ms., Countway Library of Medicine.
8 Buchan, 1769, pp. xii–xiii.
9 Tissot, *Advice to the People in General, with Regard to their Health, But Particularly Calculated for those, who are the most unlikely to be provided in time with the best Assistance, in acute Diseases,* . . . Trans. from the French . . . by J. Kirkpatrick. 3d ed. (London: T. Beckett and P. A. De Hondt, 1768), p. 16.

of Buchan's ultimate audience. Common sense and demography tell us that those who purchased and relied on his *Domestic Medicine* were not drawn primarily from the ranks of large landholders and the clergymen and schoolteachers associated with them; and there are some more specific clues in the text itself pointing toward the social location of Buchan's readers. First and most obviously, as we have seen, this book was not meant for the "peasants" and "rustics" who might benefit from the ministrations of their local betters, still less for the workers in manufacturing ("that useful set of people upon whom the riches and prosperity of Britain depend") whose health also concerned the Edinburgh physician. Buchan talks about them, not to them; landless farmers and workers were no more expected to read, reflect on, and use his *Domestic Medicine* than was a foot soldier expected to read Pringle's or Van Swieten's contemporary treatises on diseases of the army.[10] Another group of potential readers was described not in the condescending terms Buchan used in referring to peasants and workers – but in tones of moral judgment.

The idle, affected, and luxury-loving rich were a target of Buchan's repeated scorn – and exemplars of ways of living which compromised health. Premature illness was the inevitable consequence of a lifestyle which permitted grown men to be carried about in sedan chairs, to spend their nights in drinking, gaming, and overeating; their consorts at the same time could scarcely hope to bear and raise hardy children without the physical exertion demanded both by morality and the body's own design.

> How ridiculous would it seem to a person unacquainted with modern luxury, to behold the young and healthy swinging along the shoulders of their fellow-creatures! or to see a fat carcase, over-run with diseases occasioned by inactivity, dragged thro' the streets by half a dozen horses.[11]

10 The quoted phrase is drawn from p. xi, 1769. Buchan's *Proposals for Printing by Subscription an Original Work, Intitled, the Family Physician . . . in Six Parts* promised that one of the six parts would be devoted to the "Diseases of Manufacturers, Labourers, &c"; the book itself devoted far less space to the ills of working men. (The *Proposals* is an undated, sixteen-page pamphlet held by the Wellcome Institute for the History of Medicine.) Pringle was a particular influence on Buchan, who dedicated the second (1772) and subsequent editions to him. Tissot (*Advice*, 1768, p. 14) mentions Van Swieten as a specific predecessor. Pringle's *Observations on the Diseases of the Army* first appeared in 1752. Gerard van Swieten's *Kurze Beschreibung und Heilungsart der Krankheiten, welche am öftersten in dem Feldlager beobachtet werden* appeared in 1758; it was translated into English in 1762.

11 Buchan, 1769, p. 101. See also pp. 106, 576–577. In the last-cited passage, Buchan urged that if the rich and indolent ate and exercised like "the better sort of peasants" they would be little troubled by barrenness. "An Active life," Buchan emphasized, "is the best guardian of virtue, and the greatest preservation of health" (p. 107). He was, quite literally, an advocate of the work ethic; for example, he endorses the desirability

One can hardly pinpoint anything as elusive as the readership for an eighteenth-century text so widely read and reprinted, but it would seem that the purchasers of Buchan's *Domestic Medicine* represented a cross section of the literate, servant-employing, and consciously self-improving "middling orders" – men and women who would think twice before spending hard-earned shillings and pounds on a physician, and who sought a rational guide both to prudent domestic practice and to a moral and health-ensuring regimen. The growth in numbers and self-consciousness of this new class may well explain both the enormous success of Buchan's guide and the specific shape of the genre it created. His readers could not be satisfied with the general advice on regimen suited to a leisured elite; nor could they be content with the terse and unadorned recipes of a Wesley or Theobald.[12]

Far less problematic than the identification of Buchan's actual readership are the concrete insights which the Edinburgh physician casually provides into the medical thought and practice of his generation. Perhaps most surprising to twentieth-century assumptions was the broad diffusion of medical knowledge among his fellow Britons. Buchan felt no need to describe the symptoms of malaria, whooping cough, smallpox, or insanity; they were too well known. Laypeople, he noted in passing, never thought to consult a physician in treating a simple intermittent fever – unless the patient were in desperate straits. There was "not a parish, and hardly a village in Britain, destitute of some person who can bleed." Almost all rural clergymen knew "something of medicine. Almost all of them bleed, and can order a purge."[13] Buchan was aware as well that beneath the level of formal academic medicine was an elaborate and regionally differentiated tradition of folk and domestic medicine – much but not all of it herbal. As

of even the rich mastering a craft: "They would at least derive as much honour from a few masterly specimens of their own workmanship, as from the character of having ruined most of their companions by gaming, or hard drinking" (p. 106).

12 The term *middling orders* is obviously imprecise and elusive – except insofar as it underlines the role played by images of the rich and poor in defining who the middling orders were not – and in contrast to whom they defined their social identity. There are some other, more circumstantial, hints in Buchan's text as to his assumed readership. Buchan assumed, for example, that his readers employed servants (though, given the number of Britons who did, this is not too precise a socially defining characteristic). There is also evidence that Buchan assumed that a goodly portion of his readers would not be familiar with rural health beliefs and practices – implying an urban-oriented audience. His *Proposals* specified a prepublication price of five shillings (delivered to the subscriber's house); the price was to be six shillings after publication. For recent discussions of class in this period, see E. P. Thompson, "Patrician Society, Plebian Culture," *J. Soc. Hist.* 7 (1974): 382–405; Thompson, "Eighteenth-century English Society: Class Struggle Without Class?" *Soc. Hist.* 3 (1978): 133–165; R. S. Neale, *Class in English History, 1680–1850* (Oxford: Blackwell, 1981).

13 Buchan, 1769, pp. 182, 194, 282–283, 253, 338, 516; *Proposals*, p. 8.

we shall see, Buchan adopted a revealingly ambiguous position in regard to household practice; he never contemplated its entire suppression, but sought instead to limit the boundaries of lay practice and define the physician's relation to it.

In a world of widely diffused medical knowledge and a far from universal domination of practice by formally trained practitioners, it is not surprising that one of Buchan's concerns – and one presumably related to his rapid acceptance by both laypeople and physicians – was precisely the setting of plausible boundaries between medicine and its lay competitors. This is obscured somewhat by Buchan's criticism of the profession's weakness for vaporous speculation and "mystical jargon," its often mercenary character, and its pretentious Latin prescriptions and claims to exclusive authority; it is obscured as well by his acute and telling critique of folk medicine and its sometimes superstitious and always uncritical therapeutics.[14]

The treatment of women and children was a particularly controverted area – one in which the medical man's very relevance was unclear. Buchan was unrelentingly hostile toward the nurses and midwives who, in fact, still dominated care at birth and during infancy. He assailed the age-old assumptions that the physician possessed no special ability to treat children's diseases and that a regularly trained medical man need not be called in such cases. "The consequence," Buchan contended, "is that a physician is seldom called till the good women have exhausted all their skill; when his attendance can only serve to divide the blame and appease the disconsolate parents."[15] Buchan assailed as well the prevalent neglect of children's ills by physicians. Enormous sums of money and amounts of labor were "daily bestowed to prop an old rotten carcase for a few years, while thousands of those who might be useful in life perish without being regarded."[16] The often acute character and rapid course of sickness in such tiny patients, Buchan emphasized, only underlined the need for immediate medical intervention; these ills were too dangerous and infant lives too precious to be left to the doubtful ministrations of nurses, midwives, and "old women."

Historians of the Enlightenment have emphasized the growing eighteenth-century awareness of children as individuals, of childhood as a distinct and significant developmental period, and of a parallel consciousness of infant mortality as a remediable and thus inexcusable evil.[17] These themes are

---

14 Buchan, 1769, pp. viii, ix, xiv; *Proposals*, pp. 14, 16.
15 Buchan, 1769, p. 8. See also pp. 21, 40, 44–45, 440; Buchan, 1772, p. 7n.
16 Buchan, 1769, p. 9.
17 See the extremely influential study by Philippe Aries, *Centuries of Childhood: A Social History of Family Life* (New York: Knopf, 1962). Two more recent works are J. H. Plumb, "The New World of Children in Eighteenth-century England," *Past and Present* 67 (1975): 64–95; and Ivy Pinchbeck and Mary Hewitt, *Children and English*

certainly discernible in Buchan's *Domestic Medicine*; yet his emphasis on the neglected obstetric and pediatric role of physicians and his consistent hostility to "ignorant old women," nurses, and midwives, indicate another kind of motivation in his concern for child health. This lay in his desire to establish an increasing role for medical men in this traditionally female realm. Buchan's readers were of the class which would normally employ a nurse, yet for whom some personal responsibility for child care – if only a personal oversight of that nurse – was a plausible option.[18] Childbirth and child care represented an enormous potential opportunity for the expansion of medical practice among the middling and better sort; for it was an area which most mid-eighteenth-century Englishmen and women did not yet see as the physician's appropriate sphere.

Even surgery implied problems of boundary definition; laypeople, Buchan emphasized, should not be expected to employ a catheter, cut for the stone, or perform tracheotomies in diphtheria; even in cases of difficult teething a surgeon was the only practitioner appropriate for lancing the little patient's gums. And, Buchan warned, in any unnatural labor, a surgeon or "man-midwife" should be called immediately. The widespread ability of laypeople to bleed, to dress wounds, and even to set fractures did not mean that there should not be a sharp distinction between the proper spheres of lay and medical practice in surgery.[19]

More generally, Buchan warned laypeople to overcome their hesitancy in summoning physicians. "Physicians may indeed assist nature;" he urged, "but their attempts must ever prove fruitless, when she is no longer able to cooperate with their endeavours."[20] In any acute fever, for example, the physician should be called immediately. There remained, of course, a large residual category of colds and simple fevers, arthritis, and minor diarrheas which normally and legitimately engaged the layperson's medical skills; but

Society, 2 vols. (London: Routledge & Kegan Paul; Toronto: University of Toronto Press, 1969, 1973). Buchan also cites mercantilist arguments, casually referring to the value of healthy children and a low mortality rate to the state.

18 See, for example, p. 47, where parents are urged not "to trust so valuable a treasure entirely in the hands of a hireling," or p. 42, where the mother is urged to go along with the nursemaid when she is taking the child out – though "some may think this office below their dignity." This passage was deleted in the 1772 edition.

19 Buchan does concede that dislocations were frequently reduced even by those without medical education (p. 605) and that local bonesetters might be competent (p. 606). But bonesetters, he warned, should not be consulted when a competent surgeon was available. On procedures beyond the layperson's capacity, see p. 221 (chest abscess); p. 320 (opening the windpipe in diphtheria); p. 398 (catheterization); p. 413 (bladder stone); p. 571 (difficult childbirth); p. 593 (gums lanced); p. 595 (trauma). It is striking that Buchan nowhere specifically discusses the proper relationships between apothecaries – who must in reality have served as physician to many of his readers – and holders of the medical degree.

20 Buchan, 1769, pp. 184–185.

even within this accustomed therapeutic world, a line had to be drawn between the medicaments suitable for lay practice and those best left to the trained physician; he alone could make precise clinical judgments, balancing a patient's constitutional idiosyncrasies against his ailment's particular stage of development. Buchan conceded the ability of laypeople to employ an elaborate repertoire of traditional herbal remedies; he assumed as well that laypeople would purge and bleed themselves "at the usual seasons." He warned, however, against a mindless routinism in lay practice, a routinism which ignored individual differences; Buchan decried as well the excessive and unthinking use of bleeding and purging in domestic practice.[21] Practically speaking, however, it was mercury that Buchan used most frequently to draw a pragmatic line between the appropriate competences of laypeople and physicians. Mercury, he cautioned, was always dangerous when administered by untutored hands, but was particularly so when misused by those legions of quacks who employed the dramatic effects of large doses to impress the credulous.[22]

If the establishing of an appropriate boundary between lay and professional practice was a particular concern for Buchan, so also was the allied question of controlling and ordering medical knowledge. As he did with regard to practice, Buchan sought to follow a delicate course between those aspects of lay ideas he tacitly accepted and those he anathematized. Though acid in his criticisms of the vagaries of folk medicine, he was perfectly willing to incorporate folk practice into his catalogue of approved advice – so long as such remedies were not obviously in conflict with those ideas and assumptions which guided his own thought and practice.

Especially in chronic ills such as "dropsy" and rheumatism, a goodly proportion of the remedies Buchan noted were herbal and either implicitly or explicitly part of folk practice.[23] Some remedies he merely listed without comment, others – such as garlic ointment in whooping cough, jellied lamb soup in dysentery, or greased and combed wool in gout – he heartily endorsed.[24] The practices Buchan rejected most emphatically were those which invoked charms or magic, and those in which a disease-specific efficacy was attached to a particular drug. Herbs did not cure because they

---

21 On bleeding at the usual seasons, p. 406. For criticisms of lay use of bleeding, see pp. 169, 194, 244.

22 *Proposals*, p. 12, notes the proclivity of quacks for the use of mercury and antimony, "well knowing that these are the most proper for a bold stroke." For warnings in regard to the use of mercury, see Buchan, 1769, pp. 312, 444n, 489, 613–614.

23 See, for example, the herbal remedies and prophylactics suggested in "dropsy," pp. 453, 454.

24 Buchan, 1769, pp. 377–378 (jellied lamb soup); pp. 341–342 (garlic ointment); p. 459 (Lancashire use of wool in gout). See also pp. 316, 592 for similar references to folk treatments.

were administered at a certain time or because they were accompanied by a particular invocation. Drugs did not cure because they had a specific effect on a particular disease; a case in point was the popular belief that a specific antidote must exist for every poisonous substance – when, in fact, Buchan argued, remedies worked through their general physiological properties as emetics or cathartics, not because of some mystical affinity to the poison.[25] Bathing preserved the health of children because it kept their skin clean and facilitated the insensible perspiration, not because the water came from a sacred well or because the child had been dipped into it a ritually meaningful number of times. Similarly, Buchan inveighed against a persistent popular faith in *Dreckapotheke*; in jaundice, for example, he complained that many "dirty things" such as lice and millipedes were recommended. Common people assumed that such arcane substances would "act as charms" and administered them only once. Even if lice or other vermin might by chance have some useful effect, it could be exerted only through a persistent course of treatment, Buchan explained, one consistent with the body's necessarily gradual efforts to restore itself to health.[26]

The Edinburgh physician was well aware that the patient's tendency to recovery in the great majority of ills accounted for the reputation of most folk remedies. Rabies, for example, was a notorious case in point. Scores of remedies had been urged as invariably effective. Recovery was a natural consequence, Buchan explained, of the supposedly rabid dog not having been rabid at all. (One of the most vivid passages in the *Domestic Medicine* describes the typical circumstances in which a lost dog was chased and tormented, becoming gradually more frantic, and finally biting a hypothetical rabies victim.) "This readily accounts," Buchan explained,

> for the great variety of infallible remedies for the bite of a mad dog, which are to be met with in almost every family. Though not one in a thousand has any claim to merit, yet they are all supported by number-less vouchers. No wonder that imaginary diseases should be cured by imaginary remedies.[27]

More important, of course, was the fact that patients ordinarily recovered in such everyday ailments as malaria or "sore eyes"; it was not surprising that "almost every person" possessed a remedy for ophthalmia and that

25 Buchan, 1769, pp. 523–524.
26 Buchan, 1769, pp. 39–40, 448, 534. Buchan consistently ridiculed beliefs which seemed "superstitious." In this later treatise on the venereal disease, Buchan bemoaned the fact that many laypeople still entertained "absurd notions" such as that one could cure oneself of the pox by transmitting it to another. *Observations Concerning the Prevention and Cure of the Venereal Disease* (London: The Author, 1796), pp. xvi–xvii.
27 Buchan, 1769, p. 530.

hardly an "old woman" lacked an infallible cure for malaria. Popular belief in the efficacy of the royal touch in scrofula grew out of the same tendency to spontaneous remission; nature, not the physician, and certainly not some quack remedy or the king's touch accounted for the patient's cure.[28]

Although Buchan could be intellectually ruthless in questioning both the empirical basis of many folk remedies and in impugning the medical man's habits of rationalistic speculation, he never questioned his own assumptions about the way in which the human body functioned in health and disease. And these assumptions were not only widespread among laypeople as well as physicians, but so deeply internalized that they demanded little systematic exposition; they were self-evident truths. One can hardly avoid concluding that one of the fundamental reasons for the success of Buchan's text lay in the very familiarity of his ideas and language. Just as his discussions of contemporary medical practice revealed substantial overlap between lay and professional spheres, so the most fundamental conceptions which informed Buchan's thought were widely disseminated among the literate in mid-eighteenth-century Great Britain. I refer both to his general way of seeing nature and man's place in it – and, more specifically, to the way in which man's body functioned in health and disease. Both were part of the repertoire of language and agreed-upon metaphor which shaped his and his contemporaries' perception of the world.

First, Buchan resorts again and again to arguments from design – especially those of a primitivist sort. He assumes that that which is innate in man is closest to his natural condition and thus necessarily best calculated to preserve health. England's enormous infant mortality was unnatural; if it were not, Buchan argued ingenuously, other species would die in equal numbers. Contemporary modes of child rearing had much to do with England's lamentably high infant mortality: "brutes guided by instinct, never err in this respect; while man, trusting solely to art, is seldom right."[29] Women in primitive cultures experienced few problems in childbirth, Buchan argued; and after delivery such natural folk never constrained their infant's innate drive toward physical activity with swaddling or leading strings early in life – nor did they subject them to a premature classroom discipline somewhat later. Spared the "manacling" which confined most English children, savages were hardly aware of such a thing as a deformed infant; their children could shift for themselves by the time

28 Buchan, 1769, pp. 478–479. On malaria and ophthalmia, see pp. 180 and 308. Buchan concluded that there were more "charms and whimsical remedies" prescribed in "malaria" than in any other ailment.
29 Buchan, 1769, p. 2.

England's "puny infants" were ready to leave their nurse's arms.[30] Animals in the wild chose their food with unerring appropriateness and were never debilitated by man's taste for luxury and artificial stimulation. "It were well for mankind," Buchan warned as he inveighed against high seasonings, pickles, and the like, "if cookery, as an art, were entirely prohibited."[31]

An agrarian life was man's healthiest state – his closest approximation to the invigorating life of his ancestors. "Labouring the ground," Buchan explained,

> is every way conductive to health. It not only gives exercise to every part of the body; but the very smell of the earth and fresh herbs, revive and chear the spirits, whilst the perpetual prospect of something coming to maturity, delights and entertains the mind.

Much of the ill health which characterized urban life was a result of the city's unnaturally crowded conditions; such ills as scrofula and rickets, Buchan argued, had not come into existence until English farmers and cotters began their migration to the cities and exchanged active, outdoor labor for sedentary, ill-ventilated work. And the situation grew steadily worse. "Agriculture the first and most healthful of all employments," he mourned, "is now followed by few who are able to carry on any other business."[32] Man's taste in styles of work and consumption, like his taste in food, had brought artificiality, luxury, and inevitable ill health. It was not the industrial laborer and tenement dweller alone whose health deteriorated through sedentary, indoor work. The scholar as well put his health at risk in pursuing a style of life so contradictory to that of man in his natural state.

> Intense thought is so destructive to health, that few examples can be produced of studious persons who live to an extreme old age. Hard

30 Buchan, 1769, pp. 14–16, 30. Buchan cites Rousseau approvingly as author of the aphorism that temperance and exercise were the two best physicians (p. 94) and places consistent emphasis on the need for exercise (pp. 29, 34–35) in women as well as in men (pp. 35–36, 557, 559, 569). "Our love of motion is surely a strong proof of its utility. Nature implants no disposition in vain. . . . Every creature, except man, takes as much exercise as necessary. He alone, and such animals as are under his direction, deviate from this original law, and they suffer accordingly" (pp. 100–101). Man's intellect which allowed him to create an artificial civilization was the operational locus for that original sin which marked and degenerated Adam's posterity.

31 Buchan, 1769, p. 68.

32 Buchan, 1769, pp. 143 (for the longer quote), 137, 28–29, 141. Buchan also warned that nervous diseases would increase as a result of the growth in luxury and sedentary employments (p. 223). Worker cultivation of small garden plots seemed a plausible means for counteracting the effects of sedentary, indoor work: "It may seem romantic to recommend gardening to manufactures in great towns; but observation proves, that the plan is very practicable." Buchan was referring to his experience in Sheffield where he noted that the cutlers almost all tended small plots of ground (p. 144).

study always implies a sedentary life. . . . The perpetual thinker seldom enjoys either health or spirits; while the person who can hardly be said to think at all, seldom fails to enjoy both.[33]

The design immanent in man's body provided unfailing clues to the optimum conditions for maintaining that body in health – if man would only follow such guidance.

Buchan was a strenuous advocate of the healing power implicit in the body's fundamental design. Like many of his illustrious medical predecessors, Buchan assumed that the symptoms of disease were in actuality modes through which the body sought to reestablish health. Just as the body had a certain anatomical and physiological basis, so too it had a built-in tendency toward recovery and a set of mechanisms – sweating, fever, diarrhea – which brought it about. Thus there was no real distinction between a mechanism distinctly pathological and one characteristic of the body's normal physiological processes.[34] It was the physician's task to understand the nature and timing of these healing mechanisms; his practice should be calculated to support, not undermine them.

As we have seen, Buchan was careful to distance himself from the superstitious and even magical aspects of folk medicine; but he could not well distance himself from the speculative model of the body which informed his every attitude toward healing and illness. For not only his own understanding, but his plausibility as a healer rested on a faith shared by laypeople and physicians in the legitimacy of that system and the medical man's special understanding of it. Rote practice without a rationalistic understanding was a particular object of Buchan's disdain. "If half the time now spent in copying receipts and collecting nostrums were spent on rational understanding by reading," he chastised, the better sort of Britons "might be the instruments of doing much good, and prove real blessings

33 Buchan, 1769, pp. 145–146. The second half of this quotation was deleted in the 1772 edition. The diseases of the sedentary and studious had traditionally constituted a distinct subject matter. Tissot, for example, devoted a separate treatise to the subject: *An Essay on the Diseases Incident to Literary and Sedentary Persons*, 2d ed. (London: J. Nourse and E. and C. Dilly, 1769). Tissot, like many of his contemporaries, obviously assumed a class-specific as well as occupation-specific model of disease incidence and causation.

34 Buchan and his contemporaries tended to use the word "intentions" in referring to this healing process – implying both the body's mechanism and ends. "A fit of the gout is rather to be considered as Nature's method of curing a disease than a disease itself, and all that we can do, with safety, is to promote her intentions, and to assist her in expelling the enemy in her own way." Buchan, 1769, p. 460. Even in trauma: "It is Nature alone that cures wounds; all that art can do is to remove obstacles, and to put the parts in such a condition as is the most favourable to Nature's efforts" (p. 595). Still the best historical discussion of what has traditionally been called the healing power of nature is that by Max Neuburger, *Die Lehre von der Heilkraft der Natur im Wandel der Zeiten* (Stuttgart: Ferdinand Enke, 1926).

to society."[35] The enlightened and respectable might ultimately serve as a bulwark against the worst features of traditional empiricism and the insidious blandishment of quacks.

Buchan entertained an extremely – if eclectically – traditional view of the body. He saw it essentially as an equilibrium system, one in which balance constituted health, imbalance illness. Death resulted from a disequilibrium that became irreversible. Though medical historians have often referred to this as a humoral model of pathology and physiology, it might more usefully be referred to as a holistic equilibrium model; Buchan certainly does invoke humors, but in a casual and unsystematic – almost decorative – way; what is consistent is his emphasis on the body's functioning as a balanced whole, as defined and redefined in its unending interaction with a particular environment. Intake, process, and outgo determined health and disease. Diet, atmosphere, and climate determined intake; exercise, stress, and constitution, even clothing, affected process; and urine, feces, and perspiration rid the body of potentially dangerous end products. Illness was a particular state of a particular organism – not ordinarily the reaction of that organism to some specific and monolithic external cause. It is only logical that he should have placed extraordinary emphasis on the body's outgo; disordered or impeded evacuations (urine, feces, insensible perspiration) might be the cause of illness just as they might days or weeks later serve to cure the same dysfunction.[36] Even climatic and geographic factors associated with the causation of disease (the relationship of low, damp places to malaria, for example) caused sickness only through the intermediate mechanisms of humoral interaction.[37]

Just as there was little place in this speculative system for specific disease agents, so there was little place for truly localized ills or any way of separating body and mind. The passions could both cause and help cure illness – but only through the body's fundamental physiological mech-

35 *Proposals*, p. 13. Tissot (*Advice*, p. 13) makes much the same point in criticizing popular collections of recipes.

36 This rationalistic framework was not simply a rhetorical legitimation for the physician's status, but a means of structuring the relationship between doctor, therapeutics, and patient. See Charles E. Rosenberg, "The Therapeutic Rev᎐᎐.ion: Medicine, Meaning, and Social Change in Nineteenth-Century America," Chapter 1 of this volume. Buchan and his contemporaries were particularly interested in the "insensible perspiration" and its role in causing and curing disease; it would be hard to imagine a more diffuse yet effective mechanism for fostering and rationalizing health anxieties. See Buchan's comments on catching cold (1769, pp. 52–53) or on the way in which "looseness" might be a consequence of obstructed perspiration (p. 82). This concern was also consistent with a novel emphasis on cleanliness – for a dirty skin inevitably interfered with the perspiration (p. 88).

37 Malaria was, according to Buchan, caused by "moist air," watery diet, damp houses: "In a word whatever relaxes the solids, diminishes the perspiration, or obstructs the circulation in the capillary or small vessels, predisposes the body to ague" (p. 172).

anisms.[38] Man's physiological identity was not a state, but a process; it was hardly surprising that Buchan should have so forcefully dismissed the one-time administration of would-be specific cures. Only a drug which could intervene over time in the body's constitutive processes and gradually alter them could help change sickness to health.[39]

What is particularly striking about Buchan's use of this explanatory system, however, is the way in which it is carefully integrated into his therapeutics. It is not simply a reassuring rhetorical style which functions like the parsley on a roast, to be pushed aside before the serious business of eating is begun. One could cite scores of instances. Buchan, for example, emphasized the importance of not attempting immediately to allay diarrhea in dysentery; if the health process rested upon the body's ability to rid itself of morbid matter, then it was the physician's duty to observe and guide his ministrations by the integrity of that process. Diarrhea, as he put it, should not be considered a disease, "but rather a salutary evacuation." Even in "bloody flux" Buchan warned against the routine use of binding and astringent medicines "till the proper evacuations have been premised." Such overeager therapeutics might otherwise "fix" the disease instead of removing it.[40]

Buchan similarly emphasized the functional necessity of skin lesions in fevers; they were part of the body's attempt to relieve itself of the morbid end products of an unbalanced physiology. Danger always lay in anticipating this process too aggressively; one of Buchan's complaints against women who ventured to treat smallpox was their tendency to encourage the disease's characteristic eruptions prematurely.[41] Only a trained physician, Buchan contended, could know when the fever had lasted long enough for the body's humoral interactions to "elaborate" the morbid matter before its

38 Epidemics of childbed fever, for example, could be explained as a consequence of the fear induced in other women by the appearance of the first case in an area – yet that fear had to exert its effect through physiological mechanisms. "But fear seldom fails to obstruct the necessary evacuations upon which here recovery depends. Thus the sex often fall a sacrifice to their own imaginations, when there would be no danger did they apprehend none" (Buchan, 1769, p. 115). Even erysipelas (p. 293) and cholera morbus (p. 367) might be caused by the passions.

39 Buchan, 1769, pp. 532–533.

40 Buchan, 1769, pp. 370, 381–382. See also pp. 46, 368, 402, 611–612. A parallel case is that in whooping cough; Buchan suggested that ipecac might be needed to induce vomiting if it were not sufficiently copious. Buchan, 1772, p. 364, I. S. L. Loudon has recently pointed out a similar pattern of pathological assumption and therapeutic practice in the case of "Leg Ulcers in the Eighteenth and Early Nineteenth Centuries," *J. Roy. Coll. Gen. Prac.* 31 (1981): 265–266.

41 Buchan, 1769, pp. 255–256, 267. See also Tissot, *Advice*, pp. iv–v. Buchan did, however, approve in general of the "common notion" that it was always necessary to induce a sweat in the beginning of a fever – since fever was so often caused by an obstructed perspiration (p. 170).

removal by way of the skin. It was as much the *when* as the *what* that defined the physician's competence. Following a consistent logic, Buchan acknowledged that bleeding might be a necessity in measles, while it could ordinarily be avoided in smallpox. In the latter case, the characteristic eruptions helped the body to regain its health-defining equilibrium. In measles, on the other hand, the lack of running sores might suggest bleeding to aid the fevered patient in restoring an appropriate internal balance. Fever was itself, in fact, "nothing else but an effort of nature to free herself from an offending cause."[42] Even when the lesions appeared in timely fashion, there remained the danger that the disease might – in the idiom of the time – be "driven inward" by the application of too potent a plaster or ointment while the lesion remained open. Symptoms were the physician's most important clues to an appropriate therapy.

Just as a suddenly interrupted evacuation (menstruation stopped by a cold bath, insensible perspiration blocked by dirt or cold) could cause illness, so might the establishment of another, functionally equivalent, evacuation initiate the healing process. A nosebleed might serendipitously relieve madness; bleeding piles might have the same effect. A "habitual looseness" might be nature's way of compensating for an obstructed per-spiration. Buchan cited pleurisy as a striking example of this healing process: "Nature endeavours to carry off this disease either by a critical discharge of blood from the nose, &c or by expectoration, sweat, loose stools, thick urine, &c."[43] Such evacuations could not only cure, but provide invaluable clues as to the body's otherwise impenetrable interior. Bloodletting, for example, provided not only a therapeutic, but a diagnostic modality – for the appearance of the drawn blood provided insight into the patient's condition, just as did the appearance of the feces, or the taste and turbidity of the urine.[44] Gout provided another case in which symptomatology reflected the body's efforts to isolate a morbid matter at its

42 Buchan, 1769, pp. 289, 165. "At the beginning of a fever," Buchan cautioned, "Nature generally attempts a discharge either upwards or downwards, which if promoted by gentle means, would tend greatly to abate the force or violence of the disease" (p. 261). Experience, not surprisingly, seemed to provide much support for these doctrines. Skin eruptions in children, for example, were seen as attempts by "Nature ... to free the bodies of children from bad humours, by throwing them out upon the skin: By that means fevers, and other diseases are prevented" (p. 45). The continued health that characterized most cases underwrote the system; if the eruption were to "strike inward" and the child grew gravely ill or died, it might then be blamed on too active a therapy or an improper diet.

43 Buchan, 1769, pp. 193, 82, 518, 402.

44 Buchan, 1769, pp. 192–193, 234 (blood); 385, 444–445 (urine). Quacks specializing in uroscopy seem still to have been ubiquitous and Buchan warned against their deceptions, 1772, p. 154n.

periphery; this natural healing tactic could be undermined by a meddle-some therapeutics which might dislodge the gouty matter and drive it back into the body's more vital areas. Gout was primarily a systemic disease and should be treated systemically, through regimen and drugs that affected the body as a whole.[45]

Buchan's therapeutic admonitions were attuned as well to contemporary assumptions that the body bore within it an unavoidable developmental pattern – a timed blueprint through which each human being must pass between birth and ultimate death. Each stage in that individual evolution – teething, adolescence, menopause, senility – brought with it characteristic perils and Buchan was sensitive to the dangers of each (though rather less concerned with the dangers of teething than many of his peers).[46] It is not that the primacy of the body's interaction with its environment changed at such stressful periods, but rather that a new equilibrium needed to be established; and during this period of transition the body was at particular risk. Menopause was dangerous because it was by definition the cessation of a customary evacuation. Buchan warned physicians not to treat ulcers or other superficial lesions in menopausal or immediately postmenopausal women; they might be efforts by the body to compensate for the suddenly interrupted menstrual flow. Even hemorrhoids might serve the same func-tion; and they too should be left untreated. If the woman's body had not been able to establish an evacuation functionally equivalent to menstrua-tion, it might be the physician's responsibility to create a chronic discharge through the use of setons. "This," Buchan explained, "is imitating Nature, who often, at this period, endeavours to relieve herself by a fistula, the haemorrhoidal flux, etc."[47] Like most of his contemporaries, Buchan assumed as well that each individual boasted a characteristic constitutional makeup, one which placed its peculiar imprint on every aspect of life – from the individual's response to drugs to temperament. Each body defined itself in terms of the equilibrium it established with its environment; but the optimum pattern for that equilibrium was different for every person.

---

45 Buchan, 1769, pp. 343, 458, 460–461. Erysipelas is treated in much the same way, pp. 296–298. It should be emphasized, however, that Buchan, like most of his contemporaries, believed strongly in constitutional predisposition in many ills – including gout (p. 455).

46 Buchan, 1769, p. 593. For an example of a guide to regimen organized around the life cycle, see Bernard Lynch, *A Guide to Health through the Various Stages of Life*... (London: Printed for the Author, 1744).

47 Buchan, 1769, p. 566. "The diseases peculiar to women," as Buchan explained the common sense of his generation, "arise chiefly from their monthly evacuations, pregnancy, and child-birth" (p. 557). For a general discussion of this traditional view, see Carroll Smith-Rosenberg, "The Cycle of Femininity: From Puberty to Menopause," *Feminist Studies* 1 (1973): 58.

Only the physician could appropriately judge the therapeutic implications of such individuality.

Not surprisingly, Buchan was instinctively opposed to the concept of specific drug action. The most striking example is his attitude toward quinine. He was well aware that the "bark" had a peculiar efficacy in intermittent fevers, yet like most of his contemporaries, Buchan suggested an array of purges and emetics to prepare the body for its action – even in malaria. His unwillingness to accept quinine's specificity was underlined, ironically, by the fact that it was perhaps his favorite article in the entire materia medica, one which he recommended in a score of ills other than intermittent fever.[48] Scurvy presents a parallel case; although Buchan was well aware of the curative properties of fresh fruits, he still considered a "poor" diet (or one particularly dependent on salt provisions) as only one among an eclectic smorgasbord of causes for scurvy.[49] It was hard for an eighteenth-century medical man to believe that so deep-seated a systemic ill could be caused or cured by any one environmental factor.

Buchan was, in short, very much a man of his generation in terms of his most fundamental conceptions of physiology and pathology and of the therapeutics he recommended – and presumably practiced. His frequently critical judgments of contemporary medicine and his endorsement of the healing powers of nature by no means imply a noninterventionist stance in practice. He bled, salivated, prescribed the polypharmic remedies so popular among his peers. Buchan was no premature therapeutic nihilist: "a doubtful remedy," as he put it, "is better than none."[50] His often energetic therapeutics was, moreover, not at all inconsistent with a parallel emphasis on regimen and environmental circumstance. Within his basic explanatory framework, Buchan was remarkably eclectic. He was willing to suggest folk remedies when they seemed effective or recommend them in conjunction

48 Among the ills in which Buchan recommended the use of quinine were consumption (p. 219), typhus (p. 241), ophthalmia (p. 311), erysipelas (pp. 298–299), rickets (p. 486), whooping cough (p. 342), and worms (p. 442). It even aided Nature in preparing "laudable pus" in infections (p. 265). Buchan's contemporary, William Cullen, was also an enthusiastic advocate of quinine. See Guenter B. Risse, "'Doctor William Cullen, Physician, Edinburgh': A Consultation Practice in the Eighteenth Century," *Bull. Hist. Med.* 48 (1974): 349. For a more general discussion of the way in which the malaria-specific effectiveness of quinine was generalized to other conditions, see Erwin H. Ackerknecht, "Aspects of the History of Therapeutics," *Bull. Hist. Med.* 36 (1962): 389–419, pp. 410–412. In his 1772 revision, Buchan added a paragraph placing the use of quinine in a more tentative, empirical framework (p. 244).

49 Buchan, 1769, pp. 470–472. Buchan was only typical in his rejection of specifics as "irrational." Another contemporary, for example, thought "the notion of a specific inconsistent with reason, and unsupported in practice," and he prescribed none. William Smith, *A Sure Guide in Sickness and Health, in the Choice of Food, and the Use of Medicine*... (London: The Author, 1776), [p. ix].

50 Buchan, 1772, p. 375.

with more exclusively medical remedies. His emphasis on diet and regimen was entirely traditional, a prominent element in medical thought from classical antiquity down to such immediate predecessors as George Cheyne and John Armstrong.

How then *was* Buchan different? Did his success reside simply in a plausible synthesis of previously disparate genres – and the presentation of that synthesis in lucid prose? This is obviously part, but only part, of the answer. Despite the familiarity of many of the elements in his *Domestic Medicine*, both their arrangement and some of the book's specific emphases combined to create a genuinely novel cultural product.

One innovative element was Buchan's careful utilization of regimen in a disease-oriented format. The symptoms of disease and not the general prospect of future health shaped most of his admonitions. His conventional treatment of regimen was thus incorporated as one element in a pragmatic, practice-defined context. Second, his concern for children and their proper care and rearing was an element ordinarily absent from both treatises on regimen and collections of domestic remedies. Third, he sought to treat both chronic and acute ills within the same text; Tissot, for example, had explicitly refused to consider chronic ailments in his *Advice to the People*, submitting that they presented subtle problems of diagnosis and management which only a trained medical man could hope to master.[51] Fourth, Buchan's environmentalism transcended the traditional Hippocratic epidemiology of airs, waters, and places as well as the prudent counsel on house sites and the like often found in earlier treatises on health and regimen. He was willing to underline the growing dangers of crowded tenements and unventilated factories, of hospitals and almshouses which promoted death not life, of the fundamental unhealthiness of the sedentary tailor's or shopkeeper's life. Though his suggested remedies for such urban ills seem feebly inadequate, it is significant that he not only presented such observations as the fruit of his own experience, but placed them as well within an emotionally resonant agrarian ideology which assumed and deplored the unhealthiness of industrial and commercial life. Finally, Buchan put a particularly strong emphasis on contagion; dysentery, whooping cough, and other childhood ills, smallpox, malignant fevers, even tuberculosis might be spread through contact with the sick. He was force-

---

51 "Each acute Distemper generally arises from one Cause, and the Treatment of it is simple and uniform; since those Symptoms, which manifest the Malady, point out its Cause and Treatment. But the Case is very differently circumstanced in tedious and languid Diseases" (Tissot, *Advice*, pp. xxvii–xxix). Buchan modestly confessed that he would not have undertaken his *Domestic Medicine* had Tissot considered chronic ills (p. x).

ful and explicit in his warnings against contact with sufferers from such ills
– in the case of dysentery even of contact with their excreta.[52]

Some at least of these novel emphases seem particularly relevant to a
time and place; Buchan's *Domestic Medicine* was crafted for a specific
audience. His concern with children, for example, would have immediately
appealed to a class whose future prospects would inevitably be problematic;
the nobility knew what their children would be; so, unfortunately, did
Britain's peasants and workers. It was the "middling orders" who could not
easily predict their children's future. When Buchan warned that "Nature
has left so much in the power of parents, that children are, in a great
measure, what they please to make them," he was appealing to the natural
anxieties of parents whose children did indeed have options. The "ignorance or carelessness" of parents might doom their children to a future of
sickness and want. An attention to temperance and cleanliness (the latter
"necessary for supporting the dignity of human nature" and "useful and
agreeable to society") could help guarantee a future of health and social
assurance.[53] Buchan's clinical experience in Sheffield and at the Ackworth

---

52 Buchan, 1769, pp. 374–376. See also pp. 35, 208, 233, 286, 307, 314, 322. It might
be argued that this emphasis on contagion was logically inconsistent with Buchan's
more fundamental holistic model of pathology and therapeutics. In retrospect it was,
but only in retrospect. The inconsistency was never apparent to Buchan, who did not
see these ills as originating *exclusively* in contagion and who saw the "infectious virus"
as an end product of the metabolic process gone awry. What he and his
contemporaries determinedly avoided was consideration of the possibly specific nature
of the infectious morbid material – just as they failed to address the possibly specific
nature of disease. His assumptions about the cumulative dangers of the end products
of a morbid metabolism explain as well his warnings about the unhealthiness of
hospitals and slum dwellings; ills normally not infectious might well become so in such
confined circumstances. This position was widely assumed until almost the end of the
nineteenth century. And Buchan was by no means alone among his medical
contemporaries in underlining the dangers of contagion; John Pringle, for example,
was a conspicuous case in point.

53 Buchan, 1769, p. 7, 94–95. Such arguments, emphasizing the "ignorance or
carelessness" of individuals and appealing to parental guilt and anxiety, represent a
very different sort of argument from the mercantilist rhetoric which Buchan (and
Tissot) invoke at times. It would be tempting to fit Buchan into a framework
emphasizing his transitional place in a gradual shift from a traditional to a modern
world-view. Between the 1769 and 1772 editions, for example, Buchan added a
passage warning of the dangers of sordid arranged marriages and the need to marry for
love if health were to be preserved; disease sanctions could legitimate the affective
family as well as the need for cleanliness and moderation (1772, pp. 148–149;
Buchan, *Observations Concerning the Venereal Disease*, p. 228). See also note 11 of this
chapter for comment on Buchan's commitment to the work ethic. For an important
discussion of the eighteenth-century secularization of the infection concept (with its
associated emphasis on cleanliness as an aspect of morality among the middling
orders), see Owsei Temkin, "An Historical Analysis of the Concept of Infection," in
The Double Face of Janus and Other Essays in the History of Medicine (Baltimore: Johns
Hopkins University Press, 1977), pp. 456–471, especially 467–468.

Foundling Hospital reinforced his specific generational consciousness of the growing urban world and its problems – evidenced both in his depiction of the city's threats to health and in his atypical concern with contagion and its dangers.

What is ultimately characteristic of Buchan's point of view – and perhaps a key to his public acceptance – was its apparent inconsistency. Januslike, he assumed and communicated a reassuring conceptual past, while foreshadowing the future. It is not surprising that he should have embraced without question an ancient speculative pathology, while at the same time swearing allegiance to the new gods of empiricism and observation.[54] Perhaps most fundamentally, he was committed to an explanatory framework which retained human volition at the forefront of his etiology, therapeutics, and prophylaxis. "It will be allowed on all hands," he casually enjoined, "that diseases seldom come by accident, but are the effect of improper conduct in one shape or another."[55] Imprudence and moderation remained the keys to sickness and health respectively, and to controlling one's health-defining interaction with the environment; the very ability to read, to understand and submit oneself to the reasoned admonitions of medicine implied morality in the world order so important to Buchan and his readers. His *Domestic Medicine* was a book to use and to read, intended for a class which had necessarily to do both, unlike the idle rich and the working poor who served respectively as objects of Buchan's scorn and condescension. His readers occupied a social position very different from that occupied by either of these groups.

The luxury-loving and city-dwelling rich were clearly responsible for those ills which rendered them sickly and barren; they could at least define their own style of life. Buchan was far more ambivalent about the poor. Though he was well aware of the debasing circumstances which made it almost impossible for them to maintain health, he still found it difficult to see them as blameless victims. There was no excuse, even among the poor, for a lack of cleanliness. One of every ten urban dwellers died of tuberculosis, but Buchan attributed much of this mortality to alcohol. Agricultural laborers were guilty of drinking water when overheated, of sleeping the postharvest sleep of exhaustion in cold damp fields.[56] Like

---

54 For references to postmortems, see Buchan, 1769, pp. 440, 495n., 547; 1772, p. 467.
55 *Proposals*, p. 3.
56 "The peasants in most countries," Buchan explained, "seem to hold cleanliness in a sort of contempt. . . . Peasants are likewise extremely careless with respect to change of apparel, keeping their skins clean, &c. These are merely the effects of indolence and a dirty disposition" (Buchan, 1769, pp. 90–91). For other passages imputing responsibility to the poor for their ills, see pp. 59, 65, 70–71, 77–78, 98 (on alcohol and tuberculosis), 128–131, 233, 330, 482, 575, 585.

many public health thinkers in generations later than his, Buchan could neither fully blame nor fully exculpate these victims of social change and economic exploitation. Not surprisingly, he placed little emphasis upon a possible role for government in remedying the conditions he deplored. Alert magistrates might see to the more effective removal of wastes, and the government might encourage universal vaccination by offering premiums – but this was as much as he was willing to ask of the state.[57] Buchan looked to individual, not collective, remedies for health problems which seemed both social and potentially remediable.

Buchan's *Domestic Medicine* is, finally, an extraordinarily secular book – very much the product of an Enlightenment sensibility. Its author ordinarily eschews even the traditional invocation of the laudable consistency between the dictates of piety and those of prudence, of the parallel between modes of behavior which betokened eternal salvation and those which ensured health and long life in this world. In only a few passages does he explicitly mention religion; and these references are all marked by a cool and instrumental quality. In discussing man's need to control his passions, for example, Buchan concluded in his only extended reference to religion that

> Should all other means of comfort fail, the Christian religion affords an inexhaustible source of consolation. It teaches us, that the sufferings of this life are designed to prepare us for a future state of happiness; and that all who pursue the paths of virtue shall at last arrive at complete felicity.[58]

The use of disease sanctions to enforce an acceptable code of behavior is certainly implicit in his emphasis on moderation in regimen, but it is entirely removed from that explicitly theological framework into which a writer such as Cheyne still placed them in the century's first quarter.[59] A comparison of the texts of the second and third editions (of 1772 and

---

57 Buchan, 1769, pp. 90, 277–281. Buchan also suggested in a footnote that money would be better spent providing premiums for the poor who kept their children alive than in supporting hospitals. "This would make the poor esteem fertility a blessing; whereas many of them think it is the greatest curse that can befall them" (p. 32n).

58 Buchan, 1769, p. 120.

59 "The infinitely wise Author of Nature," as Cheyne explained it, "has so contrived *Things*, that the most remarkable rules of preserving Health are moral duties commanded us, so true it is, that Godliness has the promises of this Life, as well as that to come" (Cheyne, *Essay*, 1725, p. 5). Cheyne saw man's present ill health as ultimately and explicitly a consequence of original sin (*Essay*, pp. 92–94). The cultivating of physical health could also serve as a didactic analogy for a clergyman concerned primarily with the health of the soul. Benjamin Grosvenor, *Health: An Essay on its Nature, Value, Uncertainty, Preservation and Best Improvement* . . . (Boston: J. Winter, 1761), p. 112–113. The first London edition appeared in 1716.

1774) reveals Buchan's secularism; all the textual changes with religious content have secular or anticlerical implications.[60]

The basic structure of the text was set by 1774, but gradual changes were made through the edition of 1803 (presumably by Buchan himself, before his death in 1805). Later editions were edited by other hands, some anonymous, some willing to add their names to the familiar title page. William Buchan had written a book which appealed to the rapidly growing middle class of English cultural consumers; and it is no accident that he was popular (and enthusiastically plagiarized) among the evermore numerous middling sort in the United States. There was an American reprint as early as 1772; in 1795 a Philadelphia publisher issued an edition "revised and adapted to the diseases and climate of the United States of America." Two years later this edition was reprinted, at the same time as a competing Philadelphia edition; it too promised the gloss of an American medical man adapting the now standard guide to the medical realities of North America.[61] Later editions included – variously – sections on hernia, electricity, vaccination, rescue from drowning, diet for the poor, and cold bathing. A few included a brief biography of Buchan as well as the great man's portrait.

As might have been expected, other ambitious physicians created their own domestic medicines more or less in Buchan's style. He had indeed created a new subgenre – and such physicians as Richard Reece, Thomas Furlong Churchill, George Wallis, and Alexander Thomson created similar products for the growing household market.[62] In America, some of the early nineteenth-century editions began to jettison portions of the original

60 In one passage, for example, describing the Mosaic teachings on health, Buchan deleted the phrase "by the positive authority of the Almighty" and replaced it with the words "by their laws" (Buchan, 1769, p. 11; 1772, p. 10). See 1772, pp. 149–150, for warnings about the dangers to health implied by too extreme and enthusiastic a religious commitment. In the 1772 edition, every reference to Jesuit's bark was systematically changed to Peruvian bark. It is my feeling that these changes are not simply a consequence of anti-Catholicism, but are more likely the result of a rationalism which deplored the popular attribution of magical skills and arcane knowledge to the Society of Jesus.

61 The editor of the 1795 Philadelphia edition (Austin, *Early American Medical Imprints*, No. 317) was Samuel Powel Griffitts. Isaac Cathrall was his 1797 competitor (Austin, No. 318). The additions were, in sum, minor in both editions, though there are some interesting reflections on North American therapeutics and an added section on yellow fever in both. Buchan seemed so marketable in 1797 that Richard Folwell, publisher of the Cathrall edition, printed nine different issues for booksellers in Philadelphia, Baltimore, and New York.

62 Buchan complained acidly in his 1803 edition of the various forms of plagiarism and copyright evasion to which his book had been subjected (London: A. Strahan, T. Cadell, and W. Davies, 1803, pp. viii–xi). Prefaces of earlier editions dated 1785, 1789, and 1797 contain similarly indignant, if less elaborate, sentiments. Richard Reece was probably the most successful of these would-be advisers to domestic

text and simplify their product, emphasizing the recipes and trimming the
more discursive general admonitions; in a few cases, prudent publishers
added hints for veterinary practice, and in several later editions, botanic
dispensatories – reflecting the popularity of botanic medicine in both
Britain and the United States.[63]

My particular favorite is a London edition of 1825. Entitled *The Cottage
Physician*, its title page announces that it was edited by "William Buchan
and the members of a private medical society." Though catalogued under
Buchan's name, this book has nothing to do with the historical Buchan; it
is an anthology of snippets from a wide assortment of books aimed at a
variety of appealing ends. There are several recipes for abortifacients;
another page provides hints on maintaining a prosperous rabbit warren.[64]
Here Buchan found an ultimate apotheosis; he had become a sacred name,
invoked to reassure the lowest level of literate consumers of intellectual
goods. Like the hypothetical Aristotle who was the alleged author of the
seventeenth-century *Aristotle's Masterpiece* or the "Albertus Magnus" who
was the putative author of a widely reprinted assortment of "mysteries,"
Buchan had transcended the reality of his own life and become a figure
incorporating an almost sacred authority. It is not entirely clear that the
enlightened Scotsman would have approved of this particular beatification.

practitioners. See especially his *Medical Guide, for the use of the Clergy, heads of families,
and seminaries, and junior practitioners in medicine . . .* , first published in 1802 (London:
Longman, Rees, Orme, Brown, Green & Longman).

63 A London edition of 1811, for example, offered observations on the "comparative
advantages of Vaccine Inoculation, with Instructions for Performing the Operation, an
Essay enabling Ruptured Persons to Manage themselves, with Engravings of
Bandages . . . and a Family Herbal." To all of which, the reader was assured, there has
been added "such useful discoveries in medicine and surgery as have transpired since
the Demise of the Author." Purchasers were also provided a frontispiece of the good
doctor in the style of a Roman portrait bust (London: S. A. Oddy, 1811). For editions
with an added section on veterinary medicine, see *Every Man His Own Doctor . . .* (New
Haven: Nathan Whiting, 1816) and *The Complete Family Physician, or the New
Handmaid of Arts and Sciences . . .* (New York: Printed for the Publisher, 1816). Both
editions also contain herbals. *The Complete Family Physician* prints only a drastically
condensed version of Buchan's actual text – and includes "a choice collection of
receipts useful in every branch of business"; it was obviously aimed at a rural audience
rather lower in the social scale than assumed by Buchan in composing his original text.

64 *The Cottage Physician, and Family Adviser, or Every Man His Own Doctor and Herbalist, on
the Plain Principles of "Medicine Without Mystery"* (London: Sherwood and Co., 1825).

3

John Gunn: Everyman's physician

Ʒ⋆ If William Buchan's *Domestic Medicine* was a product of the Scottish Enlightenment, John Gunn's vastly popular guide to domestic practice embodied its particular time and place: Knoxville in 1830, the trans-Appalachian South in the era of Andrew Jackson. This essay was written to serve as an introduction to a facsimile reprinting of the text by the University of Tennessee Press, which was wary of publishing this seemingly arcane if widely read and often-reprinted book without an accessible introduction. I was attracted to the project because it seemed a natural extension of my work on Buchan.

Both self-help manuals shared significant characteristics, despite the six decades that separated their composition. They were products of a medical world very different from that to which we have become accustomed in the late twentieth century. It was a world in which knowledge and competence were not segregated in credentialed heads and hands. These books were not only read but used. Thus they did not simply describe but helped constitute a system of medical care and social relations now largely extinct. Despite such important similarities to its Edinburgh predecessor, the Knoxville physician's *Domestic Medicine* is a distinctively American artifact. Its rambling paragraphs tell us a great deal about the world-view and social relations prevailing in antebellum America – and about the ways in which texts formally medical can provide insight into key assumptions of the culture in which they are produced. ⋆Ʒ

On August 30, 1830, Dr. John C. Gunn of Knoxville registered the title of a book with the Clerk of the United States Court for the Eastern District of Tennessee. It was *Gunn's Domestic Medicine, or Poor Man's Friend. In the Hours of Affliction, Pain and Sickness.* Phrased in "plain language, free from doctor's terms," and aimed at "families in the Western and Southern States," it promised to reduce the practice of medicine "to principles of common sense." The book itself appeared later in the year and soon outdistanced a score or so competitors. At least nineteen separate printings appeared by 1840 – in cities as diverse as Madisonville, Nashville, and

Pumpkintown, Tennessee; Springfield and Zenia, Ohio; Louisville, Kentucky; and Pittsburgh and Philadelphia, Pennsylvania.[1] The manual's immediate popularity and widespread reprinting in the "West" indicate that Gunn, if not precisely a poor man's friend, was able to anticipate the medical needs of a good many ordinary Americans in the era of Andrew Jackson. Just as William Buchan's *Domestic Medicine* had become the prototypical guide to Anglo-American lay practice soon after it appeared in Edinburgh in 1769, Gunn's product dominated its particular and rather different market.[2] Copies of pre-1840 editions almost invariably survive in shabby, dog-eared, and often incomplete condition. Endpapers are frequently adorned with manuscript prescriptions or remedies clipped from newspapers. The majority of those who owned copies of Gunn's *Domestic Medicine* almost certainly read and used it. The question, of course, is why.

The answer must be sought in the text itself and its relationship to the Americans who purchased and, in all likelihood, consulted it in household practice. The Knoxville practitioner was able to frame his clinical advice in a rhetoric appropriate to its purchaser's expectations, package it in convenient form, and, most importantly, endorse a style of practice congenial to the habits and presumptions of his trans-Appalachian contemporaries.

Sugarcoating the pill: Common sense for common men

We know little about John Gunn's life aside from the scraps of information provided in his *Domestic Medicine*. But it is clear that he was no simple frontier doctor – though he was a doctor on the frontier. Gunn had studied in New York, traveled to Cuba, lived in France, and had begun practice in Boutetort County, Virginia, before moving to Knoxville in 1827. His

---

1 At least sixty-eight printings had made their appearance by 1920 when the last edition found its way into print. After 1839 and its first (Philadelphia) stereotype edition, almost all were reprints in an increasingly elephantine format by big-city publishers. This preliminary bibliography has been compiled from the *National Union Catalogue* and the catalogue entries of the Countway Library and National Library of Medicine; I would like to thank John Parascandola of the Historical Section of the NLM and Richard J. Wolfe, Curator of the Countway, for their cooperation.

All quotations from Gunn's *Domestic Medicine* are from the original edition (Knoxville: The Author, 1830). Parenthetical references are to page numbers in this edition.

2 Buchan was reprinted in almost 150 English-language editions in the century following its first publication. See also Chapter 2 of this volume; C. J. Lawrence, "William Buchan; Medicine Laid Open," *Medical History* 19 (1975): 20–35. Gunn never achieved the influence of Buchan's genre-defining manual but easily outstripped his chief American competitors in the regular profession such as Thomas Ewell, Horatio Jameson, and James Ewell. In terms of numbers of editions, Gunn's chief rivals were in fact sectarians Sammuel Thomson, Wooster Beach, and Horton Howard.

rough-and-ready general practice included cancer surgery, dentistry, mid-wifery, pediatrics, and the treatment of venereal disease and tuberculosis in circumstances demanding both ingenuity and intrepidity. Lacking a female catheter, he (and his patients) had to make do with a goose quill. Faced with intractable "blindness," he treated it by removing an adherent "film" from the eye with *"clean hog's lard"* introduced on a "fine Camel-hair pencil, and with much care" (295, 253).

Despite his provincial circumstances, however, Gunn's authorities remained the cosmopolitan leaders of Philadelphia and New York medicine. He referred to no author as frequently as Benjamin Rush, who before his death in 1813 was Professor of the Practice of Medicine at the University of Pennsylvania, America's preeminent medical school. Gunn also cited Rush's successor Nathaniel Chapman and contemporaries Benjamin Smith Barton and Phillip Syng Physick as authoritative sources of medical knowledge.[3] Again and again, he reassured readers that indicated treatments bore the imprimatur of such prominent academics. Gunn seems himself to have been a regular subscriber to Philadelphia's *American Medical Recorder*, the nation's leading professional journal in the late teens and early 1820s.[4] In a period marked by public hostility toward the regular profession and widespread sectarian practice, Gunn was a regularly trained physician who saw no reason to question the authority or, in general, the competence of men who had occupied the most prestigious medical chairs in America's largest cities.

Yet another and rather different set of attitudes is expressed even more conspicuously in Gunn's *Domestic Medicine*. They are appeals to the wisdom of the common people, to the beneficence and plentitude of God, to fears of academic learning, to lay suspicion of medical knowledge and motives. "Three-fourths of medicine," Gunn contended, "as now practiced and imposed upon the common people amounts to nothing but fudge and mummery" (99).

> For the common and useful purposes of mankind, the refined fripperies
> and hair-drawn theories of mere science, are of no use whatever;
> indeed they have never had much other effect, than to excite a stupid

3 He referred to "the great Dr. Rush" (84) and described Physick as "probably among the greatest men of his profession, either of this or any other age" (252). With equal generosity, Gunn described their New York rivals "Mitchill, Hossack [sic], Mott, McNeven [sic] &c" as among the "greatest medical men in the United States" (101). Samuel Latham Mitchill, David Hosack, Valentine Mott, and W. J. Macneven were prominent clinical teachers.

4 It was the printed source referred to most frequently in his *Domestic Medicine* – and the only one for which volume and page numbers were sometimes provided. I can only suppose that Gunn actually subscribed to the *Recorder*. The lack of medical libraries in rural Virginia and East Tennesee makes this a plausible assumption.

admiration for men who pretended to know more than the mass of
mankind: and it is this stupid admiration, this willingness to be duped
by the impudent pretensions of science and quackery combined, that
has led to impositions and barefaced frauds upon society, without
number. (98)

Over the centuries, greed and pride had kept medical men from sharing
knowledge with laypersons. Yet most of the so-called secrets of medicine
could easily be learned by any person possessed of common sense.

Did knowing the Latin name for a plant make one more capable of
understanding its clinical uses? Or more skilled in recognizing it growing in
the tangled brush along a stream, or better able to pick it at the right time
of the year and preserve it most effectively? These traditional skills and the
ideas that justified them were, of course, far older than the United States
itself but were particularly relevant to a generation willing to question every
aspect of professional authority.

Since at least the seventeenth century, writers of health manuals,
many of which were oriented toward the use of readily available herbs or
astrology, had appealed to the fears and prejudices of patients – as well as
to their economic needs. To base a domestic practice on herbs accessible
to "any Englishman" promised a path to the maintenance or restoration of
health free from the exactions of arrogant, formally trained physicians.
Disease in all its varieties had entered a morally imperfect world after
man and woman had left the Garden; but God in his beneficence and
abundance had provided means for curing those ills. Gunn argued that
even pulmonary tuberculosis, normally considered a death sentence, would
ultimately be "subdued by some common and simple plant." He had
always believed "that our wise and beneficent CREATOR has placed
within the reach of his feeble creature *man*, herbs and plants for the cure of
all diseases but old age, could we but obtain a knowledge of their real uses
and intrinsic virtues" (161–162). All these simple resources of meadow
and forest were available to anyone who chose to learn their ways. There
was generally no need for the elaborate prescriptions for the hundreds of
exotic drugs with which physicians justified their social role – and fees.

The "God of Nature" spoke through the natural world and it was one's
duty to understand and obey these simple commands – just as it was one's
duty to employ the universe of plants provided for one's use. If a sick man
felt no hunger pangs, then those caring for him should not stuff him with
food. "NATURE GENERALLY SPEAKS THE TRUTH" (214). Laypersons as well
as physicians could read a pulse. Man's body expressed itself in a language
understandable by any careful observer.

These were ancient ideas that Gunn reiterated, but he was able to
present them in a context of aggressive nationalism. Not only could the

North American continent provide its own materia medica, he argued, but it would obviate the need to import drugs, a need that drained millions each year from American pockets. "In the beneficence of his mercy," Gunn intoned,

> the great FATHER OF THE UNIVERSE has clothed our soil with means, powerful means, of curing our diseases.... There is, in my opinion, nearly as much folly and stupidity in importing costly drugs at enormous expenses from foreign lands while we have their equals at home, as there would be in importing *bricks* and, *timber* from Europe to construct our habitations. Industry and science alone, can develope [sic] the immense resources of this unrivalled country, and these we are personally, morally, and *politically* bound to employ. (365)

Knowledge based on experience could make each American husband or wife the primary physician and provider of drugs for his or her own family.

All these rationales for domestic practice were traditional. Equally familiar was Gunn's emphasis on moderation and control in every aspect of life. Excesses in eating and drinking, in sloth, in expression of the "passions" could all lead to sickness. Like most of his medical predecessors, Gunn emphasized the ways in which health was largely within the control of individual men and women.

The first quarter of Gunn's treatise dutifully repeats such age-old hygienic wisdom. The Knoxville practitioner, however, mobilized a number of less familiar arguments – arguments more specific to his time and place. Perhaps most striking was his emphasis on the role of women and marriage. Gunn urged the need for woman's education, stressed her primary role in child rearing, and deplored the emotionally and physically destructive consequences of loveless marriage.[5] Gunn was even more forthright in his religious views, in his anticlericalism and dislike of predestinarian orthodoxy. And if Gunn appealed to some prospective readers with his liberal, vaguely Unitarian opinions, he must have antagonized a good many of the more orthodox with his vitriolic contrast between "pure and genuine christians," on the one hand, and "bigots, hypocrites, or intolerant fanatics" on the other (70; see also 66–70).

This is not to say that Gunn eschewed moralism, as he did orthodoxy and enthusiasm. He warned, as we have seen, against excess in food and drink, in sex, and especially in the use of alcohol and tobacco. Health turned on a "due subjection" of the passions. He believed in rewards and

5 Much of this argument was framed in the age-old context of medical emphasis on interactions between mind and body. Emotional and physiological health had always been seen as interdependent. Gunn's text makes it clear that women were in practice the actual domestic practitioners (and gatherers of herbs). It was no more than prudent for him to have focused on so important a component of his prospective readership.

punishments in the temporal present as well as the eternal future; if the caustic salve applied to venereal sores was painful, the discomfort was only to be expected inasmuch as the sufferer was "on the stool of repentance" and was "only learning the salutary moral lesson, that 'the penalty always treads upon the heels of the transgression,' and that sacred laws of *nature* and her GOD, can never be violated without punishment to reform the offender!" (267). God had created the natural passion of love for man's good and not as a spur to promiscuity and the spread of venereal disease (24).[6]

Gunn devoted the first section of his book to a discussion of man's social and moral environment before turning to the more mundane task of describing and prescribing for disease. This was no more than a convention of the domestic medicine genre. It followed a formula perfected by Buchan and imitated by dozens of other physicians, American and British, who had sought to duplicate the Edinburgh physician's commercial success.

The "better sort" of reader wanted something more "improving" than an unadorned collection of recipes – yet something more practical than a generalized treatise on how to live a healthy and moral life. Gunn provided just that, for the bulk of his book constitutes a circumstantial guide to the domestic practice of medicine. And unlike most of his predecessors who had written such how-to-do-it manuals, Gunn treated almost every aspect of medicine as appropriate for lay practice. No longer did it seem necessary to define careful boundaries between lay and professional spheres and to place certain areas of practice off-limits, areas into which the nonprofessional could stray only at his or her peril.

The best poor man's practice

The practice Gunn describes is a difficult one for twentieth-century Americans to understand. We assume a fundamental distinction between physician and layperson, between lay and professional knowledge, between

6 Gunn occupied an inconsistent – or perhaps more accurately transitional – position in regard to the relationship between disease and culpable behavior. He accepted, for example, the existence of a physiological dependence so materially based that it would exculpate *some* alcoholics for acts undertaken when under the influence. These individuals did in fact suffer from liver disease and were not simply acting out the consequences of their moral choices. Such unfortunates had to be treated for that organic ailment (178–179). Although careful to warn against the dangers of excessive sexual intercourse, masturbation, and venereal disease, Gunn was atypically able to suggest that the French system of licensing and inspecting prostitutes might be appropriate to American conditions (265).

the areas of legitimate lay and professional competence. We assume as well the segregation of most medical practice in specialized, often institutional settings – certainly outside the home. We associate medicine with a complex and specialized technology and with mastery of an array of powerful drugs limited in their clinical application to highly trained and formally accredited practitioners.

Realities could not have been more different in 1830, especially among that great majority of Americans who lived on farms and in villages. There was, of course, no complex and expensive hospital-based technology and thus no compelling technical reason to remove medical care from the home. The vast majority of Europeans had always been treated in their own or their master's homes by neighbors and family members. Poverty and rural isolation meant that most medical problems were treated first in the family, then by an experienced neighbor, and, finally, and only after these options had proved fruitless, by an individual who thought of himself or herself as a physician. (And only a minority of such were formally trained and licensed; early modern Europe was doctored by a bewildering variety of practitioners.) Every wife and grandmother, many public-spirited clergymen commanded a repertoire of healing skills and in particular a knowledge of local herbs – how they were to be recognized, when they were to be gathered, how they were to be prepared and preserved, how to determine the nature of their medical "virtues," and whether such active components resided in root, leaves, bark, or stem.

Such knowledge constituted the heart of a vernacular healing tradition, preserved to some extent in printed manuals and guides, in the handwritten recipe books of prudent homemakers, and most tenaciously in oral tradition. Much of this age-old practice turned on the administration of herbal remedies, but many nonspecialists did not hesitate to bleed or perform minor surgery, set fractures, or reduce dislocations. In some areas, "bone-setting" was a traditional craft passed on in families or through apprenticeship.

By the nineteenth century, this indigenous tradition had been enriched by the availability of a wide range of highly active drugs and patent medicines, not all of native growth. In early nineteenth-century America, the most important were mercury, opium, and ipecac – all indispensable to domestic and regular physician alike. What needs emphasis here is the way in which a good portion of the actual therapeutic practices of formally trained physicians overlapped with those employed by untutored laypersons – perhaps not in the consistency and sophistication of the rationalizations that justified them but in the particular drugs, dosage levels, and social setting in which their remedies were administered. Equally striking is the fact that these drugs and even the majority of those "innocent" remedies that made up the herbal tradition exerted an obvious and predictable physiological effect.[7] Opium altered mood, alleviated pain, and checked diarrhea; ipecac induced vomiting; mercury exerted a bewildering assortment of physiological effects, all palpable. One could hardly doubt their "efficacy" – and thus the therapeutic competence of the individual who had prescribed them.

Physicians and nonprofessionals also shared a traditional understanding of how the body functioned in health and disease. The understanding was based on the classical idea of balance, on concern with the maintenance of a health-defining physiological equilibrium.[8] Not surprisingly, this led to a concern with those aspects of intake and outgo that could be observed and controlled: diet, exercise, and atmosphere, on the one hand; and perspiration, urine, and feces, on the other. It was no accident that so many of the drugs used most widely in both lay and professional practice visibly altered these bodily products. Nor was it an accident that diagnosis and prognosis placed a similar emphasis on these tangible indicators of a patient's physiological status. In tuberculosis, for example, Gunn explained that the "urine or water is highly colored, and desposits in the urinal or pot a muddy sediment" (162). Blood drawn from the arm of a patient with liver disease was marked by a characteristic color and texture.[9] No clue as to the body's internal state could be ignored by the practitioner – whether physician or family member.

Not surprisingly, disease was seen as a shifting, holistic phenomenon. Local ills might have distant and more general roots; disorders of the stomach or uterus, on the other hand, might have constitutional effects. Similarly, Gunn, like most of his contemporaries, emphasized the connection between body and mind. Thus grief could have an enormous range

---

7 "Innocent" was used by Gunn and his contemporaries to indicate an herb that was mild in its action; its administration did not imply the cost–benefit considerations posed by the use of such toxic metals as mercury or antimony. Critics of regular physicians were often quick to attack the profession's reliance on "unnatural" metallic drugs. Not all herbs were in fact "innocent," of course; one thinks of digitalis, atropine, or opium.

8 For a more detailed discussion of these age-old medical beliefs, see Chapter 1 of this volume. Popular ideas of disease causation still reflect elements of traditional holistic schemes – and late twentieth-century physicians may still interact with patients on terms shaped in part by such ideas. See, for example, Cecil G. Helman, "Feed a Cold, Starve a Fever – Folk Models of Infection in an English Suburban Community, and their Relation to Medical Treatment," *Culture, Medicine and Psychiatry* 2 (1978): 107–137; Mildred Blaxter, "The Causes of Disease: Women Talking," *Social Science and Medicine* 17 (1983): 59–69.

9 "Before it begins to coagulate or congeal, and while the red part is setting to the bottom – and before the buffy or yellow coat is fully formed, it looks of a dull green color; but, immediately after the full formation of the upper coat, it changes from a dull greenish hue to a yellow" (179).

of physical consequences. Gunn warned that disease, insanity, and even death could be caused by "moral" – that is, psychological – causes. The pregnant mother's "imagination" could impress itself on her gestating infant's future health and character. Physicians might not understand the mechanisms that underlay such interactions, but clinical experience seemed to leave no doubt of their reality (53–54). Disease had many causes and ever-shifting manifestations.

Somewhat inconsistently, however, Gunn also assumed that a number of ills were specific and "catching" – diphtheria, venereal disease, dysentery, whooping cough, and measles. But like the great majority of his contemporaries, Gunn never saw an inconsistency between his casual acceptance of specific contagion and his equally unquestioning assumption of a traditional holistic model of disease, in which neither contagion nor specificity should logically have played a role. Disease was in theory at least no more than the sum of an individual's symptoms at a particular moment in time. It was the physician's task to "subdue" those symptoms.

Gunn's therapeutic advice was firmly rooted in these traditional ideas, though it reflected, in fact, a particularly enthusiastic and not entirely traditional style of practice. It is a style referred to by contemporaries and subsequent historians as "heroic" – a term referring as much to his patient's endurance as to the physician's intrepid use of bleeding and toxic drugs. Gunn believed, for example, in the indispensability of mercury, that "SAMPSON of the Drug-shops" (264), and blandly recommended enormous dosages administered in a variety of forms ranging from metallic mercury to its far more toxic salts. In venereal disease, he assumed, like the majority of his contemporaries, that mercury exerted a specific efficacy. In most other ills, mercury was assumed to have a general "alterative effect," guiding the body to a new internal equilibrium. (And unlike Buchan and many of his eighteenth-century peers, Gunn never doubted the practicality, in fact the necessity, of domestic administration of even the most active mercury compounds.) Mercury's therapeutic powers were attested to by the symptoms of what a modern toxicologist would regard as mercury poisoning. 'You will spit freely," Gunn explained, "the salivary glands will become enlarged, and the throat sore, the gums tender, and the breath will have an offensive and peculiar odor &c."[10]

10 (183) Gunn, like any of his regularly trained contemporaries, was well aware of danger in the excessive use of mercury, especially if concentrations were allowed to build up gradually in the body. Thus he warned against the careless use of mercury-based salves in which the drug was absorbed into the bloodstream but tolerated the ingestion of massive doses of mercury salts orally, with the understanding that the drug would be largely purged before the metal could be assimilated. He was aware as well that some individuals entertained a prejudice "not to be removed" against it (184), even if mercury compounds were, in fact, "daily and commonly used" (438).

Gunn was also an enthusiastic advocate of routine "puking" – that is, the use of emetics, most frequently ipecac, to cleanse the sick person's system. Similarly, Gunn often prescribed bleeding to help combat inflammatory or violent febrile symptoms. And even more than most of his contemporaries, Gunn was an almost uncritical admirer of opium for its extraordinary ability to assuage pain, alter mood, and moderate diarrhea.[11] He questioned its indispensability as little as he doubted the ability of nonspecialists to use it to advantage. "Without this valuable and essential medicine," he explained, "it would be next to impossible for a Physician to practice his profession, with any considerable degree of success; it may not improperly be called, the monarch of medicinal powers, the soothing angel of moral and physical pain" (401).

Gunn's was an active and intrusive therapy, one that assumed the possibility, in fact the necessity, of routine and forceful intervention in the healing process.[12] Much of his domestic medicine consists of detailed therapeutic advice following rather more perfunctory guidance in recognizing particular ills. In "dysentary or flux," for example (recognizable by a *"bloody kind of mucus* – which resembles that generally scraped from the entrails of a hog"), bleeding would be appropriate at the onset of sickness if the patient were generally healthy and feverish. The next steps were mandatory. First, "cleanse the stomach by an emetic or puke of ipecacuanha." Second, the patient was to be subjected to a mercury purge. "Next: – if the disease does not abate, you must repeat the purging daily with castor oil" (190–191). Gunn provides several more paragraphs of eclectic advice including chalk, opium suppositories, a variety of enemas, blackberry syrup, flax-weed oil, and slippery-elm tea (192).

Gunn's practice thus incorporated both academic medicine and the vernacular practice of ordinary people. Its eclectic quality is particularly striking because his *Domestic Medicine* appeared at a time when many individuals felt that they had to take sides, when a not inconsiderable number of lay critics of the medical profession inveighed against its reliance on bleeding and its routine use of "unnatural" metals such as arsenic, antimony, and, especially, mercury. Such sentiments rationalized a vigorous new medical sect, Thomsonian or botanic medicine, which was spreading

11 See, for example, his euphoric comparison of the mood-enhancing and intellect-sharpening virtues of opium as compared with the unfortunate effects of alcohol (403).
12 This activism was to become decreasingly fashionable in the generation following 1830 as physicians granted increasing autonomy to the body's natural healing powers. It would be no exaggeration to say that Gunn, on the other hand, like many physicians of his generation, saw the patient's body as a battlefield on which the practitioner struggled with the symptoms constituting the disease.

in the very same Western and Southern areas in which Gunn's manual was being adopted.[13] Its success in the marketplace implies that a good many Americans saw no need to take sides, to declare themselves committed and exclusive advocates of either botanic or regular medicine.

Gunn in fact recommended a number of American herbs with particular enthusiasm. These included South Carolina pinkroot (a supposedly effective antihelminthic), Virginia snakeroot, Jamestown (jimson) weed, dogwood bark (which he considered as effective as chinchona bark in treating malaria), and Indian turnip (which bore "the highest reputation in country practice, as a remedy in pulmonary or consumptive complaints"). "Bone-set" was particularly useful, for it was, as Gunn reassured his readers, "endowed with more real and genuine virtues than any plant now known."[14]

As we have seen in the case of dysentery, many of Gunn's recommended treatments for particular ills were uncritical catalogues of remedies from the mineral and vegetable kingdoms, from folk wisdom and the pharmacopoeia. In chronic ills, Gunn's advice seems in fact often reasonable; common sense endorsed a less active therapy in nonlife-threatening ills familiar to every adult. The common cold, piles, mumps, whooping cough, and rheumatism implied discomfort but not fear.

It was in acute ills that Gunn's therapy was most active and intrusive. Violent and unpredictable symptoms demanded violent countermeasures; in retrospect such measures may seem irrational, even dangerous, but at least they reassured family and friends that something was in fact being done.[15] Drastic bleeding, puking, and purging left no doubt that the

13 Founded by Samuel Thomson of New Hampshire, Thomsonianism eschewed metallic drugs and bleeding – though its favorite herbal remedies and sweat baths were hardly bland and innocent by twentieth-century standards. The most thorough study of this phenomenon is still Alex Berman, "The Impact of the Nineteenth-Century Botanico-Medical Movement in American Pharmacy and Medicine," (University of Wisconsin, unpublished Ph.D. diss., 1954). See also, Joseph Kett, *The Formation of the American Medical Profession: The Role of Institutions, 1780–1860* (New Haven: Yale University Press, 1968), ch. IV; G. B. Risse, R. L. Numbers, and J. W. Leavitt, eds., *Medicine without Doctors: Home Health Care in American History* (New York: Science History Publications, 1977); and Madge E. Pickard and R. Carlyle Buley, *The Midwest Pioneer: His Ills, Cures, & Doctors* (New York: Henry Schuman, 1946).

14 (398, 379) The distinction between academic and vernacular medicine is blurred by both the overlap in actual practice and the interest of at least some academic physicians in native herbs and their possible therapeutic uses. Gunn, for example, could cite the authority of Philadelphia professor Benjamin Smith Barton in advocating the use of particular herbal remedies. See also Barton, *Collections for an Essay towards a Materia Medica of the United-States*, 3d ed. (Philadelphia: Edward Earle & Co., 1810).

15 It will be recalled that acute illness was normally treated in the home. Friends and neighbors often gathered to "sit up with" the patient; Gunn, in fact, warned that their constant chatter might interfere with the patient's rest (139). The physician and his prescriptions were thus constantly on stage; the sick room was a social context that could serve to focus and mobilize the patient's emotional resources.

physician was intervening in a frightening and possibly fatal situation. This was a period still ravaged by dangerous infectious ills and it was only natural for the physician to devote considerable attention to febrile and inflammatory symptoms; it was in such situations that his most active remedies were routinely employed.[16]

If the patient recovered, it was equally natural to credit the therapeutic measures "exhibited" and the physician who had prescribed them. In less severe ills, the physician could always claim that he had averted more serious consequences. A mismanaged cold might culminate in pulmonary consumption, a minor diarrhea in dysentery. In the holistic view of health and disease shared by both physician and nonprofessional it was assumed that one disease might pass imperceptibly into another. Two-thirds of the cases of consumption, Gunn warned, grew out of neglected colds (204–205). The body was always in danger of slipping out of balance; minor ills indicated a potentially dangerous tendency – and justified measures aimed at helping the body return to its normally healthy state.

The bulk of medical practice, whether lay or medical, began and ended with the administration of drugs. And neither law nor custom drew a rigid line between pharmaceutical spheres appropriate to laypersons and physicians. The layperson could buy opium and its derivatives or the toxic arsenic, antimony, or mercury just as easily as the physician (though less likely to do so in wholesale lots). Proprietors of general stores sold more drugs than did individuals who thought of themselves as trained pharmacists. As we have seen, laypersons could and did gather, prepare, and administer their own herbal remedies; it had never seemed appropriate or realistic that government intervene in the traditional realm of domestic healing.

Gunn and his contemporaries went further than a previous generation of physician-authors of manuals for domestic practice in erasing boundaries between the nonspecialist and the physician. While Buchan, for example, had been careful to draw that line at the use of mercury, Gunn simply assumed that laypersons should and would administer it despite mercury's admitted toxicity. The only problem lay in providing enough clinical description so that nonprofessionals would prescribe mercury at the right moments and in appropriate forms.

Gunn's advice was by no means limited to the administration of drugs. Parents of children born with a hare-lip were assured that they could themselves remedy the condition with the aid of pins to be procured from

16 Gunn tended, like some prominent physicians of his teachers' generation, to categorize ailments along a debility–excitement scale. So-called depleting remedies (bleeding and purging especially) were rationalized within this framework. Fever and inflammation were clinical signs of an excited physiological state and thus called for depletion.

a local silversmith (343). Gunn, assuming that laypersons would bleed
the sick, included a convenient chart of arteries in the arm to guide
the inexperienced (411). More surprisingly, Gunn provided advice on
how to catheterize both men and women; the women could practice on
themselves, while men – facing a more difficult anatomical challenge –
would have to call upon a friend or relative for help. He provided directions as well for giving oneself an enema, thus avoiding cost and, in the
case of women, damage to their modesty.[17] Only in a few instances did
Gunn emphasize the need for trained medical assistance: for example,
eye surgery, dentistry, "flooding" or hemorrhaging in childbirth, and
administering the truly enormous doses of opium contemporary medical
opinion called for in treating lockjaw (quantities that would "make even the
best physician dread his own practice" [284]). Unlike most treatises on
domestic medicine, moreover, Gunn's manual wasted little effort in attacking quacks; his strategy was clearly based on the assumption that most
"Western" families had provided and would continue to provide much of
their own medical care.

Significantly enough, he did have unkind words for midwives. The great
majority, he warned, entered the trade "from too great laziness to exert
themselves in other walks of life." Ignorant of their responsibilities, they
were motivated by a "heartless destitution of feeling and humanity, which
permits their ignorance, to entail diseases originating in mismanagement,
on thousands of women for life" (292). The preferable alternative was to
call in a skilled physician, Gunn argued, "a man of delicacy of sentiment
and feeling, tried and well-known discretion, and dignified elevation of
character." Both contemporary mores and traditional practice placed the
would-be "male-midwife" on the defensive. Nineteenth-century physicians
were extremely sensitive to the division of clinical responsibility in childbirth and early infancy; it was an emotionally intense and predictably
recurring period of crisis in which a physician could cement his relationship to a particular family or see it eroded. Competition from less expensive midwives was unwelcome indeed.

Gunn, however, was nothing if not a realist. He also provided a brief
obstetric catechism for those same midwives he had in general defamed,
urging them to consult physicians in difficult cases, if only to "relieve
yourself of dangerous responsibilities" (327; see also 308, 322–323, 326–
329). Neither a utopian nor an aggressive defender of professional prerogative, Gunn simply accepted the prevailing division of medical practice

17 At one point (202) Gunn recommends that physicians be called to insert the catheter
   but concedes that if "necessity should urge," the task could be done by nonprofessional men and women. In a number of other passages, however, he casually
   assumes that laypersons can and should catheterize.

between laypersons and trained physicians; physicians would in most instances serve in fact as consultants. And this was particularly true in the case of childbirth. Cost and distance, as well as the viability of traditional domestic practice in a period of limited technical resources, guaranteed that this would be the case. In the vast majority of instances the trained physician could offer little in the way of therapeutics different from the drugs, bleeding, minor surgery, and hygienic advice available to any self-confident adult.

The tenacious defense of sharp boundaries between lay and professional areas of competence was obviously inappropriate to the realities of medical practice in Jacksonian Virginia and Tennessee.[18] Class assumptions were similarly diffuse. Buchan and Tissot, authors of the leading domestic medicine treatises in the mid- and late eighteenth century, presented their works in the guise of advice to members of the upper orders who would be expected to provide aid to their less privileged and "intelligent" neighbors and tenants.[19] Even if this was no realistic picture of the actual purchasers of their books, it still seemed an appropriate rationale to justify the writing of a treatise for domestic practitioners. Gunn was burdened by no such qualms.

It is striking, in fact, how few clues to the social location of the book's readers the text provides. Most writers of early nineteenth-century household manuals, cookbooks, and guides to domestic medicine refer constantly and unself-consciously to the cooking, cleaning, and nursing duties of servants – the assumption being that readers would be members of the servant-employing and at least minimally leisured class. It seems clear from Gunn's text, on the other hand, that he assumed his readers would be the actual practitioners. Family members would provide hands-on care and nursing – perhaps with a copy of Gunn for guidance.[20] To our conventional picture of frontier life, we must add the prosaic images of the pioneer gathering and preserving herbs, puking, purging, bleeding, inserting catheters – and when alone and necessity called, administering enemas to him- or herself.

18 The American physician's role as purveyor of drugs and instruments constituted an important mechanism for averting conflict between lay and professional practitioners. Gunn refers again and again to the "doctor's shop" as the place to purchase the drugs, catheters, lancets, enema pipes, and other fundamentals of household practice. The lines between shopkeeper, apothecary, physician, and surgeon that at least theoretically structured British medical practice had never had any significance in America. Rural and small-town physicians have often served as apothecaries well into the twentieth century.

19 See Chapter 2 of this volume.

20 In only one instance does Gunn refer to a servant's potential role (in helping her mistress with a catheter) (421).

A medical voice on the frontier

Gunn describes a world of sickness very different from that we have come to assume in the twentieth century – though it would have been familiar indeed to physicians of any previous century. He regarded infantile diarrheas as the most dangerous ailment in Jacksonian Tennessee (353). Malaria was commonplace, along with typhoid and typhus fevers. Tuberculosis was perhaps even more feared and was regarded as incurable once pulmonary symptoms appeared. "Sore eyes," "leg ulcers," and rheumatism were less alarming but nevertheless frequent sources of discomfort; whooping cough, mumps, measles, and the common cold were unavoidable conditions of life. Venereal disease was surprisingly prevalent and associated in Gunn's mind with the "petty and filthy scale" of prostitution in frontier towns (265). If only in passing, he tells us a great deal about the time and place in which he practiced medicine.

But Gunn was not the voice of the frontier, even if he was a voice on it. And that frontier had more than a geographical meaning. As we have seen, the Knoxville physician assimilated and expressed both vernacular and high-culture traditions. He invoked the antielitist formulas of Jacksonian public discourse, yet still cited the teachings of Paris, New York, and Philadelphia as sources of authority. Both Gunn and his readers saw no need to choose between these bodies of knowledge; in his rambling yet energetic prose they reinforced rather than contradicted each other. Most of his readers presumably accepted both sources of assurance. And, as we have emphasized, professional and domestic therapeutics differed comparatively little at the level of day-to-day practice.

Contemporaries were, of course, acutely conscious of differences that seem in retrospect surprisingly small. Gunn, for example, was well aware of diversity in the medical ideas and practices he observed during his years in Virginia and Tennessee.[21] Most striking is the way in which he refers again and again to "country people" and their distinctive practices; rural–urban differences were clearly central to his conception of social identity – on the Western as well as Eastern side of the Appalachians. An educated, traveled, town-dwelling professional man, Gunn lived near but was hardly of the frontier.

On another level, Gunn expresses the same sort of Janus-faced ability to look toward both past and future. For his medicine is deeply embedded both in the marketplace of international commerce and in the self-

---

21 Gunn refers again and again to divergent linguistic practice. We learn, for example, of such ills as "tetter" (ringworm) and "hip-gout" (sciatica) and that constipation was referred to as "being bound in the body" and the vagina referred to as "birth-place."

sufficiency of traditional herbal practice. The drugs recommended most frequently – mercury, ipecac, opium, senna – were by no means products of East Tennessee. They were imported, transported by middlemen, and finally sold for cash or exchanged for crops or services by physicians and shopkeepers. Though Gunn refers again and again to the need to supplant imports with plants of American growth, the reality he describes is quite different.[22] Like many others of his generation, Gunn held views marked more by pragmatic inconsistency than by a well-defined orientation toward either frontier or metropolis, toward self-sufficiency or the international marketplace. It was an inconsistency that paralleled his casual assimilation of both vernacular and academic medical practice.

Even if key elements in Gunn's thought and practice were millennia old, his *Domestic Medicine* was oriented toward his century's men and women. Explicit recognition of class differences plays a relatively small role in Gunn's discussion of disease and its prevention (though there are a few passages inveighing in traditional terms against the debilitating lifestyles of the rich). Gunn's book on the other hand is, as we have suggested, strikingly oriented toward women. It includes lengthy sections on childbirth and the diseases of women and children (matters quarantined in separate companion volumes by some of his competitors). The Knoxville physician vigorously endorsed women's education and expressed a sympathetic understanding for the tedium of domestic life. "Place man in her situation," Gunn contrasted, "and compel him to perform the duties of woman, and he would soon either degenerate into a savage, or sink into perfect insignificance" (291). Marriage had to be based on affection as well as respect and was "cemented and powerfully strengthened by the endearments of sexual enjoyment" (45). Even female sexuality played a legitimate social role.

But Gunn was no premature feminist. His attitude toward woman and her position in the family is still fundamentally traditional, as were his attitudes toward medicine itself. One of the functions of education was to guard a woman against seduction – and thus her husband against dishonor.[23] Woman's easily stimulated imagination was always a source of danger; affection might be a necessary element in marriage but romantic novels led to "whoredom and suicide" (35). It was only natural for Gunn to

22 American as well as imported drugs had, of course, already become articles of commerce. Gunn refers, for example, to supplies of Carolina pinkroot being brought into Knoxville for sale (368). The vernacular tradition was already assimilating itself to an energetic marketplace.

23 Significantly, Gunn also promised that "a cultivated mind is a never-failing passport to the best society" (46–47). This passage and a number of others in Gunn point to connections between social change, class, and the legitimating function of class-appropriate lifestyles.

"consider the brain as the father, and the stomach as the mother of the system" (424).

Gunn was an energetic but essentially conventional man. His intellectual caution is particularly striking with respect to the world of academic medicine. Though he had visited France, Gunn was little influenced or concerned with contemporary developments in Paris, developments that had by 1830 already reshaped the conceptual world of academic medicine. His lasting impressions of France seem to have focused on the treatment of venereal disease and the Gallic attitude of reverence toward the enema. Like most American physicians, he was concerned with practice, with viable therapeutics – and not with the more abstract teachings of the postmortem room. His *Domestic Medicine* was just what it claimed to be: a friend to families in the Western and Southern states (and an advertisement for its author's clinical services).[24] If the commonsense measures it prescribed seem not so efficacious in retrospect, they were certainly a reflection of the possibilities and necessities of East Tennessee in the era of Andrew Jackson.

24 Gunn's description of his book as a "poor man's friend" implies the problem of readership and market. Evidence for the book's actual readership (especially in its first decade) is scanty, but its format and level of discourse suggest that it was intended for ordinary farmers and shopkeepers, and not for the poorest members of society.

4

Body and mind in nineteenth-century medicine: Some clinical origins of the neurosis construct

&. Contemporary physicians often file the study of relations between body and mind under the rubric of psychosomatic medicine, a mid-twentieth-century movement inspired by a self-conscious desire to counteract what its founders felt to be the profession's dominant mechanistic and reductionist tendencies. Yet interest in the relationship between body and mind is, of course, much older. Physicians have always assumed that emotional factors can induce sickness, undergird health, or – properly manipulated – bring about its restoration. The hypothetical mechanisms used to explain this interdependence have changed during the past few centuries, but the clinical reality they sought to explain has never been in doubt.

This essay was originally delivered as the Benjamin Rush Lecture to the American Psychiatric Association in 1988 – at a moment when the longtime domination of dynamic, intrapsychic models in psychiatry had waned, while somaticism had attained increasing prominence. I tried not only to suggest the antiquity of medical concern with the interaction of body and mind but also to underline a continuing and more general ambiguity. As we concern ourselves increasingly with individual lifestyle as a factor in the pathogenesis of chronic disease – in cancer and circulatory disease, for example, or alcoholism – we underline another aspect of mind: volition and thus responsibility. In that elusive and shadowy terrain between blaming and explaining, the relevance of body-and-mind relationships remains central, especially when we consider choice as well as stress. ℞

The conjunction of the words *body* and *mind* suggests a millennia-old philosophical debate. In twentieth-century psychiatry it implies a century-long discussion over the relationship between somatic and psychological factors in the etiology and treatment of sickness. The following account focuses on a rather different context: that of everyday doctor–patient interactions. It emphasizes neither theological and metaphysical issues, nor the history of psychiatry in the modern – specialized – sense. It seeks instead to understand the late nineteenth-century construction of the neurosis concept as in good measure an outcome of the needs and circumstances of medical practice and the changing structure of etiological speculation that framed clinical interactions in the period between the mid-eighteenth and early twentieth centuries. It necessarily explores the interactions between etiological thought and moral assumption, between practitioner and patient, among behavior, emotions, and seeming pathological outcomes.

At the end of the eighteenth century, most physicians were careful to avoid considering the ultimate nature of the relationship between body and mind; such speculation, as the widely read Swiss physician S. A. Tissot put it in the mid-1760s, was appropriate to metaphysics; medicine, on the other hand, was

> engaged in less abstruse, but perhaps in less uncertain researches; it does not attempt to display the first causes of this reciprocal power . . . , but confines itself to an attentive observation of the phenomena that result from it. Experience instructs the physician, that such a peculiar state of the body must necessarily produce a certain correspondent exertion of the soul; that such emotions of the soul must unavoidably be attended with a reciprocal alteration in the body.[1]

Such sentiments were no more than typical. Late eighteenth- and early nineteenth-century writings on clinical medicine ordinarily avoided categorical discussion of the problematic and theologically perilous distinctions among soul, mind, and soma – and concentrated instead on elucidating the presumed interaction between body and mind, emotions and physiological dysfunction, internal and external environment.[2]

Centuries of clinical experience seemed to endorse the ubiquity of such interactions. It was natural for physicians to explain the frequent efficacy of

---

1 Samuel A. Tissot, *An Essay on Diseases Incident to Literary and Sedentary Persons*, 2d ed. (London: J. Nourse, and E. and C. Dilly, 1769), p. 14.

This chapter, in essence, was presented as the Benjamin Rush Lecture to the American Psychiatric Association in May 1988. I should like to thank audiences at Duke, Yale, and the University of Pennsylvania, who provided useful criticisms of earlier versions.

2 The significance of such associations has, of course, been often noted by historians of medicine. "The fact that bodily diseases or symptoms are profoundly influenced by mental processes, often partially caused by them," as Erwin H. Ackerknecht put it, "was well known to all great clinicians from Erasistratos and Galen to Charcot and Struempell." *A Short History of Medicine*, rev. ed. (Baltimore: Johns Hopkins University Press, 1982), p. 235.

mesmerism and quackery as a consequence of "imagination" and "suggestion"; it was equally natural to assume that "imagination" had much to do with the action of drugs – what we would today call placebo effect in the case of presumably inert compounds and an aspect of idiosyncratic response in the case of drugs with known physiological activity. Thus music, to cite a parallel example, could prove therapeutic through its action on the emotions and nervous system.[3] Even in surgery and trauma, outcomes were assumed to be in some measure dependent on the patient's psychic state. Similarly, puerperal fever could be explained as in part a consequence of the fears that tormented lying-in women.[4] Male impotence could be the result of psychic factors.[5] Situational and emotional factors affected the onset of menstruation, to cite another widely accepted medical truism, and determined its possible dysfunction once established. Even acute ailments such as fevers or dysentery could be promoted by the "depressing passions of fear, grief, and despair. These act on the whole system," as one physician explained the etiology of dysentery in 1803, "but particularly on the alimentary canal, as is evidenced by loss of appetite, nausea, vomiting, etc."[6] No one doubted the causal relationship between situational stress and disease etiology, and, in particular, the dangers of emotions unchecked.[7] Later in the nineteenth century, physicians casu-

3 "In fevers, for instance, of great arterial action, attended with morbid excitement in the brain, inducing mania, it is very probable that music may act in a way similar to the lancet, to wit, by lessening the morbid action, and equalizing the excitement and excitability of the system, provided it be of the soft, plaintive kind." On the other hand, in diseases of debility one might presume that lively sounds would provide a healthy stimulus, "invigorating it as a cordial, or tonic medicine." Edwin A. Atlee, *An Inaugural Essay on the Influence of Music in the Cure of Diseases*... (Philadelphia: Printed for the Author, By B. Graves, 1804), pp. 17–18. Cf. Benjamin Rush, *Medical Inquiries and Observations upon the Diseases of the Mind* (Philadelphia: Kimber & Richardson, 1812), p. 211.

4 Depression and shame could, similarly, be cited as one cause for the disproportionately high mid-nineteenth-century childbed fever incidence among the prostitutes and unmarried mothers who constituted so large a proportion of women giving birth in urban hospitals. See, for example, J. Matthews Duncan, *On the Mortality of Childbed and Maternity Hospitals* (New York: William Wood, 1871), pp. 24–25.

5 William Buchan, *Observations concerning the Prevention and Cure of the Venereal Disease. Intended to Guard the Ignorant and Unwary against the Baneful Effects of that Insidious Malady*... (London: T. Chapman; Edinburgh: Mudie and Sons, 1796), pp. 225–226.

6 Lewis Creager, *An Inaugural Essay, on the Dysentery*... (Philadelphia: Thomas T. Stiles, 1806), p. 19.

7 For a contemporary marshaling of such arguments, see William Falconer, *A Dissertation on the Influence of the Passions upon Disorders of the Body*, 2d ed. (London: C. Dilly, 1791); and for an American version, Henry Rose, *An Inaugural Dissertation on the Effects of the Passions upon the Body*... (Philadelphia: William W. Woodward, 1794). Advice books aimed at lay audiences typically emphasized the physical dangers of passions unchecked. See, for example, James MacKenzie, *The History of Health, and the Art of Preserving it*, 2d ed. (Edinburgh: William Gordon, 1769), pp. 388–390; William

ally accepted (yet at the same time derided) the undoubted efficacy of homeopathy within the same framework.[8]

This was still a period of holistic pathology; specific disease entities played a relatively small role in a scheme that emphasized the body's unending transactions with its environment. Diseases shaded gradually – and dangerously – from minor to serious forms, from bronchitis to tuberculosis, for example, or from nervous habit to ultimate insanity. Physicians assumed that local ills could gradually and insidiously become systemic, that systemic imbalance induced local lesions – and that passions and emotions could and did help destabilize the tenuous balance that constituted health. One should neither repress "the desires and appetites" of one's nature, Thomas Hodgkin explained to a mechanics' institute audience, nor give in to them. The healthy man "should be like some skillful charioteer, who guides two fiery horses, and is excited by their ardour, whilst his prowess restrains their impetuosity."[9]

Until the mid-nineteenth century, in other words, all medicine was necessarily and ubiquitously "psychosomatic"; there was no need for a special term to describe the unquestioned common sense of perceived experience. Morality and clinical prudence alike emphasized the strength and thus potential danger posed by feelings uncontrolled. For emotions out of balance meant physiological function out of balance – which over time might bring about those changes pathologists had begun to find at postmortem. Thus anger, envy, or fear could be the ultimate cause of physical lesions. The hypothetical mechanisms that were used to explain this relationship varied from generation to generation – from sympathy, to William Cullen's neuropathology, to the reflex arc, to the blood's nutritive function

Buchan, *Domestic Medicine; or, the Family Physician*... (Edinburgh: Balfour, Auld, and Smellie, 1769), pp. 112–120, 145–146, 162, 293, 367, 372, 396, 460, 495, and *passim*.

8 With the conceptual aid of nature's healing power in self-limited ailments. For background, see Max Neuburger, *Die Lehre von der Heilkraft der Natur im Wandel der Zeiten* (Stuttgart: F. Enke, 1926). It is striking how physicians have for the past two centuries in general accepted the reality of such phenomena yet defined them as something categorically "other," implicitly subversive of medical authority, self-identity, and cosmology. "But of all the tricks of charlatanry, none in our day have equalled those of animal magnetism, and the more recent cheat of homoeopathy, which I may briefly allude to as tending to show the curative influence of the mind." *The Influence of the Mind on Health: A Lecture delivered to the Members of the Coventry Mechanics' Institution, by a Medical Man* (London: Effingham Wilson, 1838), p. 11.

9 *Lectures on the Means of Promoting and Preserving Health, Delivered at the Mechanics' Institute, Spitalfields* (London: J. and A. Arch, Darton and Harvey, S. Highley, and E. Fry, 1835), p. 350. Such warnings were no more than typical. For an American equivalent of such didactic admonitions, see Joseph Pancoast, *The Art of Preserving Life Briefly Considered: A Lecture, delivered before the Athenian Institute, January, 1839* (Philadelphia: Adam Waldie, 1839), pp. 30–32.

– but the phenomenon itself was never questioned. There were no categorical boundaries between the realms of body and mind in late eighteenth- and early nineteenth-century medical theory.

Nor was there a parallel boundary between doctors of the body and mind. There were no specialists in disorders of mood, cognition, and behavior.[10] Every clinician had to be something of a psychiatrist and family therapist; middle-class practice took place in the patient's home and necessarily involved family members, both as possible causes of stress and as potential factors in the recovery process. The integration of body and mind in eighteenth-century medical thought paralleled and mirrored this style and site of practice. Experienced physicians saw their regular patients over a period of years and in a particular emotional and social setting. This was a necessarily contextual point of view, consistent with traditional emphasis on the unique yet ever-changing individual as the fundamental unit of clinical analysis. The patient was more than a manifestation of the disease from which he or she happened to be suffering at a particular moment in time.[11]

Late eighteenth- and early nineteenth-century disease theory was interactive as well as holistic; health was being constantly negotiated by each individual's body *and mind* as that body moved through time. This ongoing negotiation was in fact the fundamental process in which soma and psyche interacted. An individual's life course might in this sense be likened to the voyage of a ship that must steer among shoals and navigate in potentially troubled seas. The mind was always the navigator. Education, morality, and emotions all affected decision-making; but volition – and thus responsibility – remained central to this speculative model of disease causation. Decisions had consequences. Health or sickness could be determined by what one ate, how long one slept, whether one chose to indulge in whiskey or promiscuous sex. Predisposition to disease could grow out of habitual patterned behavior as well as innate physical endowment.

Medical theory assumed a prominent role for constitution in defining temperament, and in the etiology of such ills as cancer, tuberculosis, and

10 By the mid-nineteenth century there was a small group of Anglo-American physicians who administered institutions and cared for those incarcerated within them; but even such physicians often practiced general medicine outside the asylum, while treating the somatic as well as psychiatric ills of their inmates. It should also be emphasized that even self-consciously reformist advocates of moral therapy assumed that their charges might well benefit from drugs and bleeding – and routinely employed them as part of their treatment plans.

11 This generalization does not apply as well to the inevitably more episodic and class-distanced interactions that characterized hospital practice. But such practice constituted no more than a small minority of doctor–patient interactions in the late eighteenth century.

insanity. Sensations impinged more easily and thus dangerously on the fertile soil of a hypersensitive nervous system; an ordinary diet might produce gout in individuals constitutionally predisposed. Nevertheless, one inherited tendencies, not fully developed syndromes. A "nervous diathesis" produced insanity or marked behavioral symptoms only in those exposed – or exposing themselves – to the appropriately exciting circumstances.[12] And those circumstances were often under the individual's control. The fundamental causes of chronic diseases were three, William Cadogan argued in a widely read late eighteenth-century advice book: "Indolence, intemperance, and vexation." One inherited a constitutional predisposition from one's parents, "and, if we live in the same manner they did, we shall very probably be troubled with the same diseases; but this by no means proves them to be hereditary: it is what we do ourselves that will either bring them on, or keep us free."[13]

Such relationships implied an emphasis on regimen – what we might call lifestyle today. The cause and clinical course of all chronic disease were in some measure always a matter of regimen, and regimen was necessarily a reflection of willed behavior (as well as social circumstance). Thus the tenacity of the presumed mind–body connection lay less in a concern with precise mechanism – though a speculative one could always be suggested – than in an emphasis on volition. This mode of understanding was particularly well suited to the explanation of chronic disease. Every man, as Cadogan emphasized, "was the real author of all or most of his own miseries."

> Whatever doubts may be entertained of moral evils, the natural, for the most part, such as bodily infirmity, sickness and pain, all that class of complaints which the learned call chronic diseases, we most undoubtedly bring upon ourselves by our own indulgencies, excesses or mistaken habits of life, or by suffering our ill-conducted passions to lead us astray or disturb our peace of mind.[14]

Since the body was always in the process of becoming, health and disease were incremental and additive resultants of habitual behavior patterns.

Even acute ills could be placed in the same etiological framework. The incidence of epidemics as dramatic as plague and cholera had been often explained as in part the consequence of fear. To cite another sort of

12 For a more detailed discussion, see Charles E. Rosenberg, "The Bitter Fruit: Heredity, Disease, and Social Thought in Nineteenth-Century America," *Perspectives in American History* 7 (1974): 189–235.
13 William Cadogan, *A Dissertation on the Gout, and all Chronic Diseases . . .* (Philadelphia: William and Thomas Bradford, 1772), pp. 4–5. The first edition appeared in London the previous year.
14 Cadogan, *A Dissertation on the Gout*, p. 1.

example, although we see the relationship rather differently in retrospect, venereal disease illustrated the way in which volition and physical mechanism could interact to produce disease. The mechanism of transmission was apparent, its systemic consequences obscure but undoubted – and the role of volition undeniable.[15] The gluttony which produced gout in the predisposed was paralleled by the licentiousness which resulted in syphilis or gonorrhea. The fundamental issue was controllable behavior, not predisposition in the one case or the particular sexual act in the other. From the twentieth-century psychiatric point of view what is most striking, of course, is the way in which this style of explanation allowed the casual and multidimensional integration of emotions, family and business circumstances, and individual habits into etiology and therapeutics.

Another characteristic of this style of framing disease was its parallel – if at first thought seemingly paradoxical – emphasis on ultimate somatic mechanism; even if speculative, the provision of such mechanisms provided both legitimacy and substance. Anxiety and stress did not constitute disease but could, as I have suggested, play a substantive role in causing disease through their cumulative effects on the body's physiological functions. Such assumptions were a staple of medical education as they were of the general knowledge assumed by educated laypersons. A medical student's 1836 commonplace book, for example, under the heading "mental affections," explained such interactions. "Vexation disturbs the functions of the stomach inducing Dyspepsia.... Sorrow diminishes the energy of the nervous system, lessens the force of the circulation, impedes the secretions & induces organic disease.... Joy is a powerful & Axhausting [sic] stimulus to the nervous system."[16] Sympathy and irritability could explain the connection between body and mind just as they did the connection between local and systemic pathologies. The stomach and brain interacted continuously as did the uterus and nervous system. (The longstanding belief in "maternal impressions" nicely illustrates, for example, this assumed nexus among perception, mental processing, sympathy – and, in this case, irreversible anatomical change in the gestating fetus.)

15 The presumably innocent wives and infant children of promiscuous males were, of course, an exception.
16 Allyn Hungerford, Commonplace Book, 1836. Yale Historical Medical Library, Yale University, New Haven, Conn. Such sentiments were – literally – commonplace. See, for example, Nathan Hatfield, Case Report [1825], Hatfield Papers, Historical Collections, College of Physicians of Philadelphia, Philadelphia. In elaborating the "laws of sympathy," Hatfield explained: "for instance it is well known that there is a very remarkable sympathy between the brain and stomach, and Stomach and Uterus – Should any cause whether moral or physical produce an effect on the brain the stomach in all probability will become affected sympathetically from the brain and very probably the uterus will suffer either directly from the brain or indirectly through the stomach and these effects again become the cause of other effects."

These concepts helped frame and rationalize traditional doctor–patient relationships; ideas shared by medical men and their patients constituted a fundamental aspect of their microsocial system. And by the same token, such widely accepted ideas became one element of the rationalistic framework within which the patient thought about himself or herself and constructed an understanding of the symptoms that caused pain or incapacity.

One might well emphasize the functional aspect of this explanatory style, its usefulness in providing understanding and thus a measure of reassurance to both physician and patient. Such hypothetical etiologies provided a sense of direction and potential control for individuals and a basis for confidence in their medical attendant's therapeutic and prophylactic advice.[17] Yet for certain individuals, these same ideas must have been dysfunctional and guilt-inducing; blaming oneself is as widespread and enticing as blaming others. One was in good measure responsible for one's clinical history. Decisions made or decisions not made fashioned health or pathology – brutally and directly as in the case of venereal disease, gradually and more insidiously in the case of mental illness or consumption.[18] Individual personality, particular family setting, and particular incidences of sickness combined to determine how particular men and women would evaluate their behavior and find meaning in their illness.

In many cases the central question reduced itself to simple form. Was one complicit in one's own pain and incapacity? And was it in fact illness or mere self-indulgence? Distinctions blurred. Was chronic diarrhea or mood swings syndrome or self-indulgence, disease or "merely nervousness"? "How much of my present depression is the consequence of viciously indulging in submission to the causes of it? This is an important question," a young physician reflected in his diary. "Why should I not rouze myself & determine to banish uneasiness? I will. It is but a little resolution – & bodily inquietude, & mental impatience, vanish from the view. The bare idea makes me feel better."[19] Laypersons especially seemed prone to the belief that "nervous" ills were in fact imaginary – and thus culpable. "You have mistaken me if you suppose that I believe any part of your

---

17 While for society more generally they expressed and legitimated collective values and anxieties – toward adolescence, for example, toward the disquieting pressures of market competition, toward alcohol and other stimulants, toward school stress, and toward changing sex roles.

18 Contemporaries were well aware that volition and decision-making functioned within constraints defined by social location. The poor man, for example, could not control his diet, sleep, and exercise; the wife and mother could hardly avoid the stress of childbearing and rearing. The urban worker could not easily avoid poor ventilation and filthy surroundings.

19 Entry for October 24, 1795, *The Diary of Elihu Hubbard Smith (1771–1798)*, ed. James E. Cronin (Philadelphia: American Philosophical Society, 1973), p. 80.

complaints to be *imaginary*," Benjamin Rush reassured a patient he had diagnosed as hypochondriacal. "On the contrary, I am sure that your disorder is as much a *bodily* one as the pleurisy or the gout. It is however frequently increased by certain states of mind."[20] Formal medical thought tended to emphasize the convertibility and thus moral legitimacy of ailments physical and mental; guilt and popular wisdom often conspired to make rather different distinctions.

No category of ailment was more conflict-ridden than that of the so-called "nervous ills" – especially in their more efflorescent forms such as hypochondria and hysteria. These ailments bore a particularly resonant burden of moral incapacity. Disease concepts helped not only structure the physician–patient relationship, but figured within the emotional micro-environment of individual family constellations as well; it was a particularly important factor for clinicians practicing in a family setting. Let me cite, for example, the words of an American in 1848, as he explained his decision to seek health at a water cure sanitarium:

> I am fully sensible that my mind and disposition are most materially influenced by the affections of my body, – and that my dear family are thus most unjustly, made to experience what they should by all means be wholly exempt from, the influence of my own unhappy morbid feelings.[21]

The only proper solution was to absent himself from his family and seek physical and emotional health.

Another antebellum American battled with similar problems – but seemed more resigned to his fate, if not in fact consoled by the finely

---

20 Rush to Walter Stone, January 30, 1791, *Letters of Benjamin Rush*, ed. L. H. Butterfield, 2 vols. (Philadelphia: Published for the American Philosophical Society by Princeton University Press, 1951), 2: 567. In a previous letter (of January 5, 1791, *Letters of Benjamin Rush*, 2: 574–575) Rush had diagnosed Stone's case as "the hypochondriac disorder." This fashionable diagnosis had long been surrounded with moral ambiguity. "To call the Hypochondriasis a fanciful malady," a popular mid-eighteenth-century writer contended, "is ignorant and cruel. It is a real, and a sad disease: an obstruction of the spleen by thickened and distempered blood; extending itself often to the liver, and other parts." John Hill, *Hypochondriasis, A Practical Treatise on the Nature and Cure of that Disorder; Commonly called the Hyp and Hypo* (London: Printed for the Author, 1766), p. 3.

21 John Knight to My dear wife [Frances], July 9, 1848, Knight Papers, Manuscript Division, Perkins Library, Duke University, Durham, N. C. Physicians too felt the same potential burden of guilt and responsibility. A mid-century Boston physician, for example, explained to his parents that he had hesitated to write of his illness because "it might trouble you or ... you might think I was becoming a hypochondriac" and "Thinking it to be mere fancy I at first forced myself to go to lectures, operations &c." Clarence Blake to Dear Pater and Mater, January 10, 1866, and Blake to Dear Pater, January 21, 1866; Clarence Blake Papers, Countway Library of Medicine, Harvard University, Boston.

tuned sensibility they implied. He had consulted Dr. Valentine Mott, the prominent New York clinician, who concluded that he was not a dyspeptic, but that his problems stemmed from a defective or broken-down nervous system. "I am & always have been inclined to that opinion," the patient confided to his diary. "The truth probably is that I suffer in both ways each operating to produce the other disease. The nervousness is at the bottom of both." His chronic bowel complaints, he explained, were the result of "intense suspense in all matters public and private." When the same anxious gentleman consulted Granville Pattison in 1836, the prominent Philadelphia practitioner reported that his "complaints are dependent on *Functional*, not organic disease."[22]

Physicians had always to distinguish between nervous, or functional, ills and the physical ailments they mocked and masked. "The *symptoms* were rather alarming," a New Jersey physician noted in his journal in 1852, "but seemed to be nervous rather than febrile."[23] The need to make such differentiations was a routine challenge in every practitioner's day. Such clinical judgments are well illustrated in the correspondence of James Jackson, the prominent Boston consultant and teacher. "One of the difficulties in the case," a Salem physician explained to him, "is that his wife considers him hypochondriachal & his family disguise a great deal of sympathy and not a little terror under the [affectation] of not believing he is affected with any bodily disease." Another patient writing directly complained that he was "rather costive" but his physician thought "nothing of it and treats me as if I am only nervous." In another case a fifteen-year-old girl's family sought to learn whether the young lady's pain was a consequence of "deep-seated structural disease" or "functional or nervous head-ache."[24]

The tensions are obvious. The burden of diagnosis in the physician's

22 Granville Pattison to James Henry Hammond, April 19, 1836; Hammond, "Medical Diary," Entry for May 3, 1837, Hammond-Bryan-Cumming Papers, South Caroliniana Library, University of South Carolina, Columbia; Hammond to William Gilmore Simms, September 21, 1858, James Henry Hammond Papers, Library of Congress, Washington, D.C. I should like to thank Drew Gilpin Faust for these references. Obviously laypersons did not necessarily accept the view that *functional* ills were, in fact, physical and that they transformed themselves over time into anatomical form.

23 Entry for June 30, 1852, Samuel W. Butler Diary, Historical Collections, College of Physicians of Philadelphia.

24 A. L. Pierson to James Jackson, November 12, 1823, A. L. Pierson Letterbook, Countway Library of Medicine; Elisha Bartlett to James Jackson, April 17, 1838; Henry Van Wart to Jackson, January 8, 1845, James Jackson Papers, Countway Library of Medicine. There are a good many similar letters in the Jackson papers. For another example of this traditional dilemma, see Guenter B. Risse, "'Doctor William Cullen, Physician, Edinburgh': A Consultation Practice in the Eighteenth Century," *Bulletin of the History of Medicine* 48 (1974): 346.

case or self-perception in his patient's could, as I have suggested, be particularly stressful at just this point. Was one's disease legitimate or illegitimate, culpable or random? Such dilemmas had always shaped not only self-image but doctor–patient interactions. Recall Benjamin Rush warning young physicians that they must not show boredom during the hypochondriac's recounting of "tedious and uninteresting" symptoms. Recall the harsh therapeutics, psychological and physical, often meted out to hysterics or other "nervous" patients. "My last call was to an hysterical Hybernian damsel," a mid-century practitioner noted in his diary, "who had summoned the neighborhood to witness her speedy operation of shuffling off this mortal coil. The exhibition I suspect will be postponed until some organic disease gets a chance at some of her viscera."[25] The thin line between the therapeutic and punitive, the sympathetic and judgmental, was easily crossed.

Physicians were well aware of the difficulty of making proper distinctions in such cases. "You are not to suppose," as one medical school professor warned his class, "that nervous patients cannot have real disease. It may supervene and you must be careful not to mistake the real for the imaginary, as you so often may the imaginary for the real."[26] At mid-century, nervous ailments like emotional stress remained ever-present yet elusive realities in everyday practice. Even the most trivial-seeming of such ills could provide help in prognosis and – at the same time – constitute a substantive factor in the development of more serious ailments in the future.

The problem lay in the ambiguous status of emotional ills. For even if they enjoyed a plausible and traditionally accepted place in medical theory, they constituted an occasion for the imposition of moral judgment. Sickness and identity were not easily distinguished. Moreover, such emotional ailments inhabited a liminal status in medical thought – significant not because of what they were, but for what they might become. Ills did not

---

25 Entry for February 1, 1855, William H. Holcombe, Diary, Southern Historical Collection, University of North Carolina, Chapel Hill; Rush, *Medical Inquiries*, p. 106.

26 John B. S. Jackson, *An Introductory Lecture, delivered at the Massachusetts Medical College, November 1, 1848* (Boston: William D. Ticknor, 1848), pp. 17–18. Similarly, an evaluation of "recent progress in materia medica" in 1864 underlined the role of "mind, or mental influence, as coming legitimately within the province of Materia Medica. The mind is a remedy. Our modern science claims it as a potent therapeutic agent." Edward H. Clarke, *Recent Progress in Materia Medica* (Boston: D. Clapp, 1864), p. 9. At almost the same time, the anonymous reviewer of a monograph on diseases of the stomach could criticize it for failing to consider "the matter to a greater extent from a psychological point of view." Every clinician knew "from experience, how greatly the function of digestion is influenced by the mental organization of the individual, or by some temporary derangement, or shock received by the nervous system." *New York Medical Journal* 2 (1865): 142.

become legitimate until and unless they became somatic, no matter what the interpenetration of psychic and situational factors in bringing about the physical lesions or irreversible physiological changes that ultimately constituted disease.

It was an ambiguous situation that was not to change in general until the last third of the nineteenth century, when emotional ills, altered mood states, and even patterns of behavioral deviance were for the first time widely advanced, if not universally accepted, as legitimate diseases in and of themselves. We associate this change with the expansion of sickness categories generally and the development of the neurosis concept more specifically – in parallel with the development of outpatient neurology as a specialty. This is not to say that there were not earlier advocates for broadening diagnostic categories. Control and responsibility were central, if not always explicitly articulated, issues. Isaac Ray, for example, argued in 1863 that

> the man who goes through life creditably performing his part, though oscillating between the two states of excessive depression and excessive exhilaration, is as clearly under the influence of disease as if he believed in imaginary plots and conspiracies against his property or person.[27]

A half-century's debate over the appropriate criteria for legal responsibility, for example, illustrated the tenacity of such vexed issues as the clinical legitimacy of moral and nondelusional insanity.[28]

What is as striking as the expansion of borderland categories in the last third of the nineteenth century – such as the neurasthenia described by the American neurologist George Beard or the cerebral hyperemia suggested

27 Isaac Ray, *Mental Hygiene* (Boston: Ticknor and Fields, 1863), p. 32. The second half of the nineteenth century saw, in fact, the growth of a subgenre of "mental hygiene" tracts aimed at laypersons; most emphasized the insidious slippery slide that led from "overworked" nerves to full-blown mental illness. See, for example, J. Leonard Corning, *Brain Exhaustion, with Some Preliminary Considerations on Cerebral Dynamics* (New York: D. Appleton, 1884), p. 114 and *passim*, which argues that adequate sleep is a first step in averting the slide toward insanity. Cf. Barbara Sicherman, *The Quest for Mental Health in America 1880–1917* (New York: Arno Press, 1980), especially pp. 78–152.

28 See, for example: Nigel Walker, *Crime and Insanity in England, Volume 1: The Historical Perspective* (Edinburgh: Edinburgh University Press, 1968); Roger Smith, *Trial by Medicine: Insanity and Responsibility in Victorian Trials* (Edinburgh: Edinburgh University Press, 1981); Charles E. Rosenberg, *The Trial of the Assassin Guiteau. Psychiatry and Law in the Gilded Age* (Chicago: University of Chicago Press, 1968); Janet A. Tighe, "A Question of Responsibility: The Development of American Forensic Psychiatry, 1838–1930" (Ph.D. diss., University of Pennsylvania, 1983); John S. Hughes, *In the Law's Darkness: Isaac Ray and the Medical Jurisprudence of Insanity in Nineteenth-Century America* (New York: Oceana Publications, 1986). And, of course, debates over criminal responsibility also reflected assumptions in regard to an appropriate somatic basis for exculpatory mental states.

by his rival W. A. Hammond – are the relentlessly somatic etiologies that
legitimated these innovative diagnoses.[29] This was a period when heredity
and an assortment of other somatic mechanisms were presumed to underlie
such novel disease entities as homosexuality and neurasthenia. This may
well have been a serviceable solution, useful to the self-referring patient
and necessary to the "scientific" status of the neurologists who treated and
described these conditions, and concerned themselves with what one of the
most prominent among them termed "the moral world of the sick-bed."[30]
Nervous ills could be construed as clinical entities in themselves and not
simply factors in the ultimate development of some more marked condition, whether "physical" or "mental."

At the same time, however, a growing emphasis on somatic mechanisms
dulled the traditional interest in situational factors in etiology. At one level,
it was a style of explanation that reflected the neurologist's episodic referral
practice, one rather different from a more traditional family-sited practice.
At another, this style of explanation assumed a more deterministic and
often hereditarian cast; these borderland ills needed to be clothed in
somatic garb if they were to be understood as legitimate by patient and
practitioner alike.

Even if psychosomatic ills still maintained a place in the post–germ
theory era, their etiologies were framed in increasingly reductionist and
materialist terms. An authority on asthma, for example, noted in 1889 that
the disease was "essentially a neurosis."

29 While studying Beard's neurasthenia construct some years ago I could not help but be
struck by the relentlessly somatic framework within which he sought to legitimate this
"borderline" condition. Charles E. Rosenberg, "The Place of George M. Beard in
Nineteenth-Century Psychiatry," *Bulletin of the History of Medicine* 36 (1962): 245–
259. Thus it was natural for a late nineteenth-century psychiatrist evaluating Benjamin
Rush's contribution to "claim for him ... that he distinctly recognized the corporeal
nature of insanity; that to his students and in his writings he taught that it is a disease
that must be submitted to medical as well as moral treatment." D. Hack Tuke, *The
Insane in the United States and Canada* (London: H. K. Lewis, 1885), p. 7. A mid-
twentieth-century historian of psychiatry would, of course, have been far more likely to
have commended Rush for his concern with "moral" causes and treatments. There
has been much recent interest in these questions. See, for example, among an
abundant scholarly literature: Michael J. Clark, "The Rejection of Psychological
Approaches to Mental Disorder in Late Nineteenth-Century British Psychiatry," in
Andrew Scull, ed., *Madhouses, Mad-Doctors, and Madmen. The Social History of
Psychiatry in the Victorian Era* (Philadelphia: University of Pennsylvania Press, 1981),
pp. 271–312; Nathan G. Hale, Jr., *Freud and the Americans: The Beginnings of
Psychoanalysis in the United States, 1876–1917* (New York: Oxford University Press,
1971); F. G. Gosling, *Before Freud: Neurasthenia and the American Medical Community,
1870–1910* (Urbana and Chicago: University of Illinois Press, 1987); George F. Drinka,
The Birth of Neurosis. Myth, Malady, and the Victorians (New York: Simon and Schuster,
1984).
30 The phrase is S. Weir Mitchell's: *Doctor and Patient*, 3d ed. (Philadelphia: J. B.
Lippincott, 1889), p. 10.

Medical science has not yet reached the stage where it can tell us in what neurosis consists, or what essential pathological lesion constitutes the nervous habit. That it is dependent on some structural change, I think can not be questioned, as all so-called functional disorders are, the term "functional" being simply one which we use to cloak our ignorance of true pathological conditions.[31]

The only difference, that is, between somatic and functional was that in the latter, science had not as yet demonstrated an underlying mechanism. It was no more than an instance of the aggressively scientistic character of late nineteenth-century medical thought, the rhetorical price paid to legitimate nervous and psychosomatic ills and the increasingly specialized practitioners who treated them. "The spirit of the age is upon us," as an advocate of "psychic treatment" contended in 1901, "inductive biological science has sounded the death-knell to speculative dogmatism." Progress in psychiatry would come only along the paths cleared by all those sciences that could relate to its clinical task. "Should," for example, "micro-chemical investigation succeed in proving the process underlying dementia paralytica to be one of specific toxaemia, serum therapy may offer us means to stay the ravages of this fatal malady."[32]

It is perhaps no more than to have been expected that the last third of the nineteenth century should also have seen the growth of Christian Science, Seventh-Day Adventism, and other manifestations of faith healing. For they expressed and acted out another strain implicit in attitudes toward sickness before mid-century: this was the traditional conflation of body and mind and its logical and emotional emphasis on volition and control – implicitly on self-perfection. It was the other half of the delicately balanced marriage of speculative mechanism and moral responsibility so characteristic of the first two-thirds of the century. The self-confident somaticisms of late nineteenth-century neurology were paralleled in at least some individuals by an equally self-confident emphasis on the power of mind over body and soul over mind.

Equally significant was another, and less explicitly articulated, continuity among many physicians and laypersons. This was a deep skepticism toward the bearers of "neurotic" symptoms. One must avoid thinking about one's ailments, conventional morality emphasized; keep a stiff upper lip and do not succumb to the universal temptation toward "constantly dwelling upon every slight disturbance of mental or bodily action." The consequences of succumbing could be dangerous indeed:

31 F. H. Bosworth, "On the Relation of the Nasal and Neurotic Factors in the Aetiology of Asthma," *New York Medical Journal* 44 (1889): 57.
32 Edward C. Runge, "Psychic Treatment," *American Journal of Insanity* 58 (1901): 287.

The individual body or the mind may soon seem to the perverted imagination of its possessor to assume such transcendant importance, that all other minds, bodies, and outside things are completely over-shadowed, or blotted out. Environment is obliterated, horizon is lost, and the unsatisfiable ego is all in all.[33]

And many practitioners of clinical medicine made an instinctive moral triage as they evaluated particular patients, consigning their neurotic patients to a lower status. Night duty, a Hopkins house staff member explained to his fiancée in 1894, "means to stay up all night with a very sick patient, or to hold the hand of some neurasthenic."[34] Such attitudes are by no means extinct today.

Freud's work played a role in recasting these attitudinal and diagnostic categories – even though he grew to intellectual maturity in this reduc-tionist and mechanism-oriented generation.[35] He came to accept the emotional and functional as aspects of identity, significant in themselves and still appropriately the purview of the clinician and not merely signs or portents of prospective states – or clues to spiritual worthiness.[36] Chronic anxiety or depression was, that is, not simply a failure of will or significant fundamentally in its relation to a possible supervening condition – but the revealing outcome of a particular individual's development through time. As we are all aware, this point of view has not always been popular in the medical profession; *functional* can still be a dismissive and pejorative term. Dynamically oriented psychiatry remained substantially marginal to main-stream medicine even in its era of greatest twentieth-century influence. It is not surprising that the term *psychosomatic* and the interests it stood for could seem in fact novel and reformist in the late 1930s and 1940s.[37] Nor is it surprising that illness without a demonstrable physical mechanism

33 Lionel S. Beale, *Our Morality and the Moral Question: Chiefly from the Medical Side* (London: J. & A. Churchill; Philadelphia: Presley Blakiston, 1887), p. 17.
34 John S. Billings to Katherine Hammond, December 3, 1894, Hammond-Bryan-Cumming Papers, South Caroliniana Library, University of South Carolina, Columbia.
35 It should be emphasized that *all* students of ills such as hysteria in the 1880s and 1890s were of necessity somaticists – differing fundamentally in style (and, in particular, in their emphasis on physiological/functional as opposed to anatomically sited etiologies). This is a complex and ambiguous subject, but see, for example, Kenneth Levin, "Freud's Paper 'On Male Hysteria' and the Conflict between Anatomical and Physiological Models," *Bulletin of the History of Medicine* 48 (1974): 377–397.
36 In the early years of this century many influential leaders in academic medicine called for the integration of psychological and emotional factors into the normal sphere of clinical judgment. But the widespread internalization and institutionalization of such well-meaning programmatic statements was something else again.
37 See, for example, Robert C. Powell, "Healing and Wholeness: Helen Flanders Dunbar (1902–59) and an Extra-Medical Origin of the American Psychosomatic Movement, 1906–36" (Ph.D. diss., Duke University, 1974).

should still present a potential burden of ambiguity and guilt for those bearing its symptoms.

It is particularly significant that we have in some ways come full circle in this era of concern with chronic disease – and what we now call risk factors. A life as lived has once again become a subject of analysis and policy debate; constitution, environment, and volition are once again speculatively configured as we evaluate the etiology and prophylaxis of important ills. Cigarette smoking, a fat-laden diet, inappropriate exercise patterns, and, one could hardly forget, promiscuous sexuality all loom prominently in both medical and lay considerations of the public health. The debates over AIDS, anorexia, and lung cancer, for example, all reflect in their particular ways the persistence of this explanatory style. The movement from propensity to habit to pathological mechanism has once again become a central concern of moralists as well as epidemiologists and clinicians. Body and mind, constitution and lifestyle, choice and responsibility, are not easily banished from the world of pathogenesis and public health.

5

Florence Nightingale on contagion: The hospital as moral universe

❧ While collecting materials some years ago for a history of the American hospital, I became increasingly interested in Florence Nightingale – one of the few individuals who exerted a peculiar and indispensable influence on that history. At first that influence seemed as difficult to understand as it was undeniable; her ideas were typical of the accepted wisdom of her generation, but were anachronistic by the 1880s and 1890s. An explanation seemed in order. And that explanation, I became convinced, lay in her ability to invoke a language of shared moral and conceptual reference, to articulate a world-view that at once explained the hospital's present evils and demanded their reform. It was in some ways her power as rhetorician as much as her social position and skill in bureaucratic infighting that explained Nightingale's enduring influence in nursing and hospital reform. But her ways of thinking about the world are very different from those we have come to accept in the twentieth century. As in understanding traditional therapeutics, understanding Nightingale's social impact means taking ideas seriously, no matter how alien and even inconsistent they may seem (or in her case how transparently they express a seemingly self-serving and hegemonic vision of social control). It means seeing their ultimate consistency, their ability to function as an explanatory, monitory, and hortatory system. Only then can a historian begin to appreciate her ability to mobilize the sentiments of so many of her contemporaries. ☙

We prefer our heroes to be not only heroic, but consistent – consistent, that is, with our preconceptions, not necessarily theirs. Students are still taken aback to discover that Harvey's experimental studies of the circulation were influenced by a bewildering neo-Platonic concern with the body as microcosm, or that otherwise liberal statesmen could advocate a disquieting racism. One instance of such apparent inconsistency is the lack of understanding, even hostility, displayed toward the germ theory in the last third of the nineteenth century by certain individuals prominent in the mid-century movement for public health reform.[1]

None of these reformers is better known to posterity than Florence Nightingale. Her two most widely read books, *Notes on Nursing* and *Notes on Hospitals*, had an extraordinary success in the second half of the century; it would be hard to overestimate her influence in the shaping of modern nursing and the reordering of hospitals. Nevertheless, there is a curious gap in our understanding of her work. Though historians have told us a good deal about the dramatic events of Nightingale's life – her struggle to escape the stylized routine of upper-class life, her heroic work in the Crimea, her commitment to reforming army hospitals and bringing public health to India – almost nothing has been written about her medical ideas, concepts which informed and justified her well-known program of reform.[2]

Yet the content of these ideas tells us much about their appeal to many of her contemporaries. Florence Nightingale's medical views were based on a deeply internalized and little questioned view of the world and on a consequent model of relationship between behavior, individual responsibility, and disease. These views demand explanation, for they are radically

1 For a pioneering attempt to explain the unwillingness of such reformers to deal with the implications of the germ theory and experimental medicine (as manifested in vivisection), see Lloyd Stevenson, "Science down the Drain," *Bulletin of the History of Medicine* 29 (1955): 1–26, which contends that a strongly felt "pietistic commitment" shaped the unwillingness of certain mid-century sanitarians to accept a range of novel ideas ranging from germ theory to vivisection. The present author's feeling is that "pietistic" is perhaps too inclusive a category; the interpretation suggested in the following pages is closer to a reflection in a footnote in Stevenson's paper (p. 4n): "Possibly the unwillingness to break down the conception of filth, to acknowledge dirt to be the mere vehicle of pathogenic micro-organisms, was unconscious resistance to the recognition and analysis of a metaphor which gave satisfaction in the moral realm." A significant parallel argument emphasizing the "secularization" of the concept of infection was formulated by Owsei Temkin in 1953 in "An Historical Analysis of the Concept of Infection," reprinted in *The Double Face of Janus and Other Essays in the History of Medicine* (Baltimore: Johns Hopkins University Press, 1977), pp. 456–471. See also Temkin's "Metaphors of Human Biology," in *Janus*, pp. 271–283. For a useful introduction to the problem of hospital infection, see Erna Lesky, "Hospital-acquired Infections – a Historical Survey," *Hexagon-Roche* 5 (1977): 1–10. Research for this paper was supported by a grant from the National Library of Medicine (LM 02826-02) whose assistance is here gratefully acknowledged.

2 For details of Nightingale's life, Edward Cook's standard biography is in some ways still the most complete: *The Life of Florence Nightingale*, 2 vols. (London: Macmillan, 1913). More successful as a biography is Cecil Woodham-Smith's *Florence Nightingale 1820–1910* (London: Constable, 1950). Neither of these studies critically discusses her medical ideas and their relationship to those of her contemporaries. Indispensable for any student of Nightingale's work is *A Bio-Bibliography of Florence Nightingale*, compiled by W. J. Bishop with the assistance of Sue Goldie (London: Dawsons, 1962). For a recent attempt to interpret Nightingale in psychological terms, see Donald R. Allen, "Florence Nightingale: Toward a Psychohistorical Interpretation," *Journal of Interdisciplinary History* 6 (1975): 23–45.

different from concepts of illness which have come to be accepted in the twentieth century. We must not allow the alienness of her ideas to blind us to their internal consistency, a consistency which bound together Nightingale's view of the world generally with her personal needs and career as reformer of hospitals and nursing.

The idea that disease could be induced by a specific contagion was anathema to Nightingale. It seemed to contradict her belief that filth, disorder, and contaminated atmosphere were responsible for hospital fevers and infections. To assume the reality of contagion was, as she saw it, to deny the possibility of improving hospital conditions and perhaps even to question the need for the hospital's existence. The idea of specific particles causing disease also conflicted with an even more fundamental way of understanding the body, its functions, and their relationship to health and disease. Contagion seemed morally random and thus a denial of the traditional assumption that both health and disease arose from particular states of moral and social order. To understand Nightingale's medical views is to understand how a sanitarian of her generation could find both contagionism at mid-century and the germ theory a quarter-century later similarly uncongenial. Her ideas, finally, tell us something more general about perceptions of society in mid-nineteenth-century England.

Florence Nightingale's ideas on the hospital and of the nurse's role within it were based logically on a view of the body so familiar to educated Englishmen that its fundamental aspects needed little formal or systematic exposition. It was in essence an ancient view, but one whose very antiquity underlines its usefulness in explaining health and disease.

The body was visualized in terms of a central metaphor, one in which the organism was seen as a dynamic system constantly interacting with its environment.[3] Diet, atmosphere and ventilation, psychic stress, all interacted to shape a patterned but continuously reestablished reality. Within this framework of explanation, disease was no specific entity – even if local lesions characterized a particular ailment – but rather a general state of disequilibrium. Health, on the other hand, was synonymous with balance in the body's physiological state. Though physicians in the late eighteenth and early nineteenth centuries did tend to accept the specificity and infectiousness of smallpox and of a few other ills, these seemed at first atypical and only gradually helped undermine the plausibility of this older explanatory system. By the mid-nineteenth century, however, changing views of pathology had begun to shift medical opinion toward a gradual acceptance of

3 For a more elaborate exposition of this argument, see Chapter 1 of this volume.

the assumption that most ills had a specific course, characteristic lesions, and – by implication – a specific cause.[4]

But at mid-century such attitudes toward disease specificity were neither universally accepted nor thoroughly consistent. Most medical men still assumed that ailments could shift subtly from one form to another, that all reflected a basic underlying state. Nightingale, like many such physicians, emphatically disavowed the reality of specific disease states. Sickness, she contended, should be seen – in her own words – as an "adjective," not as a "substantive noun." It must, that is, be considered as an aspect or quality of the body as a whole, rather than as an entity somehow separable from the state of a particular body at a particular moment in time. Nightingale left no doubt about the firmness of her commitment to this view. Some physicians, as she phrased it, taught that diseases were like cats and dogs, distinct species necessarily descended from other cats and dogs. But she considered such views misleading. Dogs did not change into cats, nor cats into dogs, while disease shifted its manifestations in precise response to environment. Not only had she seen disease arise spontaneously, without any possible contact with previous cases, she had also seen its characteristics change in response to altered environmental circumstances. She had seen filth produce remitting fever in a particular ward, a greater accumulation of filth change prevailing symptoms to those of typhoid, and, finally, still more dirt aggravate these symptoms into those of typhus.[5] Could she deny the evidence of her own senses? Or need she, at a time when sophisticated clinicians still found difficulty in distinguishing between some of the more common fevers?

Nightingale expressed an atypically strong aversion to the specificity of disease – a position far more categorical than that articulated by most of her medical contemporaries. Even smallpox, she believed, might emerge

4 For a study of the context in which this took place, see Erwin H. Ackerknecht, *Medicine at the Paris Hospital, 1794–1848* (Baltimore: Johns Hopkins University Press, 1967). Ordinary physicians, however, were still far more comfortable at mid-century with less specific disease concepts. See also Oswei Temkin, "The Scientific Approach to Disease: Specific Entity and Individual Sickness," *Janus*, pp. 441–455.

5 Florence Nightingale, *Notes on Nursing: What it is, and What it is Not* (New York: D. Appleton, 1861), pp. 33n, 32–33. "For diseases," as she put it, "as all experience shows, are adjectives, not noun substantives." Some years later Nightingale repeated this argument in an edition of her *Notes on Nursing* addressed to "labouring men": "Is it not living in a continual mistake to look upon diseases, as we do now, as separate things, which must exist, like cats and dogs? instead of looking upon them as conditions, like a dirty and a clean condition, and just as much under our own control; or rather as the reactions of a kindly nature against the conditions in which we have placed ourselves." *Notes on Nursing for the Labouring Classes* (London: Harrison, 1876), p. 33.

anew in an appropriately untoward environment. The stagnant air, for example, of a room long shut up could cause such sickness. "It is quite ripe," she warned, "to breed smallpox, scarlet fever, diphtheria, or anything else you please."[6]

Disease must not be seen as a response to a discrete external stimulus, but as an effort by the body to recover that normal state compromised by a particular set of unfavorable circumstances or personal habits. Recovery could only be effected by the body's normal homeostatic processes. Disease, as she put it, was simply a "reparative process," and the same laws which maintained health in the well applied to nursing the sick.[7] Thus, the heat and sweating which characterized fevers could be seen as efforts by the body to rid itself of "excrementitious" matter through its normal channels. The same was true of discharges from the bowels in dysentery or the surface eruptions which characterized smallpox or typhus.[8] But in such natural patterns of recovery, Nightingale and many of her contemporaries believed, lay danger to the patient himself – and in a hospital to those unfortunate enough to occupy neighboring beds. A continued state of health and efforts to regain it depended alike on a careful monitoring of the body's intake and outgo and on the immediate removal of any discharged metabolic products. A hospital atmosphere contaminated not only with the undifferentiated filth resulting from inefficient housekeeping and short-sighted frugality, but with the peculiarly dangerous excretions and emanations of the sick, would certainly impede normal recovery and in especially close conditions breed such ills as hospital gangrene, erysipelas, and puerperal fever. This explains her seemingly obsessive concern with the cleanliness of bedding and the regular emptying of chamber pots. The dangers she sought to avoid were not simply aesthetic. An unchanged bed, for example, meant that a patient would have "re-introduced into [his] body the emanations from himself which day after day and week after week saturate his unaired bedding."

6 *Notes on Nursing* (1861), p. 13.

7 *Notes on Nursing* (1861), p. 8. "The reparative process which Nature has instituted and which we call disease, has been hindered by some want of knowledge or attention, . . . and pain, suffering, or interruption of the whole process sets in. If a patient is cold, if a patient is feverish, if a patient is faint, if he is sick after taking food, if he has a bed-sore, it is generally the fault not of the disease, but of the nursing."

8 Nightingale, *Notes on Hospitals*, 3d ed. (London: Longman, Green, Longman, Roberts, and Green, 1868), pp. 15–17; *Notes on Nursing* (1861), pp. 74, 79–80. Similarly, Nightingale could assure her close friend and associate, Sidney Herbert, dying of renal disease, that the protein in his urine might be a sign of Nature working out its healing course: "The presence of a large amount of albumen is not proof in itself, of anything but that Nature is getting rid of something which ought not be there." Cited in Woodham-Smith, *Nightingale*, pp. 357–358.

If you consider that an adult exhales by the lungs and skin in 24 hrs three pints at least of moisture, loaded with organic matter ready to enter into putrefaction; that in sickness the quantity is often greatly increased, the quality is always more noxious – just ask yourself next where does all this moisture go to? Chiefly into the bedding. . . . Must not such a bed be always saturated, and always the means of re-introducing into the system of the unfortunate patient who lies in it, that excrementitious matter to eliminate which from the body nature had expressly appointed the disease?[9]

Adequate ventilation was similarly important. All those fevers and infections which seemed inevitably to infest the mid-nineteenth-century hospital's wards were preventable, Nightingale argued, through proper management; the very existence of such ills was a compelling argument for hospital reform.

Contagion and personal infection, on the other hand, seemed antisocial specters, "affording to certain classes of minds, chiefly in the Southern and less educated parts óf Europe a satisfactory reason for pestilence, and an adequate excuse for non-exertion to prevent its recurrence."[10] To entertain the possibility of personal contagion as the mode of transmitting hospital infection seemed, as Nightingale saw it, both to deny the need for improving hospital administration and nursing, and to replace the logic of personal responsibility with a fatalistic determinism which regarded fever and wound infection as inevitable in hospitals. This was simply unacceptable; Nightingale's emotions and intellect alike rejected such fatalism. On the contrary, she was convinced that controllable aspects of the environment, and especially the atmosphere, ordinarily caused hospital

9 *Notes on Nursing* (1861), p. 80. Thus the seemingly obsessive emphasis by mid-century hospital reformers on ventilation as an all-sufficient goal. See, for example, John Watson, *Thermal Ventilation, and other Sanitary Improvements, Applicable to Public Buildings, and Recently Adopted at the New-York Hospital* . . . (New York: Wm. W. Rose, 1851). Even after tentative acceptance of the germ theory as explanation for hospital infection, most physicians still interpreted the role of germs as – in effect – an explanation of the mechanism through which the atmosphere could be contaminated and spread infection. The germ theory seemed to many such physicians in the 1870s and early 1880s simply another argument which emphasized the need for hygiene and cleanliness within the hospital – goals endorsed vigorously by Nightingale. For revealing examples of such positions, see Charles Langstaff, *Hospital Hygiene being the Annual Address to the Southampton Medical Society. February, 1872* (London: J. & A. Churchill, 1872); John Simon, "Contagion," in Richard Quain, ed., *A Dictionary of Medicine* (London: Longmans, Green & Co., 1883), I, pp. 286–294. —

10 *Notes on Hospitals* (1868), pp. 8–9. Nightingale's emphasis on the "primitive" aspect of belief in contagionism and its association with less "advanced" cultures is consistent with Erwin H. Ackerknecht's interpretation of anticontagionism in this period: "Anti-Contagionism between 1821 and 1867," *Bulletin of the History of Medicine* 22 (1948): 562–593.

infection. "All my own hospital experience confirms this conclusion," she affirmed in emphasizing the ability of pure air alone to prevent infection. "If infection exists it is the result of carelessness, or of ignorance."[11]

The atmosphere, as Nightingale and many of her physician contemporaries believed, was the single most important medium for the transmission and causation of acute illness. The distinction between transmission and causation could not be truly meaningful for them; disease, they assumed, would inevitably develop in a sufficiently contaminated atmosphere, while that same atmosphere served as its mode of transmission. The only explanatory difficulty, an increasingly intractable one at mid-century, was whether a *specific* element in the atmosphere was needed to produce a specific disease. Nightingale could not accept such specificity. She endorsed the traditional and seemingly commonsensical notion that a sufficiently intense level of atmospheric contamination could induce both endemic and epidemic ills in the hospital's crowded wards (with particular configurations of environmental circumstance determining which). The lowered vitality and the fevers and infections which resulted from such contaminated states were morally compelling arguments for improving conditions within the hospital. Florence Nightingale was a formidable activist, and she marshalled a framework of medical doctrine which not only explained the cause of hospital infection, but indicated a possible and thus necessary mode of prevention. That sickness had always haunted the hospital's wards seemed to her hardly a justification for tolerating the conditions which seemed to breed it. "In what sense," as she put it, "is 'sickness' being 'always there,' a justification for its being 'there' at all?"[12]

As striking as the substantive aspects of this position was the language in which Nightingale expressed her arguments. They were based on the use of a special vocabulary and a series of related and emotionally compelling images. First, as has been suggested, Nightingale's etiology assumed a certain way of visualizing the body and its physiological processes – a vision structured around an ancient and accepted metaphor. Other specialized uses of language and related imagery helped communicate and legitimate her understanding of the hospital and the ills which infested it. One was the idea of *zymosis*, the concept that infectious ills spread through a process analogous to fermentation; another was a peculiar use of statistics. The

11 *Notes on Hospitals* (1868), p. 22. In the first edition of her study of hospitals, Nightingale was similarly emphatic in dismissing the notion that contagion made disease inevitable among hospital workers. "Ignorance and mismanagement lie at the root of all such presumed cases of 'infection.'" *Notes on Hospitals: Being Two Papers Read before the National Association for the Promotion of Social Science...* (London: John W. Parker & Son, 1859), p. 19.
12 *Notes on Nursing* (1861), p. 29; Woodham-Smith, *Nightingale*, p. 258.

hospital itself, finally, was not only a dismaying reality, but in her writings was also a didactic microcosm illustrating the interdependence of health and order in the larger world.[13]

But a word of explanation seems unavoidable. I have been using the terms *image, metaphor,* and *language* loosely, although I hope usefully. Much of man's perception of the world and communication of that perception comes not through his capacity to see things afresh and with a value-free neutrality, but through his capacity to shape his perceptions by means of a repertoire of conventionalized images and emotionally charged language. Language is obviously affective as well as denotative, and Florence Nightingale was in her analysis of hospital infection more rhetorician than scientist. Her understanding of bodily function and of the nature of contagion bound together perceptions of particular realities – the sickness, the filth, the disorder of mid-nineteenth-century hospitals, the everyday realities of yeast rising or beer brewing – within a language of explanation which incorporated both the prestige of science and moral certainties of a more traditional sort. Her language also communicated the perceptions of a particular class and time. In such diversity of reference lies the key to Nightingale's contemporary appeal. She expressed herself in a language rich in layers of meaning – all emotionally if not logically consistent.

Since the 1840s, students of disease had, following the influential example of William Farr, England's Statistical Superintendent of the General Register Office, categorized epidemic and infectious ills as zymotic.[14] The logic of this usage and the etiological model it implied seem

13 The use of the hospital or asylum as metaphor has a long and complex history. The connection between disease, dirt, and disorder is even more ancient and complex – as is the use of metaphor to communicate such beliefs. Since at least the work of Evans-Pritchard, anthropologists concerned with health and healing and the relationship of both to particular belief systems have sought to evaluate such questions, but ordinarily in non-Western contexts. Historians of Western science and medicine have conventionally assumed that such anthropological perspectives apply only to Third World cultures. For a recent and influential discussion of the use of symbolic forms in the shaping of particular relationships between health and world-view, see the work of Mary Douglas, especially *Purity and Danger* (New York: Praeger, 1966) and *Natural Symbols: Explorations in Cosmology* (New York: Random House, 1972).

14 For important studies on Farr and his relationship to contemporary etiological ideas, see John M. Eyler, "Mortality Statistics and Victorian Health Policy: Program and Criticism," *Bulletin of the History of Medicine* 50 (1976), pp. 335–355, and "William Farr on the Cholera: The Sanitarian's Disease Theory and the Statistician's Method," *Journal of the History of Medicine* 28 (1973): 79–100. Eyler emphasizes Farr's ability to shift gradually to a hesitant acceptance of the germ theory, using the zymotic mechanism as a basis for this shift. In general, he emphasizes the consistency between the moral values endorsed by Victorian lay social reformers and the program of medically trained sanitarians. "In short then, the environmental theories of disease causation and the social or political interpretation of morbidity and mortality provided the theoretical basis for agreement between segments of the medical profession and a

clear enough in retrospect. The scientific debate surrounding the nature
and possible specificity of fermentation was still fresh in the minds of
Florence Nightingale's medical contemporaries; even educated laypersons
could not have been unaware of this learned controversy.[15] Scientists had
disputed energetically for a generation whether the process of fermentation
was "chemical" or "vital" – whether some living organism was necessary to
initiate the changes which constituted fermentation. But to Nightingale and
to many of her medical associates, this distinction was of little practical
moment; for the essential elements of the model seemed little subject to
change whether the ferment should prove ultimately chemical or vital.
Since the seventeenth century, at least some medical men had suggested
that the phenomenon of fermentation provided a plausible explanation for
the "portability" of infectious matter. As in the process of fermentation
itself, a minute quantity of some "virus" seemed to be able to induce a
particular change in a much larger volume of material. Thus it explained
how the atmosphere could serve as a medium for the transmission of
disease; ubiquitous and necessary to man's existence, the air could become
the source of illness through its very indispensability. Contaminated by a
minute quantity of putrefying matter, it might transmit cholera or yellow
fever; within the confined walls of a hospital or tenement house, a contaminated atmosphere might cause any one of a score of ills as the exhala-
tions from human bodies acted as a kind of yeast in this vitiated culture
medium.[16]

more heterogeneous group of Victorian reformers," "Mortality Statistics," p. 339. Farr
was an associate of Florence Nightingale and their exchanges reveal not always
consistent attitudes. See Zachary Cope, *Florence Nightingale and the Doctors*
(Philadelphia: J. B. Lippincott, c. 1958), ch. 8, and "Dr. William Farr, the Medical
Statistician," pp. 98–107; Michael J. Cullen, *The Statistical Movement in Early Victorian
Britain*... (New York: Barnes & Noble, 1975).

15 William Bulloch, "Fermentation," *The History of Bacteriology* (London: Oxford, 1938),
pp. 41–63; Joseph S. Fruton, *Molecules and Life, Historical Essays on the Interplay of
Chemistry and Biology* (New York: Wiley-Interscience, 1972), pp. 22–86. To
contemporaries, "it was Liebig who first expounded the resemblance of contagious
diseases to the process of fermentation. In both, an infinitely small germ gives rise
to successive changes which propagate surprisingly the material produced –
a circumstance which makes their virulence greater than that of material poisons."
E. Mapother, *Lectures on Public Health* (Dublin: Fannin & Co., 1864), p. 245.

16 Charles E. Rosenberg, *The Cholera Years: The United States in 1832, 1849, and 1866*
(Chicago: University of Chicago Press, 1962). When empirical evidence pointed
toward the possible analogous role of water in the transmission of cholera and typhoid,
contemporary epidemiological thought had little difficulty in transferring this zymotic
process to water from its more familiar site in the atmosphere. For a brief discussion of
a seventeenth-century use of the fermentation idea and something of its origins, see:
L. J. Rather, "Pathology at Mid-Century: A Reassessment of Thomas Willis and
Thomas Sydenham," in Allen G. Debus, ed., *Medicine in Seventeenth Century England*
(Berkeley: University of California Press, 1974), pp. 79–83.

This explanation of the origin and transmission of disease seems to us speculative and, as I have suggested, in an important sense metaphorical. But, of course, it seemed anything but that to Nightingale and to many of her mid-century medical contemporaries. The very familiarity of fermentation underscored its relevance in explaining the unfamiliar and the threatening. The plausibility of this model was based in part on the very concreteness of the associations it suggested; anyone who had seen bread rise could understand how a small amount of a deleterious substance might pervade and contaminate the atmosphere.

Let me suggest, moreover, that at the same time an even deeper and still more compelling dimension of meaning helped inform Nightingale's use of the fermentation metaphor: the idea of filth as contamination, as embodying an absolute moral otherness which implied the capacity to pollute absolutely. This antithesis added emotional immediacy to Nightingale's analysis of the hospital and of the generation of infection within it. She was hardly unique in feeling and articulating this attitude toward contagion. For example, a committee of the New Jersey Medical Society in 1864 explained the communicable quality of "hospital gangrene" as

> like begetting like; the offspring of an unclean embrace that sullies the virgin purity of the blood by a detestable impregnation; a mysterious, propagable, depraved, terrible something, we know not what.[17]

Even the smallest "impregnation" could initiate those linked changes which constituted disease.

Perhaps most fundamentally, Nightingale's conception of the hospital and the generation of disease within it emphasized the role of volition and behavior in the causation of infection. This applied not only to the hospital, but to society generally. If civic authorities, she suggested, were only to monitor carefully the atmosphere of schoolrooms, Englishmen would hear no more of scarlet fever or of other seemingly unavoidable childhood ills. They would hear no more of "Mysterious Dispensations" – of disease being in the hands of God – when the responsibility lay squarely in man's own hands and brain. We must, she reiterated, look first to our own habits in seeking to explain disease.

> God lays down certain typical laws. Upon His carrying out such laws depends our responsibility (that much abused word), for how could we

---

17 Cited in David L. Cowen, *Medicine and Health in New Jersey: A History* (Princeton: D. Van Nostrand, 1964), p. 25. Owsei Temkin has emphasized not only the ancient origins of "infection" in the image of a dye polluting a much larger and previously unsullied substrate, but the moral dimensions as well. Temkin, "Concept of Infection," *Janus*, pp. 456–457.

have any responsibility for actions, the results of which we could not
forsee – which would be the case if the carrying out of His laws were
not certain. Yet we seem to be continually expecting that He will
work a miracle – i.e. break His own laws expressly to relieve us of
responsibility.[18]

For hospital hygiene, the meaning was clear enough: if we allowed contamination of the very air patients breathed, then fevers and infection must
inevitably result. Only hard work and careful planning could avert them.

Nightingale's belief in the primary role of the atmosphere in causing
disease was far more than a plausible speculation, simply one among
several intellectual options certified as respectable by the world of medical
conjecture. It was a necessity. Her etiological views didactically underlined
the connection between behavior, environment, and health. For, practically
speaking, Nightingale's emphasis on atmosphere was an emphasis on
environment – environment construed so that hospital morale was as much
a determinant of that atmosphere as was the placement of windows and
fireplaces or the frequency with which walls and floors were scrubbed. Her
explanation of disease causation in terms of fermentation was effective in
emphasizing the polarity implied by the absoluteness of the gap between
the original purity of God's atmosphere and the necessarily culpable role of
man in polluting it. As compelling justification for the social activism
demanded by her personality, the image of zymotic disease could hardly
have been more appropriate. (Significantly, she used the image of putrefaction in parallel fashion. Like fermentation, it was a progressive change
familiar to the senses, yet incorporating intense emotional and moral overtones. Consistently enough, Nightingale's use of images of fermentation
and putrefaction are almost interchangeable.[19])

Nightingale's use of statistical arguments related closely – if seemingly
paradoxically – to her use of the fermentation concept. No student of her
work and of that of her contemporaries in mid-century sanitary reform can
doubt the centrality of their appeals to "objective" statistical data.[20] (One

18 *Notes on Nursing* (1861), pp. 25n, 17n, 26–27.
19 In this casual confounding of the processes of fermentation and putrefaction,
   Nightingale was typical of many medical people at mid-century. The dangers implicit
   in the disintegration of once-living matter were vivid, not only embodying a compelling
   moral meaning, but incorporating sensory experience. Whose senses had not been
   assailed by the offensive odors and sights of putrefaction?
20 See, for example, the articles on Farr by Eyler cited in note 14. Eyler emphasizes the
   social and moral dimension of Farr's use of statistical evidence. "Medical statisticians
   assumed that disease phenomena were regular and orderly not only in the individual
   but also in their progress within a community. Health, disease, death, and physical and
   moral conditions were believed joined in an indissoluble link." Eyler, "Mortality
   Statistics," p. 336. As Farr himself wrote in 1875: "There is a relation between death

thinks, for example, of comparisons between urban and rural mortality rates or of the comparative incidence of puerperal fever in different kinds of hospitals and in private practice.) But again, let me suggest that Nightingale's use of statistical description and analysis was as much rhetorical as it was instrumental. Despite her well-deserved reputation for tactical acuteness in the service of pragmatic reform, Nightingale's mind ultimately saw things not in additive terms, but instead in morally resonant polarities: filth as opposed to purity, order versus disorder, health in contradistinction to disease. Hospital infection was thus a consequence of disorder in a potentially ordered pattern. Statistics defined the place of a particular ward along the continuum shaped by these polarities. Given her unwillingness to accept the specificity of disease and her tendency to correlate incidences of fever and surgical infection with levels of atmospheric contamination, it was only natural for her to point with indignation to correlations between particularly untoward hospital conditions and atypically high levels of hospital infection.[21] Thus the aggregate incidence of zymotic disease served as a seemingly objective index of human failure. The strength of Nightingale's statistical arguments lay not simply in their form, but in the assumed and unspoken polarity between filth and cleanliness, sickness and health, which they dramatized. They served, that is, to underwrite her ultimately moral understanding of disease causation.

The central image which at once communicated and legitimated her program of reform was a vision of the hospital itself; her picture of the hospital can hardly be described as figurative, for it incorporated a careful analysis of existing realities and a blueprint for consequent reform. On the other hand, it was hardly a value-free rendering of these realities. The hospital seemed to her quite literally a microcosm of society, every part interrelated and all reflecting a particular moral order. Just as order in the

and sickness.... There is a relation betwixt death, health, and energy of body and mind.... There is a relation betwixt the forms of death and moral excellence or infamy." Nightingale employed statistical arguments frequently and prominently in her own works. In addition to her *Notes on Hospitals*, she participated forcefully in the contemporary debate on puerperal fever and the possible dangers of lying-in hospitals, a debate which turned to a significant degree on statistical evidence. *Introductory Notes on Lying-In Institutions. Together with a Proposal for Organising an Institution for Training Midwives and Midwifery Nurses* (London: Longmans, Green & Co., 1871).

21 The first edition of her *Notes on Nursing* (1859), for example, begins with a discussion of the uses of mortality and morbidity statistics. Coupled with such habitual references to statistics was a characteristically gratuitous precision of statement. When Nightingale suggested, for example, a distance of at least three feet between the beds of fever patients, she found it easy to explain: "Miasma may be said, roughly speaking, to diminish as the square of the distance. With good ventilation, it is not found to extend much beyond 3 feet from the patient; although miasma from the excretions may extend to considerably greater distance." *Notes on Nursing* (1859), p. 58.

body and an appropriate physical and psychological equilibrium constituted health for the individual, so order in the hospital implied a low incidence of fever and wound infection for its inmates. Similarly, in society at large, ill health, poverty, and depravity all sprang from a sequence of remediable human acts. The hospital was a part of that society, a microcosm of the moral and social relationships which determined the individual's health, on the one hand, and that of society generally on the other. Within this framework, one could hardly distinguish between the moral and the material, the individual and the community of individuals. Social health and individual health were bound together by a similar set of moral relationships and responsibilities; life on the ward illustrated these truths with didactic clarity. If a man failed to obey the dictates of God immanent in the organization of his body, he could only expect disease; if a hospital were contaminated by filth, administrative irresponsibility, and immorality, the fevers and infections which arose were equally unavoidable.

And for Florence Nightingale the hospital of her day was indeed a place of disorder. No woman of her class and education could well have encountered that would-be healing institution without finding it menacing and alien. It is no accident that her new-model trained nurses were responsible as much for discipline as they were for overseeing proper diets or dressing ulcers. Indeed, the emphasis in Nightingale's etiological and pathological thought on the interaction of the patient as a whole with every aspect of his environment implied that the distinction between moral and physical well-being, between mind and body, was hardly meaningful.[22] It was of little use in explaining the causation of disease generally and certainly not applicable in understanding hospital infection. The mid-nineteenth-century hospital was a lower-class institution in many ways, organized in theory according to the moral assumptions of its lay trustees and administrators, but dominated in reality by values and behavior antithetical to those Nightingale saw as the only appropriate basis for a moral society. Zymotic images were also ideal for describing the hospital's fermenting and disorderly life – a below stairs without an above stairs to control it. We need not be surprised to learn that Nightingale's model ward arrangements placed the nurse's room so that she might observe all its inmates from a single vantage point.[23] It was equally logical that closets and

22 The unwillingness to distinguish between the psychic and physical was typical of medical thought at this time; Nightingale, however, integrated such assumptions into her analysis of the hospital and the nurse's role with extraordinary effectiveness.

23 At this time it was still assumed that the ward nurse would sleep in proximity to her patients. Nightingale's concern both with the hospital's ventilation specifically and with the allocation of space more generally is entirely consistent with this interpretation of her moral and medical views.

stairwells where "skulking" might occur or where convalescents might "play tricks" must be avoided.[24] These were to be eliminated by the enlightened hospital architect, just as he avoided corners in which dust might accumulate or sewers which allowed dangerous fumes to escape.

Since her etiological views were, as we have emphasized, fundamentally holistic and since she was unwilling to accept the specificity of disease and the possible existence of specific causative agents, Nightingale saw the nurse's role as both multifaceted and indispensable. It was also fundamentally moral. Nightingale explicitly contended that a trained nurse's endowments must be ultimately spiritual; the technical abilities which she might acquire were, if not precisely subordinate to her moral powers, at least subsequent to and dependent upon them.[25] Not the least of these moral qualities was – and here Nightingale obviously made a personal plea – activism itself. As she put it, "patience and resignation" in a nurse "are but other words for carelessness or indifference – contemptible, if in regard to herself; culpable, if in regard to her sick."[26]

That same holistic pathology and hygiene which explained the incidence of health and disease also explained the numerous ways in which the nurse could help to effect the patient's recovery. Like many of her forward-looking mid-century peers, Nightingale wrote comparatively little of drugs and bleeding, of therapeutics generally; discreet enough not to antagonize physicians on seemingly marginal issues, she generally ignored their potential for therapeutic intervention. Medicine, she explained, was not part of the essential curative process.

> Pathology teaches the harm that disease has done. But it teaches nothing more. . . . It is often thought that medicine is the curative process. It is no such thing; medicine is the surgery of functions, as surgery proper is that of limbs and organs. Neither can do anything but remove obstructions; neither can cure; nature alone cures. Surgery removes the bullet out of the limb, which is an obstruction to cure, but nature heals the wound.[27]

All nursing could accomplish – and it was no small achievement – was to put the patient into the best possible condition for nature to effect its plan of cure. But although a hospital could not *cure*, it seemed self-evident to Nightingale that it could and must avert the spread of infection and more generally promote the body's internally directed efforts to regain health. At

24 *Notes on Hospitals* (1863), pp. 49, 52, 114.
25 Woodham-Smith's discussion of Nightingale's training school policies emphasizes her minute concern for the probationer's moral health. *Nightingale*, p. 347 and *passim*.
26 *Notes on Nursing* (1861), p. 93.
27 *Notes on Nursing* (1861), p. 133. For parallel arguments, see pp. 72, 131.

least a well-run hospital could prevent a patient from being poisoned by the
emanations arising from his own excretions and those of his ward-mates.
Drugs and bleeding were marginal in her ideal hospital.[28]

The possibility of effective hospital administration implied its necessity.
Translated into behavior, Nightingale's point of view emphasized the certainty of improvement through carefully directed activity. It is not surprising that Florence Nightingale was so resolutely hostile to the idea of
specific contagion, and so skeptical of the existence of specific disease
entities. Hospital infection reduced itself to the consequence of untoward
behavior. Poor planning of windows, slovenly nursing, cold and ill-prepared
foods, drains and sinks placed where they might contaminate the atmosphere, inadequate ventilation, chamber vessels unemptied for hours, were
all remediable, all consequences of incompetence or irresponsibility. Will
and the assurance of humane accomplishment were closely related in
Nightingale's thought as she at once explained the world she saw about her
in the hospital and justified the social role she sought to fill.

In this interrelated world of volition and pathology, contagion seemed
arbitrary, random in its moral implications. It was not simply an inability to
comprehend the germ theory which made her hesitate to accept it, but its
irrelevance – if not, indeed, its destructiveness – to her complex way
of visualizing the nature of disease and its relationship to environment
and behavior. If chance alone determined whether an individual should
intersect with a disease-causing microscopic particle, then sickness was
bereft of meaning; it could play no monitory role in a world of moral order.

It is easy enough to feel removed from many of the seemingly quaint
arguments which characterized mid-nineteenth-century anticontagionism.
How are we, for example, to regard the oft-repeated contention that a
belief in contagion during an epidemic would make nursing impossible,
that the fabric of social obligation would be rent were laypersons to regard
infectious disease as contagious? These arguments were reiterated by
anticontagionists in the first two-thirds of the century. Yet they are more
than examples of obsolete casuistry. Such warnings vividly represented the
dangers contagionism seemed to pose to the carefully elaborated relationship between health, behavior, and social environment which had been so
prominent in traditional medical thought and so central to mid-nineteenth-
century public health advocacy. On a practical level, moreover, it threatened
the future of nursing as a profession; if prudence, proper regimen, and
good general health could not protect against contagion, then nursing must
be a perilous trade indeed.

28 *Notes on Nursing* (1861), pp. 8, 13. Not surprisingly, Nightingale – as we have seen –
    emphasized that disease was a normal reparative process, one which could be aided but
    never directed or demanded.

As late as 1894, Florence Nightingale could still warn that a willingness to look into drains was at least as important as a knowledge of bacteriology in the mental equipment of a district health officer. "Mystic rites," she had complained the year previously, such as "disinfection and antiseptics, take the place of sanitary measures and hygiene."[29] Nightingale's highly atypical quest for achievement in the public sphere only exacerbated her need for an explanatory system which would justify her zeal and the program to which she had dedicated her life. It was a framework she had espoused with enthusiasm; she could not easily adapt to new and seemingly less relevant modes of explaining disease.

In outlining this interpretation of Nightingale's medical views, I have in some ways constructed an overly stylized antithesis between the depiction of real pain, real filth, and real infection in the form of symbol and metaphor, on the one hand, and of rationalistic speculation on the other. The problem, however, in emphasizing the rhetorical structure of her argument is our tendency to equate the use of figurative language with a denial of the real, and our tendency to assume a categorical distinction between the rational and irrational in social discourse. Yet Nightingale's medical views illustrate the difficulty of defending such distinctions. Her descriptions of the hospital are entirely consistent with much of the surviving evidence. Even the intensity and peculiarity of the mid-century hospital's smells seemed viscerally to endorse the accuracy of her atmosphere-oriented etiological scheme.[30] It is difficult to overstate the impact which the hospital's bleak precincts must have had upon a woman of her class and previous experience. Nightingale's use of statistics, her measured dis-quisitions on ventilation and heating provided an idiom which could not only communicate specific information, but promised control while creating a reassuring emotional distance. To label certain of her characteristic modes of assimilating and expressing experience as metaphorical is not to imply that they were arbitrary (except insofar as they were necessarily

29 Nightingale, *Health Teaching in Towns and Villages. Rural Hygiene* (London: Spotswoode & Co., 1894), p. 21. The quotation is drawn from "Sick Nursing and Health Nursing," in John S. Billings and Henry M. Hurd, eds., *Hospitals, Dispensaries and Nursing* (Baltimore: Johns Hopkins University Press, 1894), p. 449. This essay, contributed by Nightingale to the International Congress of Charities, Correction and Philanthropy, held in conjunction with Chicago's Columbian Exposition in 1893, provides a remarkable capsule presentation of her views and their consistency over a half-century.

30 Contemporaries all agreed that there was a peculiar "hospital smell" which characterized the wards of mid-century institutions; it seemed obvious that it must be associated with a contaminated atmosphere. "All foul smell indicates disease," Nightingale warned working men. "Never live in a house which smells. Either don't take it, or examine where the smell comes from, and then put a stop to it; but never think of living in it until there is no smell. A house which smells is a hot-bed of disease." *Notes on Nursing for the Labouring Classes* (1876), p. 24.

expressions of individual need and perception). They were that, of course, but the very power and plausibility of Nightingale's arguments arise from their multileveled interaction with a particular reality and their peculiar appropriateness to time and place.

Perhaps we have already overemphasized the characteristic mixture of scientific and more traditionally spiritual arguments and sources of authority in Nightingale's medical and administrative program. But this is hardly surprising; nor was this emotionally resonant amalgam of ideas and images peculiar to Nightingale. Changes in world-view are presumably always syncretic and gradual, not abrupt, self-conscious, and categorical. The arguments I have sought briefly to outline constituted indeed a characteristic aspect of a more general adaptive strategy congenial to the educated and articulate in mid-nineteenth-century Great Britain and the United States. In approaching a variety of social problems, intellectuals such as Nightingale incorporated in their discussions both the legitimacy and characteristic verbal forms of two seemingly disparate realms of authority, that of traditional moral assumption and that of science as dispassionate analysis.[31] Nightingale's generation played in some ways a key transitional role in the shift from an older world-view based on the rationalization of a complex and textured relationship between behavior and its consequences – personal, spiritual, physical – of a world in which every event and relationship was tinged with moral significance, to a very different one which found impersonal and reductionist modes of social explanation more congenial and increasingly appropriate to an ever more specialized, impersonal, and bureaucratic society. Since at least the time of Marx, social thinkers have grappled with this problem of fit between social structure and world-view.

Ideas formally medical and scientific have played comparatively little role in such debates. In general, historians of science and medicine have tended to accept past medical and scientific ideas on their own terms – that is, as self-contained, value-free systems of ideas. In medicine particularly, however, such formal and intellectualistic interpretations of past thought have in the past generation come to seem increasingly one-dimensional. It is difficult, for example, to draw a categorical distinction between science and imagination, between the heuristic use of metaphor and a seemingly distinct process of ordered, disciplinarily defined investigation. The more we understand about the development of biology and medicine in the West, for example, the less enlightening seem the distinctions so frequently made

31 For a more general statement of this position, see Charles E. Rosenberg, "Introduction: Science, Society, and Social Thought," in *No Other Gods: On Science and American Social Thought* (Baltimore: Johns Hopkins University Press, 1976), pp. 1–21 and 109–131.

between scientific and nonscientific modes of thought. Substantive insights often result from the previous elaboration of an illuminating metaphor which organizes accumulated data in a novel way.[32]

Even the diffuse concept of zymotic etiology could play such a creative role in hands more disciplined – and discipline-oriented – than those of Florence Nightingale. Let me refer by way of illustration to the case of John Snow, the mid-nineteenth-century English physician deservedly and securely installed in the pantheon of medical history for demonstrating that cholera was a water-borne disease. Snow showed extraordinary epidemiological ingenuity in demonstrating the role of water in spreading the disease. He not only traced individual cases to particular sources of contamination (most dramatically, a popular well), but revealed a striking differential in cholera incidence among subscribers to two different water companies (one of which drew its water from the Thames above London and the other from the river after it had been contaminated by the city's sewage). Snow's work seems in retrospect both elegant and systematic. Yet the inspiration for his empirical investigation was drawn from a previously enunciated – and generally unsupported – analogy between the way in which a specific ferment could predictably alter an enormous substrate through the inducing of a "continuous molecular change," and how a pathogenic material might effect a similar change in a city's water supply.[33] Is Snow's work an example of the empirical style or a creative use of metaphor? To formulate the question is to suggest the awkwardness of making such absolute distinctions.

32 "The use of metaphors in human biology," as Owsei Temkin argued as early as 1949, "is not an aberration from which even great men have failed to escape. On the contrary, by using metaphors which they believed to represent adequate and true concepts, Aristotle, Galen, Paracelsus, Harvey, Descartes, Virchow, and Helmholtz shaped concepts of human biology which conformed with their own thoughts and feelings and with the thoughts and feelings of their times." "Metaphors of Human Biology," *Janus*, p. 283. Though he does not employ the language of anthropology, Temkin's substantive understanding of this medical use of metaphor is consistent with the suggestions of such contemporary advocates of "symbolic anthropology" as Victor Turner and Mary Douglas. For parallel and more detailed interpretations of the role of metaphor in the shaping of early modern science, see Walter Pagel's important work: *The Religious and Philosophical Aspects of van Helmont's Science and Medicine, in Supplements to the Bulletin of the History of Medicine*, No. 2 (Baltimore: Johns Hopkins University Press, 1944); *Paracelsus: An Introduction to Philosophical Medicine in the Era of the Renaissance* (Basel: S. Karger, 1958); *William Harvey's Biological Ideas* (Basel: S. Karger, 1967).

33 John Snow, *On Continuous Molecular Changes, More Particularly in their Relation to Epidemic Diseases: Being the Oration delivered at the 80th Anniversary of the Medical Society of London*. (London: John Churchill, 1853). This is conveniently reprinted with Snow's other major essay on cholera, a biographical memoir by B. W. Richardson, and an introduction by W. H. Frost: *Snow on Cholera*... (New York: Commonwealth Fund, 1936).

There are endless difficulties in attempting to defend the categorical distinction between the rational and the irrational, the scientific and the intuitive. To return, for example, to Florence Nightingale's own work: many of her practical suggestions must have proved efficacious despite their basis in a formal rationale that we consider mistaken. Many of the goals she sought to achieve were entirely consistent with policies dictated a generation later by the implications of the germ theory. Certainly her influence pointed toward a cleaner and in general more humane hospital environment – toward better sanitation, adequate ventilation, improved diet, competent nursing. That we cannot share all of Florence Nightingale's convictions, that we may find some of them alien or even repellent should not obscure their power to motivate or the reality of the misery she sought to ameliorate.

It must be confessed, in conclusion, that Florence Nightingale was hardly representative as an individual; indeed, her very prominence and her almost improbably melodramatic career as self-willed secular saint remind us of her very uncommon aspect. Though the term *charismatic* has been subject to much casual misuse, it does apply to a Florence Nightingale. But the specialness of her life does not imply a specialness for her ideas. Nightingale's very deviance and the intensity of her motivation – admittedly personal and idiosyncratic – made her all the more dependent on the articulation of a rationale broadly plausible to her educated and influential peers. Thus, a central aspect of her historical significance hinged upon her rhetorical ability, her skill in shaping a compelling montage of emotionally rich and intellectually plausible images, and her use of these figures in the advocacy of new institutional forms. Nightingale's career is symbolic not only of woman's emergence from the strictures of traditional roles, or the parallel emergence of perhaps equally constricting but certainly more novel bureaucratic roles, but of a fundamental reordering of English society, of its forms and self-conceptions.[34]

34 This essay has avoided the so-called woman's question, a significant matter in interpreting Nightingale's work and social impact, but one inappropriate for this brief discussion.

6

Cholera in nineteenth-century Europe: A tool for social and economic analysis

ટ૱ This paper was written for an occasion and with an agenda reflecting disciplinary politics. It was solicited for a session on health and economic development at an international meeting of economic historians held in August of 1965. Designed to attract the interest of economists, my argument underlined the importance of soft – intellectual and cultural – variables in understanding economic growth and change. Cholera, I contended, was not significant in demographic terms, but could be seen as a sampling device, a way of gaining access to particular configurations of demographic and economic circumstances, ideas, and institutional relationships illuminated in the course of the nineteenth century's successive cholera pandemics.

Written in the mid-sixties, this essay will seem dated in some ways. Perhaps most conspicuous is the way in which economic growth models seemed at the time the most plausible context in which to "sell" the intellectual and social history of medicine to an audience of economic historians and economists. Development economics, with its formal discussion of the stages and necessary preconditions of growth, its implicit evolutionary and teleological structure, has come to seem dated, ethnocentric, and arbitrary. A generation marked by relativism, antiauthoritarianism, anticolonialism, and ecological sensitivity – not to mention the accumulation of a great deal of intractable data – has made us a great deal more tentative in discussing the nature and consequences of economic growth.

With the expansion of interest in social and cultural history during the past quarter-century, moreover, epidemic disease has become an increasingly well-cultivated research area; the historian of disease no longer needs to feel defensive in seeking to demonstrate the relevance of his or her subject matter. Despite these changes in the academic climate, I still think the argument that follows remains persuasive. ટ૱

Economists have, in the past generation, become deeply concerned with the problem of economic growth. Of late years, as traditional economic models have demonstrated inadequacies, economists have become increasingly interested in the social and cultural inputs necessary for growth in economic productivity. Human, value-related factors, particularly education, role definition, and the place of science and technology, have taken a place beside the more traditional categories of the economist and economic historian.[1] But these human factors, important though all admit them to be, are, especially in historical contexts, not usually amenable to quantitative methods of data gathering. It is difficult, on the one hand, to evaluate and sample such elusive factors, and on the other hand to define their precise role in social change.

An epidemic disease, I suggest, provides an excellent sampling device for studying the numerous yet organically related factors which underlie increases in economic productivity. An epidemic, if sufficiently severe, necessarily evokes responses in every sector of society. A study of the responses to the same sharply focused and unavoidable stimulus should provide materials for the construction of a cross section of cultural values and practices at one moment in time. Values and attitudes, especially in the areas of science, religion, and traditionalism and innovation, for example, are inevitably displayed during an epidemic. Medicine itself is, of course, a social context, one in which science pure and science applied necessarily function together; the nature of their interaction during a crisis situation should provide clues to their ongoing relationship. Thus the behavior of society during an epidemic and of medicine as a social function provides an organic context in which the structural configuration of attitudinal and institutional factors may be discerned. This is, of course, not meant to imply that each of the factors mentioned could not be studied alone or by using other indices. An epidemic simply provides a convenient and effective sampling device for studying in their structural relationship some of the fundamental components of social change.

There is no human crisis more compelling than an epidemic of plague, yellow fever, or cholera. These phenomena are, indeed, so dramatic and so terrifying that most physicians and historians have tended to view them as something alien, something outside of society and contending with it.[2] This

---

1 For a recent discussion of these trends in the context of econometric production models, see R. R. Nelson, "Aggregate Production Functions and Medium-Range Growth Projections," *American Economic Review* 54 (1964): 575–606.

2 One may compare these differences in approach to the two basic orientations which have always defined man's approach to disease. One sees disease as an invading entity, attacking the body from without, while the other views disease as a resultant of the sum of the individual's responses to certain patterns of stimuli. Cf. Owsei Temkin, "The Scientific Approach to Disease: Specific Entity and Individual Sickness," in A. C.

frame of reference has served well to dramatize the history of the great epidemic diseases, and most discussions of the social and economic consequences of epidemic incidents have assumed this form. They attempt, that is, to demonstrate the direct impact of the disease upon the society attacked, either in terms of productivity curtailed or labor force reduced. (This is a position particularly congenial to physicians writing of the historical effects of disease, for it serves – seemingly – to demonstrate the importance of medical factors in history.) For more than a century, however, a variant approach, one which sees diseases as a function of social organization, has been available. Since at least the time of Virchow, physicians and historians of disease concerned with "social medicine" have tended to view disease, endemic as well as epidemic, not as an alien visitation, but rather as the consequence of social organization and especially of social inequity and social change.[3]

This strongly humanitarian and environmental approach has often placed little emphasis upon the individuality of disease entities. From this point of view, disease is essentially a pathognomonic sign, a symptom of underlying social pathology, and the history of disease becomes a weapon for social criticism as well as social analysis. Yet the individuality of disease is an indispensable aid in increasing the value of historical studies of epidemics. Differences in symptoms, for example, imply differing magnitudes of social response; differences in modes of transmission imply the ability to study different economic and ecological relationships. Influenza, for example, is not ordinarily studied by the social or economic historian; it is too easily transmitted, too universal, and insufficiently lethal or disfiguring. (Though its usual mildness, it should be noted, implies something of the values and capacities of a society which has undertaken to combat it.) At another extreme are the deficiency diseases in which the biochemical mechanisms underlying the clinical manifestations are so specific that the presence of the disease is virtually a test for certain factors in the patient's environment. Most infectious diseases fall somewhere between these two extremes. Malaria and cholera, for example, are clearly, though complexly, related to stages of economic development. Malaria receded from large areas of the

Crombie, ed., *Scientific Change, Historical Studies in the Intellectual, Social and Technical Conditions for Scientific Discovery and Technical Invention from Antiquity to the Present* (London: Heinemann, 1963), pp. 629–647.

3 For a brief historical statement of the position of "social medicine," see George Rosen, "Approaches to Social Medicine: A Historical Survey," in *Backgrounds to Social Medicine* (New York: Milbank Memorial Fund, 1949), pp. 9–23. For a discussion of Virchow's classic statement of this standpoint, see Erwin H. Ackerknecht, *Rudolf Virchow* (Madison: University of Wisconsin Press, 1953), pp. 124–130, and the same author's *Beiträge zur Geschichte der Medizinalreform von 1848* (Leipzig: J. A. Barth, 1932).

Western world before any knowledge of its mode of transmission was known. Screening, drainage of marshes, careful cultivation practices, an abundance of cattle – all products of economic development considered broadly – cumulatively interact to reduce the mosquito population and to decrease the chances of human beings being bitten.[4] The correlation between economic growth and decrease in malaria seems, in general, to have been clearly established. The relationship, however, between economic growth and changing disease conditions is, because of the individuality of disease, no simple one; measures which seem to imply increased productivity do not always bring a decreased incidence of infectious disease. Consider, for example, the cases in which the construction of irrigation and drainage canals for dry-land farming have actually increased the incidence of malaria and bilharziasis – an inevitable sequence when this specific artifact of economic growth comes into being in a society in which the evolution of medicine and public health have not organically paralleled this innovation.[5] (Irrigation canals can provide, of course, excellent breeding places for the mosquitoes which transmit malaria or the snails which help transmit bilharziasis.) The proper approach to a study of malaria or cholera lies not in attempting to state with actuarial zeal their economic costs, but to allow their individuality as biological phenomena to help illumine the socioeconomic features of the world in which they do, or do not, occur.

Cholera was the classic epidemic disease of the nineteenth century, although – in all probability – it did not reach Europe until the 1830s.[6] No disease of the nineteenth century can be compared with it in terms of immediate emotional impact; cholera kills roughly half of those infected and kills them, moreover, in a particularly unpleasant manner. And cer-

---

4 Erwin H. Ackerknecht has provided an excellent exposition of this interpretation of malaria: *Malaria in the Upper Mississippi Valley 1760–1900* (*Supplements to the Bulletin of the History of Medicine*, No. 4) (Baltimore: Johns Hopkins University Press, 1945).

5 J. N. Lanoix, "Relation between Irrigation Engineering and Bilharziasis," *Bulletin of the World Health Organization* 18 (1958): 1011–1035; Paul F. Russell, "Public Health Factors. Malaria and Bilharziasis," in L. Dudley Stamp, ed., *A History of Land Use in Arid Regions* (Paris: UNESCO, 1961), pp. 363–372.

6 A recent and inclusive outline of cholera's history can be found in R. Pollitzer, *Cholera* (Geneva: World Health Organization, 1959), pp. 11–50. Still important are August Hirsch, *Handbuch der historischgeographischen Pathologie*, vol. I: *Die allgemeinen akuten Infektionskrankheiten* (Stuttgart, 1881), pp. 278–348, and Georg Sticker, *Abhandlung aus der Seuchengeschichte und Seuchenlehre*, vol. II: *Die Cholera* (Giessen, 1912). For an account of cholera in the United States, see Charles E. Rosenberg, *The Cholera Years: The United States in 1832, 1849, and 1866* (Chicago: University of Chicago Press, 1962). Charles Creighton's is still the best general history of cholera in Great Britain, though it has been superseded in its treatment of certain incidents. Creighton, *A History of Epidemics in Britain*, vol. II (Cambridge: Cambridge University Press, 1894), pp. 796–862.

tainly cholera killed hundreds of thousands in each of its pandemic visitations upon Europe. Yet it was indirectly, as a catalyst in the development of the public health movement, that cholera played its essential role in affecting European economic and demographic patterns. That is, it is not the men actually dying of cholera who are significant, but rather those who did not die because of the public health measures instituted in fear of the disease. It is impossible, so far as I know, to discover in the literature a single instance in which urban growth or a pattern of local economic development was lastingly influenced by the immediate mortality from cholera.[7] Though the disease did play a central role in crystallizing sentiment in favor of public health and environmental reform, it could only have done so in a society in which the appropriate attitudinal, economic, and technological means were at hand.

When cholera arrived in Western Europe in 1831–1832, it was subjected to the scrutiny of a rapidly maturing scientific community. In the 1830s the disease was a mystery; by the 1860s, however, the medical profession – or at least its more advanced members – possessed a workable empirical knowledge of its mode of transmission. In 1883, Koch discovered the specific causative organism. Western Europe's last significant brush with cholera took place in the 1890s. (Certain areas, like the British Isles, never allowed the disease a substantial foothold after the 1870s.) A study of Europe's initial encounter with cholera demonstrates the existence of a relationship already well-defined between science, medicine, and social values; its visitations later in the century – for cholera was never endemic in Europe – demonstrate with equal clarity the rapid development of this society in a parallel and interrelated pattern of economic, technological, scientific, and institutional growth.

Before the 1830s, cholera had been seen only by physicians in India. In the late 1820s, as it moved West, it attracted increasing interest. As soon as the disease appeared in Russia, Poland, and Germany, medical commissions from England and France were appointed to report on this seemingly new and certainly appalling disease. Not surprisingly, however, considering their inadequate etiological knowledge, the explanations of these medical commissioners and those of their contemporaries were based

---

7 Morbidity statistics in the 1830s, even in the larger cities, were reported and recorded in a somewhat tenuous fashion, partially as a reflection of the formlessness of most physicians' diagnoses. For an example of the difficulty of determining even so relatively uncomplicated a fact as comparative class and occupational death rates from cholera, see Louis Chevalier, *Le Cholera. La Première Épidémie du XIXe Siècle* (Bibliothèque de la Révolution de 1848, Tome XX) (La Roche, Imprimerie Centrale de L'Ouest, 1958), pp. 1–45. Chevalier's demographic study of Paris during the 1832 cholera epidemic – a study, it should be noted, based on atypically full records – represents what is probably the most complete study of any community during this epidemic.

as much upon moralism as empirical analysis. And, indeed, the twentieth-century observer will be struck not only with the moralistic elements in the hypothetical etiologies of medical thought, but equally by the orthodox religious interpretations of the epidemic so prevalent throughout Western Europe and the United States, both in Catholic and Protestant areas. The individual who succumbed to cholera, both physicians and ministers agreed, had predisposed himself to disease, had somehow weakened his constitution. And the means by which one could accomplish this were as varied as the occasions of sin. Drinking, overeating, or sexual excess, for example, might all dissipate one's vital forces and thus leave one defense-less against the cholera-causing principle in the atmosphere. Ministers and moralists in general, moreover, tended to see and interpret the epidemic not as a consequence of individual transgression alone, but as the result of a national failing in morality. In a sense, however, the significance of these traditional supernaturalistic interpretations lies not in their pervasiveness, but in the manner in which such thought had been segregated; it was no longer a dominant sphere of values, but a domain supplementary and alternative to that of science and empirical knowledge. It is impossible to find instances in the 1830s in which theological imperatives clearly impaired the autonomy of medical thought. Both ministers and physicians accepted the emotional relevance of both reference areas – hence the ingenuity with which clergymen explained the moral lessons of cholera in terms of physiological mechanisms, while the physician with equal facility expressed in his etiological theory the accepted moral teachings of his generation. That cholera had been sent by the Lord in punishment of sins individual and collective did not imply the impossibility, the impiety, or even the undesirability of attempting to explain and prevent the disease.[8] Indeed both theologians and physicians agreed that it was man's duty to employ God's temporal means to preserve human life; prayer could not be expected to prevail if man did not alter the second causes through which cholera acted. No amount of prayer would clean filthy streets and tene-ments. One could not expect miracles in the nineteenth century. Growing secularism paralleled scientific progress and by the 1860s, the theological and moralistic explanations of the disease so prominent in the 1830s had, with increasing medical knowledge, become a clearly marginal theme.

The relative autonomy of medical and scientific values characterized a community of medical thought and practice in some ways surprisingly mature. In pathology, in therapeutics, even in public health practice,

8 Rosenberg, *Cholera Years*, pp. 40–54, 121–132, and *passim*. Though the preceding reference is based on American sources, subsequent research has indicated that these conclusions hold true, on the whole, for England and the Continent.

intimations of cholera's ultimate conquest were already apparent in the early 1830s. More enlightened physicians in Europe and North America had already come to accept pathological anatomy as a necessity in the understanding and defining of disease entities. (And, indeed, the first general acceptance in medical circles of the idea that diseases were specific, discrete entities is connected with this period and this approach.) As soon as cholera reached Russia and as it moved West, pathologists began to study the physical changes which it wrought in its victims. A number of physicians, for example, made detailed examinations of the stomach and intestinal linings and contents of cholera victims. Such studies, of course, could not prevent the disease, nor were they pursued by more than a small minority of physicians. Yet one cannot deny the sophistication of a community which produced such patient studies and had nurtured a flourishing clinical school, one which emphasized the correlation of disease symptoms in life with pathological findings after death.

Let me suggest another, and I think particularly striking, illustration of the relative maturity of Western medicine in the 1830s. It is an episode, moreover, which suggests the relationship already subsisting between scientific progress and change in medical practice, and as well the willingness of at least some members of the medical profession to innovate and experiment with any technique promising socially meaningful results. When cholera first appeared in Europe, a centuries-old tradition had already created an interest in pathological changes in the blood of the sick; in the early nineteenth century, this traditional interest in humoral pathology had been given a new impetus and content by the application of knowledge originating in experimental chemistry. It was inevitable that a number of physicians, attracted by the alluring certainties of the new chemistry, would study the chemical and physical changes in the blood of cholera victims. It was soon announced that the blood of patients succumbing to cholera exhibited drastic physical and chemical changes. The proportion of serum to solids was clearly reduced, while the acidity of the blood seemed to have altered as well. (Though there was disagreement among the several investigators publishing on the subject as to the precise nature of these chemical alterations.) All the symptoms of cholera, the argument followed, proceeded from these hematological changes and, logically enough, it was concluded that patients might be cured by injecting saline solutions into their veins and thus restoring the blood to its proper chemical and physical makeup.[9] And indeed this technique was experi-

9 There is no detailed modern study of this incident. For useful summaries, however, see Pollitzer, *Cholera*, pp. 611–615; A. B. Garrod, *On the Pathological Condition of the Blood in Cholera* (London: Richards, 1849), pp. 2–11, 29. Garrod's summary is particularly useful as it embodies the author's already more critical view of the

mented with relatively widely by physicians willing to look anywhere for help in treating cholera – or at least to any source bearing the imprimatur of science.[10] These pathological conclusions and the therapeutic measures deduced from them did not actually succeed in curing patients; the technique was neither sterile nor otherwise appropriate and was tried only on patients *in extremis*.

This episode demonstrates the conjunction of a number of developments. One was the manner in which science had already begun to become part of medicine – and to some physicians at least an indispensable part – and how in a crisis situation, at least some physicians turned naturally to investigation and to experimentation. Another novel reality was the ease with which information was diffused within the European medical community – including its provincial outposts in the Western Hemisphere. Within the space of less than a year, experiments with saline injection were tried from Russia in the East to North America in the West. Even though the international community of medicine was limited to the better educated, more critical, often urban physicians, its presence and integrity cannot be denied. One might well argue on the basis of such instances that a scientific and technological "takeoff" stage had already been attained by the early 1830s. Certainly it would seem to indicate a stage which non-Western countries have been unable or unwilling to reach without an input of intellectual and economic capital from without their own society. Hence the difference between cholera – or malaria – in India and in the West. Means were clearly evolving within Western society which would ultimately limit such ills, while nations not participating in the West's economic, technological, scientific, institutional, and attitudinal development have not organically developed within their own societies the means to banish these pestilences.

The manner in which cholera dramatized and justified existing demands for public health and municipal reform could only have taken place in a

rough-and-ready methods and conclusions of the medical chemists of the 1830s. The English discussion of saline injection and its rationale may be followed in the London *Lancet* and *London Medical Gazette* for 1832; for parallel work done in Russia, see R. Hermann, *Analyses chimiques: contenant l'exposé des alterations qui subissent le sang et les sécrétions du corps humain pendant le cholera* (Moscou, 1832).

10 For an enlightening contrast between the appeal which novelty, if clothed in the prestige and style of science, makes to the Western mind, and the place of supernatural values in the mind of a Chinese village during a cholera epidemic, see Francis L. K. Hsu, *Religion, Science and Human Crises* (London: Routledge & Kegan Paul, 1952). Equally relevant to the same consideration is the somewhat undignified struggle for priority in the discovery and popularization of this new mode of therapy. See, for example, Thomas Craigie, *Statement of Facts with Observations* (Edinburgh, 1832). It is important to remember that many physicians were already quite conscious of their place in an international structure of knowledge and status.

society in which the possibility of meliorism seemed plausible and the attempt to achieve it was an imperative in at least some minds. Obviously a complex set of attitudes and influences conditioned European and American responses to cholera: humanitarianism, evangelical religion, utilitarianism, and so forth. Central to all, however, was a faith in means and in the assumption that a mixture of social organization and scientific inquiry would inevitably provide a means of vanquishing cholera.

It is these attitudes which are significant, though the specific medical theories which justified public health measures were in detail wrong. The idea, for example, that the availability of an adequate supply of pure water might prevent cholera is one which we find it natural to accept. Public-spirited physicians and reformers in the 1830s generally supported the idea that water was necessary primarily to keep the streets clean and thus prevent the accumulation of miasma-breeding filth. (Almost all physicians at the time assumed that the presence in the atmosphere of deleterious miasmatic substances played an essential role in the causation of the disease, either by debilitating the individual or by acting as a specific causative factor.) Water should be not only abundant, but pure, not because some "virus" might be spread through it, but because the consumption of contaminated water would weaken the body's natural power of resistance and thus predispose it to disease. The important thing is not the accuracy or inaccuracy of the particular formulation, but the concern for environmental factors which these ideas implied and as well the parallel conviction that something should – if something could – be done to change living conditions which seemed to breed cholera as well as other infectious ills.

Most dramatically, an explanation of cholera was made available in mid-nineteenth century, an explanation which not only provided some under-standing of the etiology of the disease, but implied as well the creation of effective preventive measures. John Snow, a London physician, suggested as early as 1849 that cholera was a contagious disease caused by a poison reproducing itself in the bodies of its victims. The poison was to be found in the excreta and vomitus of cholera patients and, according to Snow, it was these substances that spread the disease, most frequently through a contaminated water supply.

From the point of view of this discussion, we must consider Snow's argument as an artifact peculiar to the generation which produced it. Like other cultural artifacts, it incorporated diverse yet characteristic elements.[11]

11 William Farr, another pioneer English epidemiologist, came to very similar conclusions at almost the same time. For the sake of convenience, however, I shall refer in succeeding passages to these new ideas as Snow's, though he was not alone in holding them. Snow's major publications have been reprinted by the Commonwealth Fund,

Even a generation previously, Snow's reasoning would have been improbable, if not impossible. His argument subsumed advances in chemistry, in pathology, in technology, and in public health practice. Snow's first logical step was the assumption, based on certain pathological findings of the first epidemic, that changes in the stomach and intestines indicated that the alimentary canal was the true seat of the disease and that changes in the blood and other organs were epiphenomenal in nature. Thus it seemed likely, Snow submitted, that the disease-causing substance was taken into the body by way of the mouth – and considering contemporary personal and public hygiene it was not difficult to suggest the channels by which this substance might find its way from one alimentary tract to the next. Nor did the ability of this hypothetical substance to reproduce itself (or to induce continuous molecular change, as Snow put it) seem unlikely. The fermentation controversy had been raging for several generations and in Snow's day the issue was an urgent one. But whether one accepted the biological or the chemical explanation of fermentation, it required little imagination to find in the process itself an analogy by means of which epidemic disease might be explained. It required, that is, little imagination to visualize a disease-causing microscopic substance which might act as a ferment, reproducing itself continuously and in doing so bringing about changes in the surrounding medium. Scientific experience with inoculation and vaccination had also shown the ability of minute quantities of morbid material to reproduce themselves in the human body and thus cause disease. (Similar conclusions followed from experiments in the transmission of syphilis.)[12] It had, moreover, been shown conclusively by the 1840s that fungi could cause disease in man, in plants, and in insects. It was only to be expected that simultaneously with Snow's early publications on cholera, other investigators were announcing that they had found microscopic fungi in the excreta of cholera patients, fungi which they argued were the cause of the disease.[13]

Snow's epidemiological reasoning is equally revealing. His original pamphlet, published in 1849, caused no immediate stir. It was one among

---

with an introduction by Wade Hampton Frost: *Snow on Cholera* (New York: The Commonwealth Fund, 1936). The best brief discussion of Snow's work, though perhaps overly antiheroic, is P. E. Brown, "John Snow – The Autumn Loiterer," *Bulletin of the History of Medicine* 25 (1961): 519–528.

12 *Snow on Cholera*, pp. 156–157.

13 These investigators were, not surprisingly, wrong in their identification of particular fungi. But their interest is symbolic of a steadily increasing interest in the study of microscopic phenomenal. A recent reviewer, for example, accepts the claims of at least four different investigators to have actually seen the cholera vibrio by 1867 – that is, sixteen years before Koch's discovery. S. N. De, *Cholera: Its Pathology and Pathogenesis* (Edinburgh: Oliver & Boyd, 1961), pp. 14–15.

dozens of hopeful theories published at the time. Anyone could, and many did, compose a fanciful etiology of cholera; the problem was to prove it. Snow, unlike the others, did. Most striking is his demonstration that cholera was spread through a contaminated well by tracing individual cases to use of water from the suspected pump. Equally striking is Snow's use of the Registrar-General's records to show a difference in the cholera case rate between customers of one London water company that drew its water from the Thames above the point at which it would be contaminated with London sewage and another company that drew its supply from below that point.[14]

Just as Snow's ability to posit an appropriate etiological agent was a product of changes both scientific and technological, so equally was his epidemiological reasoning a product of the multiple aspects of change which had taken place in the first half of the nineteenth century. Indeed both water companies and the Registrar-General's office itself were created in this period. It would be hard to imagine a mid-eighteenth-century student of epidemic disease determining individual cases and then plotting them on street maps. By the mid-nineteenth century, Snow was only one among a number of physicians who carefully mapped individual cholera cases in recording and analyzing the history of local epidemics.[15] Snow's attitudes were, in general, characteristics of the scientism and utilitarianism which he shared with so many of the scientific leaders of his generation. Rationalistic and "imponderable" considerations he simply dismissed. The problem of predisposition to disease, a concern of physicians since Hippocrates, he casually rejected as a hypothesis required

14 Snow found that, despite the help of the Registrar-General's Office, it was in many cases difficult to discover which of the two companies had serviced particular houses. Significantly, Snow also tested the actual water with a silver nitrate solution, finding that the sewage-polluted water of the Southwark & Vauxhall Company had a much higher sodium chloride content than that of the Lambeth Company's water. *Snow on Cholera*, pp. 77–78.

15 E. W. Gilbert ("Pioneer Maps of Health and Disease in England," *Geographical Journal* 124 [1958]: 172–183) has emphasized the role of cholera in first stimulating the application of cartography to problems of epidemiology. For examples of such mapping by contemporaries, see Henry Acland, *Memoir on the Cholera at Oxford in the Year 1854, with considerations suggested by the epidemic* (London, 1856), and Thomas Shapter, *The History of the Cholera in Exeter* (London and Exeter, 1849). It should be noted, however, that mapping cases did not guarantee one's accepting some theory of infection or contagion. The often erratic pattern of distribution of cholera cases frequently seemed to preclude contagion. Lloyd G. Stevenson has argued that the first use of spot maps came in the discussion of yellow fever in the 1790s and in the first decades of the nineteenth century; see his "Putting Disease on the Map: The Early Use of Spot Maps in the Study of Yellow Fever," *Journal of the History of Medicine* 20 (1965): 226–261. It seems clear, however, that the first *general* use of such maps came in the study of cholera; certainly their widespread use by mid-nineteenth century would indicate an increasingly pervasive empiricism.

by ignorance alone. ("The alleged predisposition," Snow caustically remarked, "was nothing visible or evident: like the elephant, which supports the world, according to Hindoo mythology, it was merely invented to remove a difficulty." The difficulty, of course, being the immunity of some to epidemic influences supposedly in the atmosphere though all were equally immersed in this same atmosphere.)[16]

If Snow's reductionism has a narrow and perhaps even ruthless tinge, it is a characteristically modern ruthlessness. Cholera could not have been understood in 1832. Yet the conditions that nurtured and spread cholera already did exist. An urban and industrial society had come into being, a society with comparatively rapid and frequent modes of transportation; for a brief period cholera could thrive in this material culture, but only for the relatively short period during which the same processes of change which created this material culture produced as well the medical and administrative advances which would inevitably banish the disease.

Needless to say, Snow's ideas and those of his like-thinking colleagues did not meet with immediate and universal approval.[17] But by the mid-1860s, when cholera next appeared in Western Europe, his studies of the mid-1850s had already won many converts. In the 1860s sporadically and in the 1870s more generally public health authorities were putting into execution the admonitions of medical spokesmen who felt with Snow that the disease was spread from person to person by some microscopic living organism.[18] (This, of course, was before Koch's discovery of the cholera vibrio in 1883.) After the 1870s, Western Europe and North America were spared widespread and devastating epidemics of the kind which had been so destructive earlier in the century.

To apply Snow's prophylactic conclusions, moreover, changes would have to be made in the evolving pattern of municipal government. (And, of course, as an instance of feedback, the existence of these new medical concepts and the necessity of implementing them provided at once occa-

---

16 *Snow on Cholera*, p. 159. Compare Snow's equally casual dismissal of the problem of vitalism, *Snow on Cholera*, p. 146.

17 For a discussion of the reaction to Snow's ideas, see Rosenberg, *Cholera Years*, pp. 196–200. Particularly striking was the example of John Simon, the great organizer of English public health; despite what would seem to be Snow's detailed and overwhelmingly elaborate proof of his contention that cholera was essentially a waterborne disease, Simon himself could, in the 1850s, consider contaminated water to be only one among several possible causes of the disease. Royston Lambert, *Sir John Simon 1816–1904 and English Social Administration* (London: Macgibbon & Kee, 1963), pp. 247–249.

18 Particularly illuminating is the United States Government's report on *The Cholera Epidemic of 1873 in the United States*; this report shows in exhaustive detail the general acceptance of these new ideas even in small, semirural communities (Executive Doc. No. 95, 43d Cong., 2d sess. [Washington, D.C.: Government Printing Office, 1875]).

sion and justification for such increases in municipal power.) Let us outline
in this connection another and final illustrative example. The United States
in 1866 was in terms of world science at best provincial, and in terms of
municipal administration chaotic. In 1866, however, public-spirited New
Yorkers made the threat of cholera an occasion for successful agitation for
the creation of a board of health with powers appropriate to its task.[19] And,
as the New York medical profession generally accepted Snow's conclusions, it was these newer ideas which defined the appropriateness of the
board's powers. Means of disinfection had to be provided if clothing and
infection, for example, were central. Even before the first case of cholera in
New York, the city's new board of health procured a building for the
storage of chemicals to be used in disinfection of the excreta and personal
effects of cholera victims. A number of wagons were purchased; and these,
together with a sufficient complement of horses, were kept in a stable close
by. Also quartered nearby and in constant readiness were details of men
especially trained in the use of disinfectants. When the first cases appeared,
each was reported to the closest police precinct station. The victim's
address was immediately telegraphed to the board's central office, which
quickly dispatched a wagonload of disinfectants to the infected premises.
Within an hour of the report's having been received, a team of well-trained
men would be at work disinfecting the clothing, house, and effects of the
victim.

This particular example need not be pursued in detail; its meaning
seems clear enough. The chemicals, the telegraph, the efficiency and care
of organization were, like Snow's ideas themselves, characteristic products
of the material development of Western society. If, in 1831, when cholera
first appeared in the West, we could discern the formative elements in the
development of modern technological society – the close relation between
science pure and science applied as seen in medicine, the autonomy of
scientific and economic motives, the faith in meliorism, and the assumption
of the necessity and meaningfulness of human actions – we can see by the
1860s a far more mature stage in the development of this society. In each
case, however, epidemics of cholera provide a cross-sectional phenomenon
in terms of which the structural relationships among these aspects of
change may be studied.

19 The most detailed account of the Metropolitan Board of Health's fight against cholera
in 1866 is to be found in its first annual report (*New York State, Annual Report of the
Metropolitan Board of Health, 1866* [New York, 1867]).

PART II

Institutions and medical care

7

The practice of medicine in New York a century ago

&~ This essay with its breezy title was in fact originally conceived of as an after-dinner talk – an accessible chat intended for a banquet meeting of the Society of Alumni of Bellevue Hospital. I had casually agreed to speak on medicine in New York City a century ago; it seemed like an appropriate theme for a group of nostalgic black-tie-clad physicians. But as I actually began to collect material to document the talk, I realized how very little I knew about "medicine a century ago." Or to phrase it somewhat differently, I began to realize how little the existing scholarly literature addressed the history of medicine in terms of care, how small a proportion of it had been devoted to the medical profession as practitioners in an everyday world of sickrooms and unpaid bills, of competition for status and hospital appointments as well as patients. My preliminary research revealed the inadequacy of thinking of the profession in monolithic terms; there were clearly many professions, not just one, and many kinds of physicians, not just the elite and the innovative. While attempting to expose a cross section of medicine during one arbitrarily chosen year, I discovered a variety of surprising interconnections between intellectual, ethical, institutional, and economic factors in an already complex world of urban medicine. The very arbitrariness of my task dictated an approach rather different from the accepted canon of problems, data, and subject matter in the history of medicine. I was influenced a great deal by this exercise in reconstructing medicine in a particular time and place, as will be apparent in subsequent chapters. ~&

I

According to the census of 1865, New York City and County had a population of 723,587. Well over 90 percent lived on Manhattan Island's southern half. The northern half of Manhattan Island, in a day before really convenient public transportation, was for all practical purposes empty and served indeed as a summer resort into the 1880s. South of these hills and meadows, New Yorkers lived in conditions more cramped than those of any other American city. New York, a contemporary estimated, was ten times as crowded as Philadelphia. A housing census taken late in 1865 reported 15,357 tenements containing 501,327 persons – over two-thirds of the city's population.[1] New York was as crowded as any city in the Western world.

A congested, jerry-built city, New York was notoriously unhealthy. It had the highest death rate (one in thirty-five) of any major American city, a rate higher than that of either Paris or London. Whereas one child in six born in London died before its first birthday, one in five New York infants died before reaching this milestone. Indeed, in the half-century since 1810 when the first more or less accurate statistics were published, New York's death rate had increased steadily. Sewage and sanitation arrangements were primitive. Fewer than half the city's inhabitants lived in houses or apartments containing bathing facilities; summer and the rivers provided the poor with their only opportunity to wash thoroughly.[2] Accidents were common, and the large amount of outdoor work in the city's streets and on its piers meant exposure to cold in winter, heat and sun in summer.

Food supplies reached the city's markets in poor condition, a trial even to prosperous New Yorkers, and a good portion of New York's tenement population suffered from chronic if marginal malnutrition as well. "These decaying animal and vegetable remains," one physician wrote of the food purchased by the poor, "are daily entombed in the protuberant stomachs of thousands of children, whose pallid, expressionless faces and shrunken limbs are the familiar attributes of childhood in these localities."[3] Far more

1 For tenement house statistics, see New York *Evening Post*, January 6, 1866, which reprints the annual report of the Board of Police Surgeons. For other statistics, see New York State, *Annual Report of the Metropolitan Board of Health, 1866* (New York, 1867), Appendix C, pp. 61, 97, 102. The best general survey of tenement house conditions is to be found in the *Report of the Council of Hygiene and Public Health of the Citizens' Association of New York upon the Sanitary Condition of the City* (New York, 1865). The manuscript copy-books kept by the Council of Hygiene's district physicians, upon which this published report is based, are deposited in the manuscript division of the New-York Historical Society; they contain somewhat more detail than is available in the published version. Until the end of the nineteenth century the northern reaches of Manhattan Island were regarded as dangerously malarious. Simon Baruch, "Malaria as an etiological factor in New York City," *Medical Record* 24 (1883): 505–509. This investigation was supported by U.S. Public Health Service Research Grant LM-00013-02.

2 L. Emmett Holt, "Infant Mortality and Its Reduction, Especially in New York City," *Journal of the American Medical Association* 54 (1910): 682–690; W. F. Thoms, "Health in Country and Cities. Illustrated by tables of the death-rates, sickness-rates, etc...," *Trans. A.M.A.* 17 (1866): 431–434, esp. p. 422; *Annual Report of Metrop. Bd. of Health*, p. 65. On inadequate bathing facilities in the city, see *Annual Report of Metrop. Bd. of Health*, p. 157, and Robert Ernst, *Immigrant Life in New York City, 1825–1863* (New York: King's Crown Press, 1959), p. 51.

3 Ezra R. Pullen, *Citizens' Association Report*, 1865, p. 59. Much descriptive material on the markets is to be found in the work of Thomas F. DeVoe, *The Market Assistant*

than in the twentieth century, New York's physicians were faced with acute infectious diseases, with cases demanding frequent visits, anxiety, and intimate personal contact.

It is hardly surprising then that medical men placed so great an emphasis upon the peculiarity of city practice. Not only the poor, but New Yorkers generally were exposed to dirt and overcrowding. Though the poor were particularly debilitated by inadequate food and poor ventilation, the city, contemporary physicians believed, held dangers almost as great for the well-to-do. The idle wealthy and especially women of this class suffered, doctors assumed, from lack of exercise coupled with improper diet and clothing. "Among the American ladies brought up in our dark parlours and rooms," one health enthusiast wrote, "crooked spines, decaying teeth, a pale sickly color of the skin, flabby muscles, weak digestion, tender spines and irritable nerves, are the rule."[4] Businessmen too suffered from improper diet and lack of exercise – both exacerbated by the anxieties of trade. Logically enough, textbooks of medicine and materia medica warned that city dwellers could not tolerate dosages in strengths necessary for the hardy country dweller. Milder, less heroic measures were appropriate for city folk.

If there were doubts in 1866 as to the healthfulness of city life, there could be none as to the vigor of the city's growth. New York's medical community was equally vigorous – or at least numerous. With practically no control of licensing, with even the best medical schools enforcing relatively lenient requirements, the number of physicians in proportion to the population was high and their competition for the available, paying clientele correspondingly intense. The *Medical Register for the City of New York for 1866* listed 806 regular practitioners, while the Homeopathic Medical Society counted some seventy active members.[5] One must, moreover, include a good number of irregulars in order to arrive at the total number of practitioners. It would probably be a safe guess that about 1,500 New Yorkers treated the sick in some manner, a ratio of one physician to roughly 500 inhabitants.

Much of the treatment of sickness was not overseen by men calling themselves physicians. Midwives and "old ladies" (the latter a term favored by medical contemporaries in describing all laypersons who routinely pro-

(New York, 1867) and *The Market Book, Containing a Historical Account of the Public Markets in the Cities of New York,* ... (New York, 1862).

4 John Ellis, *Suggestions to Young Men, on the Subject of Marriage and Hints to Young Ladies, and to Husbands and Wives* (New York, 1866), p. 9.

5 *The Medical Register of the City of New York for the Year Commencing June 1, 1866,* Guido Furman, ed. (New York, 1866), pp. 217–243; *Trans. Homoeopathic M. Soc. State of New York,* 1866, pp. 268–270.

vided advice and simple remedies to family and neighbors) provided a good deal of informal practice. It is apparent as well from the number and generous claims of patent medicine manufacturers that these remedies with, as many physicians complained, the advice of a none-too-scrupulous breed of pharmacist, provided the first line of medical attention for many New Yorkers regardless of social class. Patients too casually refilled prescriptions if they thought them appropriate for what seemed to be a recurrence of the illness for which they had originally been prescribed.[6] Such casual self-prescribing was estimated by contemporaries to be the source of a majority of all prescriptions compounded.

Even assuming that we limit our discussion to medicine as practiced by persons calling and thinking of themselves as physicians and earning their livelihood exclusively by treating the sick, we will see that the situation was by no means a simple one. Ideological and ethical differences, in the absence of any governmental control, created a number of subcommunities within the medical world. Most confusing was the duplication of professional organization and function between homeopathic and regular physicians, groups in some ways more similar than either would have admitted. But similarities in attitude toward education and ethics could not modify the peculiar therapeutic doctrines which kept homeopaths apart from the main camp of regular practitioners.[7] In addition to these groups, there were many other healers in the city, some practicing without benefit of diploma or medical education of even the most perfunctory sort. A flourishing group of "pox doctors," for example, specialized in venereal disease, sterility, and sexual problems generally.[8] There were herb doctors

6 See, e.g., John H. Griscom's casual reprinting of a letter in which a patient reported giving several friends similarly afflicted "the apothecaries No. of your prescription." "Essay on the therapeutic value of certain articles in the materia medica," *Trans. Med. Soc. State of New York*, 1868, p. 10.

7 Attitudes assumed by the leaders of the homeopathic medical community toward matters such as ethics, educational reform, and specialization were remarkably similar to those of regular medical men. This partially accounts, I think, for the longevity of homeopathy and the eventual assimilation of its remnants by regular medicine in this century.

8 Prostitution, the prevalence of venereal disease, and social condemnation of the sexual license such ailments implied conspired to make these specialists in "secret diseases" both popular and successful. Modesty and fear made many patients suffering with other sexual problems also unwilling to turn to their family physician. The ads of these specialists in matters sexual were everywhere in New York newspapers a century ago. The more popular hired assistants and published books advertising their services and providing information and advice on sexual problems. A few of these treatises – all going through a number of editions – were: Edward B. Foote, *Medical Common Sense; Applied to the Causes, Prevention and Cure of Chronic Diseases and Unhappiness in Marriage* (New York, 1864); Frederick Hollick, *A Popular Treatise on Venereal Disease...* (New York, c. 1852); L. J. Kahn, *Nervous Exhaustion: Its Cause and Cure...with Practical Information on Marriage, its Obligations and Impediments...* (New York, c. 1870). Such

and "electricians," specialists in cancer and lung complaints. Such practitioners, though certainly active, are difficult to trace and were in a real sense outside the medical profession – allied perhaps in performing the same function but alien in values. One can, I think, without danger of distortion, simply acknowledge these irregulars' existence and devote the rest of these remarks to the better-educated, "regular" practitioners of medicine.

Though not as intricately organized as in the mid-twentieth century, New York's physicians a century ago had already begun to show signs of differentiation. Both knowledge and status were distributed unevenly among New York's medical men. Institutional power especially was concentrated in comparatively few hands.

This can be easily demonstrated. The Medical and Surgical Society of New York, limited in membership to thirty-four, was the most exclusive of the city's informal medical associations.[9] In 1866 seventeen of the Society's members held teaching positions in the city's three regular medical schools. Even more significant was the dominance of Society men in hospital appointments. They held collectively ninety-seven consulting and attending appointments at the city's hospitals and dispensaries, roughly half the total number available. Members of the Society were also active in the councils of the New York Academy of Medicine – though conspicuously inactive in the County Medical Society. Gurdon Buck, for example, held eight hospital appointments and served as vice-president of the New York Medical Journal Association and of the Alumni Association of the College of Physicians and Surgeons, as trustee of the College of Physicians, and as a member of the Academy of Medicine's Committee on Medical Education. Willard Parker enjoyed ten hospital appointments as well as being active in the Metropolitan Board of Health and serving as Professor of Practice at the College of Physicians. Only six members held no hospital appointments. One of these, however, Robert Watt, was Professor of Anatomy at the College of Physicians, and two, C. R. Agnew and Fessenden

books ordinarily offered advice by mail, Dr. Kahn even urging patients to send samples of their urine by express for "microscopic examination." Regular physicians always charged extraordinarily high fees in cases of venereal disease and, contrary to their usual practice, demanded advance payment. George Rosen, *Fees and Fee Bills* (Baltimore: Johns Hopkins University Press, 1946), pp. 21, 44, 59; D. W. Cathell, *The Physician Himself* (Baltimore, 1882), pp. 71, 186. Cathell's remarkably revealing and popular book provides, to my knowledge, the most vivid single picture available of American medical practice in the late nineteenth century. I have relied more upon it than any other single work in my general description of medical practice.

9 *Medical Register, 1866*, pp. 54–56, provides a list of the members of the Medical and Surgical Society. Data on appointments and positions were gathered either from the rosters published in the *Medical Register* or from the annual report of the appropriate institution. For a history of the Society, see Philip Van Ingen's *A Brief Account of the First One Hundred Years of the New York Medical and Surgical Society* (n.p., 1946).

Otis, offered specialty clinics at the same medical school; two others, W. M. Blakeman and John G. Adams, were influential in the affairs of the Academy of Medicine. These were in the idiom of the time "the hospital men," the social and institutional leaders of the profession. And the dominance of these professors and attending physicians was clearly understood and resented, especially the favoritism which seemed to rule hospital appointments.[10]

The Medical and Surgical Society was, of course, only one among a number of medical societies, all representing status and knowledge in some proportion. The New York Academy of Medicine, for example, with its membership of 273, probably included almost all of the city's well-trained and financially secure physicians. Those with scientific pretensions belonged to the New York Pathological Society and, very likely, the Medical Journal Society as well. There were, of course, other roads to status and success outside the exclusive confines of the Medical and Surgical Society's membership. No immigrants, for example, were members of this establishment organization, yet a number of the city's leading medical scholars were Europeans, men like Abraham Jacobi and Ernst Krackowizer. These émigré physicians were highly respected for their specialized skills, active in the Society of German Physicians, and prominent in the affairs of New York's sizable German community. Within New York's specialty societies as well, knowledge and ability provided avenues to leadership and recognition.

I do not mean to imply that social and intellectual status were unrelated. For the opposite, of course, is true. Twenty-two of the Medical and Surgical Society's thirty-four members – to return to our example – could be classified as specialists. Among them were some of the country's leading teachers of medicine, men like Austin Flint and Alonzo Clark. Clearly, however, intellectual and institutional leadership, while overlapping, were hardly coincidental – a fact which J. Marion Sims discovered abruptly some years earlier when he received a cold reception from the leaders of New York's medical establishment.[11] Among physicians in ordinary practice, of

10 [George F. Shrady], "Medical appointments," *Medical Record* 1 (1866): 477–478; E. P., "Hospital appointments," *Medical Record* 1 (1866): 459; Stephen Smith, *Doctor in Medicine: And other Papers on Professional Subjects* (New York, 1872), pp. 247–250.

11 J. Marion Sims, *The Story of My Life*, ed. H. Marion-Sims (New York, 1894), pp. 269, 295; Thomas Addis Emmett, "Reminiscences of the Founders of Woman's Hospital Association," *New York J. Gynec. & Obst.* 3 (1893): 366. Of the seven prominent physicians mentioned specifically by Emmett as having opposed Sims, four (Willard Parker, Gurdon Buck, William Van Buren, and Alfred Post) were leading members of the Medical and Surgical Society. And the influence of the Society was, of course, a continuing one. When Edward Trudeau competed in the early 1870s for a position on the house staff of the newly opened Stranger's Hospital, he was quizzed by

course, the drop in knowledge was immense. Much of ordinary practice was undoubtedly bad, even when judged by the flexible standards of the day. Knowledge trickled slowly down to the majority of practitioners. A Boston physician, for example, quoted approvingly a pathologist friend's cynical opinion that "if what is really *known* of the laws of disease were told to the members of the profession, more than half of them would indignantly discredit it."[12]

With so many doctors, competition was correspondingly intense, and although the rewards of success could be great, an established physician's income was probably somewhere in the vicinity of $1,500 to $2,000 a year. Valentine Mott, New York's most eminent surgeon of the previous generation, died late in 1865 and left an estate of almost a million dollars. But physicians beginning practice in the 1860s probably averaged close to $400 a year, a bit less than the $416 paid resident physicians at Bellevue and Charity Hospitals. The salary of the sanitary superintendent of the Metropolitan Board of Health was set at $4,000 a year, that of police surgeons at $2,250. These were adequate but not munificent salaries in an economy still affected by the inflation of the Civil War.[13]

II

There were, essentially, two kinds of medical practice in New York a century ago, charity and pay. The ideal practice, however, was one performed by a regular practitioner in the middle-class home – in contemporary terms, a "family practice." An office clientele was, at least in theory, considered something quite distinct and indeed a vaguely marginal kind of endeavor, one in which a hard-working physician might make useful

the entire visiting staff, all four of whom (H. B. Sands, W. H. Draper, T. Gaillard Thomas, and Fessenden Otis) were members of the Society. Trudeau, *An Autobiography* (Garden City, N.Y.: Doubleday, Doran, 1930), pp. 59–62.

12 Quoted, apparently, as having been said in 1865. Benjamin Cotting, *Medical Addresses* (Boston, 1875), p. 109n. Dr. A. K. Gardner, a well-known New York obstetrician, described, for example, in the summer of 1866 the tribulations of a female patient, delivered of two successive children by two different but equally "stupid" physicians whose ignorance verged on malpractice. New York Academy of Medicine, Rare Book Room, Section on Diseases of Women and Children, "Minutes," Entry for June 18, 1866, p. 307.

13 S. D. Gross, *Memoir of Valentine Mott, M.D., LL.D.* (Philadelphia, 1868), pp. 87–88. The salary of Bellevue house-staff members is noted in: New York City, Commissioners of Charity and Correction *7th Ann. Rep.*, 1866, p. 19. *Medical Record* 1 (1866): 120 reported the Police Surgeon's salary and the *Annual Report of the Metropolitan Board of Health, 1866*, p. 62, the Sanitary Superintendent's salary. The estimate of a beginning practitioner's income was made by A. D. Rockwell, who began practice in New York City in 1866. *Rambling Recollections* (New York, 1920), p. 181.

contacts and acquire some much-needed cash. (An office practice, as opposed to a family practice, was usually conducted on a cash basis.) It was not, however, considered to be the basis of a completely sound "business."[14]

A family practice was that in a very real sense. The physician attended father and mother, children, even servants. (It must be remembered that the presence of servants in a respectable household a century ago was considered as much a necessity as a refrigerator today; when a servant lived in, it was assumed that medical care would be his or her employer's responsibility.) Bills were commonly sent on an annual basis, perhaps semiannually by the more efficient. As we have noted, this family practice was middle-class. A casual glance at any textbook of children's diseases in this period makes this clear – its discussion, for example, of the proper means of choosing a wet-nurse, or its assumption that nursery maids were in many if not most cases the proper repository for directions in infant care.

A comparative superfluity of physicians in the still-compact city helped maintain the visit as the basic unit of the physician's work day; the doctor's slate was still standard office equipment. One visited nice persons in their homes; they did not ordinarily come to one's office. It was considered, indeed, a matter of good planning to visit frequently enough to oversee the progress of a case, but not so frequently as to give the impression that one was padding the bill. Respectable persons did not ordinarily enter hospitals for treatment; nor did the truly upright allow their servants to be sent to one. Thus, what is today the physician's hospital practice was, a hundred years ago, the heart of his daily round of visits – and this in a generation during which acute and protracted infectious diseases were still common. Physicians charged a special fee for overnight visits and expected to be awakened from their sleep to make calls. At the same time it was considered quite normal for a physician to visit homes for relatively minor complaints, to vaccinate, for example, and in theory even to advise on matters such as the location of a new house, proper plumbing, or an appropriate diet.

14 There are a number of indications that this "ideal" practice was, even in 1866, more accurate as a description of practice in small towns and rural areas than it was for a large city. Office practice, for example, in a city like New York with its shifting population and its many consultants, must have been more important than in rural areas. Even the most successful practitioners held generous daily office hours, usually in the morning or late afternoon, many three times, morning, afternoon, and evening. Most had office hours on Sunday as well. *The Medical Register for 1866*, pp. 217–243, provides the addresses and office hours of New York's regular practitioners. There was, of course, no such thing as a physician without a private practice or established office hours. Some of the more successful physicians seem, however, to have had younger graduate physicians associated with them in their office practice, whose task it was to screen incoming patients.

Theory explained and justified this pattern of practice. Etiological thought still emphasized the role of constitutional and environmental factors in the causation of disease. It followed logically that the best physician was the one most familiar with individual circumstances and constitutional patterns of reaction to illness. If a model practice was that in middle-class homes, an ideal practitioner was the experienced physician who had come to know a family through several generations, becoming familiar with its characteristic strengths and weaknesses, its peculiarities in regard to the action of medicines or to changes in regime. As Oliver Wendell Holmes put it:

> The young man knows his patient, but the old man also knows his patient's family, dead and alive, up and down for generations. He can tell beforehand what diseases their unborn children will be subject to, what they will die of if they live long enough, and whether they had better live at all, or remain unrealized possibilities.[15]

Both the regular and homeopathic codes of ethics reflected the acceptance of a paradigmatic family practice, one in which it was assumed a personal as well as professional relationship would subsist between patient and physician. Both codes, for example, urged patients not to dismiss a physician without some formal explanation. It was hoped that there would be no bitter feelings. Somewhat similar considerations underlay the codes' emphasis upon the formal etiquette of consultation. This was a situation which the unethical consultant might turn to his advantage, through casual slights and innuendoes discrediting the family physician and perhaps seducing away his patients. The emphasis of medical theory, however, upon the regular attendant's unique knowledge sanctioned the prominent role he was to play in the elaborately formalized ritual of consultation.[16]

15 Oliver Wendell Holmes, "The Young Practitioner," *Medical Essays* (Boston: Houghton Mifflin, 1911), p. 377. This passage is excerpted from an address originally given in March 1871 to the graduates of Bellevue Hospital Medical College. Some years later, S. Weir Mitchell pointed acidly to the clichéd faith bestowed upon the hallowed but often undeserving figure of the "family physician." *Doctor and Patient* (Philadelphia, 1889), pp. 28–29. In keeping with this emphasis was the insistence of insurance companies upon certificates from family physicians in addition to the reports of their own medical examiners in evaluating risks. A clear-headed medical man would, it was believed, even when treating acute symptoms, acquire an understanding "of the tendencies toward a particular form of death." J. Adams Allen, *Medical Examinations for Life Insurance*, 2d rev. ed. (Chicago, 1867), p. 50.

16 The A.M.A.'s 1847 Code of Ethics (Ch. I, Art. II, Par. 3), in discussing the duties of patients, urged that one particular physician be chosen, for a medical man acquainted with the "peculiarities of constitution, habits, and predispositions of those he attends is more likely to be more successful in his treatment, than one who does not possess that knowledge." See also Ch. I, Art. II, Par. 8, and American Institute of Homeopathy, *Code of Medical Ethics, Constitution, By-Laws, and List of Members . . .* (Boston, 1869), pp. 8, 10, 13.

This emphasis upon the ethics of consultation and the frequency of such occasions emphasizes another quality of the profession a century ago. I refer to its still essentially "horizontal," undifferentiated structure. Despite what has been said concerning the distribution of status within the profession, the organization of American medicine a century ago was still largely geographical and social, corresponding to the location and class of patients attended, only partially dependent upon education and institutional ties. Since almost all physicians did the same sort of things, consultants were ordinarily potential competitors. The general practitioner today sees, of course, little danger in referring cases demanding specialized knowledge to another physician; the functional differentiation of the profession within the past century has defined and thus limited the specialist's activities.[17] (And referral, of course, is infrequently an occasion for the formal consultation so common a century ago.) Medical theory too has changed and these intellectual developments have in some ways paralleled the structural changes within the organization of the profession. Decreasing emphasis – at least until the relatively recent past – on familial, diathetical, and environmental factors in etiological and therapeutic thought has removed much of the theoretical justification for personal interaction between the general practitioner and the specialist.

Without benefit of any generally convincing or specific etiology, medical attitudes toward disease causation a century ago were broadly inclusive. Practicing physicians cannot well afford the habitual luxury of confessing ignorance; models of disease causation were shifting schemes, equations in which the factors of heredity, habit, and environment could be judiciously balanced to explain either health or disease. Although heredity was emphasized, as we have seen in the words of Dr. Holmes, it provided only one given in the disease equation. And perhaps *given* is too strong a word, for heredity itself was a variable and constantly shifting attribute. "Hereditary tendency to disease," as one contemporary put it, "is one of the most certainly established facts in pathology; yet its operations and manifestations are most singular and uncertain." Heredity was not fixed, but could be altered by external influences at any point between conception and weaning. It was, for example, part of the physician's task to warn against emotional excitement during pregnancy, or other stress which might mark the child. Even during lactation, it was believed, maternal impressions might be transmitted to children. It was the physician's task, similarly, to warn against sexual intercourse while under the influence of alcohol or

---

17 Those processes, moreover, which have brought about this specialization have at the same time raised standards and limited access to the profession – thus tending to remove a basic component of economic competition in medicine.

drugs; even a momentary indiscretion of this kind might balefully affect the constitution of a child conceived under such unfavorable circumstances.[18] The open-ended quality of etiological thought provided abundant opportunity for medical men to articulate and justify the moral convictions of their contemporaries.

Though heredity was a potent cause of illness, such ills might never manifest themselves if the individual were protected from "cooperating" causes in the environment; for disease was considered the product ordinarily of an interaction between such environmental causes and hereditary attributes. "Herein," Austin Flint, probably New York's leading teacher of clinical medicine, wrote in 1866, "lies a truth of great practical importance." Diseases, he explained, "thus are preventable, notwithstanding a predisposition to them, insofar as they depend on the union of cooperating causes."[19] It was the task then, of the family physician to avert through wise counsel the dangers posed by hereditary predisposition. Within the shifting etiological world, the physician's theoretical responsibility was far broader than mere diagnosis, prognosis, and treatment.

The practicing physician had to understand not only variations in individual constitution; the physical environment too was fluid, climate and temperature constantly changing, constantly interacting with human strengths and weaknesses. The idea of "epidemic constitution" was still generally unquestioned. Fatal epidemic diseases were, for example, still assumed to be preceded by the prevalence of similar but less serious ills. (A cholera epidemic might thus be expected to follow the prevalence of nonspecific diarrheal complaints.) General patterns of disease incidence were as well affected by changes in climate; in certain seasons or localities bowel complaints, in others neurological disorders, might be peculiarly

18 The quotation is from John J. Elwell, *A Medico-Legal Treatise on Malpractice and Medical Evidence* . . . (New York, 1866), p. 40. As late as 1870, a critical physician noted acidly the prevalence of belief among the medical profession in the ability of maternal impressions to cause any degree of malformation. G. J. Fisher, "Does maternal mental influence have any constructive or destructive power in the production of malformations or monstrosities . . . ?," *Am. J. Insanity* 26 (1870): 241–295. See also Edward Seguin's *Idiocy: and its Treatment by the Physiological Method* (New York, 1866), pp. 41–42. New York specialist Augustus K. Gardner warned in a popular treatise on sex not only against sexual intercourse when intoxicated, but also with old men, and when grief-stricken, despondent, or irate. *Conjugal Sins against the Laws of Life and Health and their Effects upon the Father, Mother and Child*, rev. ed. (New York, 1874), pp. 174, 175, 194.

19 Austin Flint, *A Treatise on the Principles and Practice of Medicine* (Philadelphia, 1866), p. 95. Insurance companies at the time, however, unanimously urged medical examiners to be wary of applicants with a clouded hereditary background; tuberculosis was especially feared and its occurrence in near relatives was an automatic cause of refusal to insure. See also *Instructions to the Medical Examiners of the Mutual Insurance Company of New York* (New York, 1866), p. 19 and *passim*.

prevalent. The action of remedies was also modified by climactic changes. The Committee on Diseases of the Medical Society of the County of New York pointed out, for example, in the spring of 1866 that mercurials seemed to be losing their effectiveness, that it was increasingly difficult to salivate patients.[20] Thus, in prescribing, transitory climatic conditions as well as more permanent environmental factors had to be considered in conjunction with known constitutional differences, including those of sex, profession, temperament, and age. An educated and experienced regular physician, the argument inevitably followed, was the only one capable of understanding and evaluating this multiplicity of protean factors.

With such a kaleidoscope of etiological and therapeutic variables, it was only to be expected that general pathological designs were most popular with New York practitioners. Only in the most egregiously local lesions – those, for example, resulting from trauma – was there any general feeling that an exclusively local process might be involved.[21] From hysteria to carbuncles, all man's ills were made to fit a similarly open-ended pattern. Local affections exerted a general effect either through the blood or "reflex-action," while general influences might through the same agencies create local inflammations. In this scheme, of course, emotional and psychological influences played a significant role. Fear or anxiety, for example, might have so debilitating an effect on the nervous system or the blood's nutritional qualities as to cause physical or mental ills of the most varied sort.[22] Particularly striking was the manner in which the uterus in women and dentition in infants were presumed capable of inducing through these speculative mechanisms almost every conceivable patho-

20 M. Soc. County of New York, Committee on Diseases, "Minutes," Entry for meeting of June 4, 1866, Rare Book Room, New York Academy of Medicine. On the epidemic constitution, see Committee on Diseases, "Report of Committee on Diseases for Month ending April 2, 1866," p. 13, which describes the month as being marked by a tendency to neurological complaints. "Persons suffering with very different forms of sickness seem often to be afflicted alike in this respect."

21 John J. Elwell in a popular text on medical jurisprudence explained in such terms the difficulties encountered even by the surgeon in producing consistent results. "Where a surgeon undertakes to treat a fractured limb, he has not only to apply the known facts and theoretical knowledge of his science, but he must contend with very many powerful and hidden influences; such as want of vital force, habit of life, hereditary diathesis, climate, the mental state, local circumstances, and a thousand other agencies..." Elwell, *A Medico-Legal Treatise on Malpractice and Medical Evidence*, p. 23.

22 In 1866, blood disorders were particularly popular as pathological mechanisms with which to explain disease; well-nigh all infectious diseases, for example, were presumed by progressive physicians to be blood conditions, spread from person to person by a substance or agency capable of bringing about some alteration in the patient's blood. J. Lewis Smith could, for example, define diphtheria as a "blood disease, which, like measles or scarlet fever, has a local inflammatory manifestation." *A Treatise on the Diseases of Infancy and Childhood* (Philadelphia, 1869), pp. 439, 450.

logical condition. (The more critical had indeed already come to the defense of the uterus, making light of the blanket charges habitually leveled against this hapless organ.)[23] The point, of course, is that physicians cannot well fulfill their social function without offering some explanation of the ills they treat; in the absence of knowledge they necessarily adopted the most flexible of etiological and pathological designs – ones in which explanations of health and disease could readily be cast.

Thus far we have been sketching a rather schematic description of private practice and the medical theory which paralleled and in some ways justified it. To illustrate this pattern in concrete, individual terms is a difficult matter. Numberless memoirs and autobiographies describe medical careers in this period; almost all lack the immediacy and often the accuracy of the contemporary diary or letter. I have been able to locate only one detailed diary kept by a New York practitioner in 1866. The diarist was John Burke, a prosperous and responsible physician, a member of the Academy of Medicine, a founder of the East River Medical Association, but by no means a member of the city's medical elite.

Dr. Burke worked very hard. This was especially true during the summer of 1866, when he lost sixteen pounds.[24] On the evening of July 30, for example, he recorded having already made "28 outdoor visits besides prescribing for innumerable office patients, and I have some calls to make to night yet for it is now only 7 OC PM." His normal day, Dr. Burke noted on December 15, began when he rose soon after seven, saw his office patients, and then read his paper.

> If I have time, [he continued,] have breakfast so that I may leave the house by $8\frac{1}{2}$ OC I visit the lower part of town and get back to the house by $10\frac{1}{2}$ – I then visit patient [sic] between this and [illegible, but presumably a dispensary] by 12 or $12\frac{1}{2}$ noon. It takes me nearly an hour there – I then visit the calls left at [illegible]. I try to get home from 3 to 4 P.M. I attend patients in the office. I have my dinner at $4\frac{1}{2}$ or 5. I then try and have a snoose [sic] for an hour or so – I come down to the office by 7 OC – I attend there until $8\frac{1}{2}$. After that hour I go out and visit more patients – I generally have from 3 to 5 to visit – I

23 Smith, "The age of uterine disease," in *Doctor in Medicine*, pp. 104–108; S. D. Gross, *Then and Now: A Discourse*... (Philadelphia, 1867). On dentition, see Abraham Jacobi, *Dentition and its Derangements* (New York, 1862).

24 The following passages, located by date, are from Burke's diary, in the possession of the Rare Book Room of the New York Academy of Medicine. The New York Academy also contains the "Diary and Case-Book" of Henry G. Cox for the period 1851–1866. Dr. Cox, who died early in 1866, kept only brief accounts of financial matters. They do, however, indicate a number of aspects of his practice: the infrequent settling of accounts by his patients, the inclusion of servants in the accounts of their employers, his staying overnight with difficult cases.

reach home for the night from 10 to 12. I lie down then after reading for an hour or so.

Dr. Burke's cases were enormously varied. In the summer, for example, there were large numbers of sunstroke and intestinal complaints; winter brought an entirely different pattern of cases. On December 2, he noted visiting in their homes two cases of scarlatina, seven bronchitis, four typhoid fever, one pneumonia, two tuberculosis, one vomiting and diarrhea, one sore throat, one scald from porridge, one retention of urine, one injury to hip joint from fall on ice, one dysentery, one threatened miscarriage, one remittent fever, one "pains in abdomen – local peritonitis." This, he observed, "for one day and not a very busy one." Despite these wearing rounds, Dr. Burke did try to keep alert to professional developments. It was no easy task, however. When he prepared a paper, for example on pneumonia, for his friends in the newly-founded East River Medical Society, Burke had to find the time in the few hours he normally devoted to sleep.[25]

Dr. Burke may indeed have been somewhat atypical, and perhaps our delineation of a general pattern of medical practice has been excessively schematized. There were many different kinds of practice in New York a century ago. New York did have its specialists, its practitioners for the rich, for the simply well-to-do, and, as well, for those families only marginally established in the middle class – artisans, small shopkeepers, and the like.

The poor were treated on a different plan entirely. They were the beneficiaries of what today might be called public medicine, and what a hundred years ago was called medical charity.

The basic unit in this system was the dispensary. These were independent, private charities, by 1866 scattered liberally throughout the city. Somewhat over 184,000 new cases were treated in eleven of these dispensaries during 1866, and, of these, more than 30,000, or roughly a sixth, were visited in their homes.[26] New York's first dispensary was founded in the 1790s and by 1866 their administration had become standardized. All had a salaried resident physician, available at the dispensary roughly from nine to five (though hours varied from institution to institution) and for

25 Entry for January 14, 1866.
26 The eleven dispensaries mentioned were those dedicated to general medicine; there were others, of course, founded for the treatment of specific classes of disease. Where the annual reports of these dispensaries have not been available, statistics have been taken from *The Medical Register of the City of New York and Vicinity...for the Year Commencing June 1, 1867*, John Shrady, ed. (New York, 1867). Homeopathic statistics were drawn from the annual reports of the New York Homoeopathic Dispensary and the Bond Street Homoeopathic Dispensary, both published in the *Trans. Homoeopathic Med. Soc. State of New York*, 1866.

several hours on Sunday. An apothecary was on duty during the same hours to make up prescriptions and in most cases to pull teeth as well. Treatment was administered by a staff of volunteer physicians, each available at stated hours during the week in clinics corresponding to the developing specialties of the day: diseases of the chest, diseases of women and children, diseases of the eye and ear, skin diseases, diseases of the genito-urinary system, surgery, and diseases of the head and abdomen. These consultants were not salaried. The resident and visiting physicians, however, normally somewhat younger men, did have regular if modest salaries. It was the task of the resident physician to treat simple emergencies, to vaccinate, and – most importantly – to screen incoming patients, sending them to the appropriate clinic and entering the names of patients unable to leave their rooms on the visiting physician's ledger.

The visiting physician's task was particularly difficult. These young practitioners had to make their way through the dark and reeking halls of crowded tenements, at times unable even to find would-be patients; tenement dwellers, they explained, often did not know their neighbors' names. They had as well to deal with a poorly educated clientele who, they found, shunned fresh air as a major cause of disease and who took little interest in cleanliness, even when facilities for washing were available. It was also difficult, the visiting physicians complained, to see patients on a regular basis or to follow them even through the course of an acute disease. If a patient should die, there was, of course, almost no chance of obtaining permission for an autopsy. And the conditions they encountered were truly appalling. William Thoms, active in medical work for several dispensaries and a city mission, described, for example, one alley harboring an inordinate number of typhus cases. In a slanting attic room measuring 14 by $7\frac{1}{2}$ by 7 feet, Thoms reported finding twelve human beings; there were five typhus cases among them. There was no real furniture; the "inmates" slept on pallets arranged on the floor. During one of his visits, Thoms recalled, he found all the children in the group stripped and lying naked under the same bedclothes and on the same mattress, though several were suffering with active cases of typhus. The children's only clothes were, it seemed, being washed. The room itself was so crowded that on several calls, Dr. Thoms found it almost impossible to force a way to the corner where his patients lay.[27]

Not surprisingly, it was dispensary physicians such as Dr. Thoms who

---

27 Thoms, "Sanitary condition of Fish Alley and surroundings," *Trans. Med. Soc. State of New York*, 1866, p. 151. For other descriptions of the difficulties faced by these visiting physicians, see: *14th Annual Report of the Board of Managers of the North-Western Dispensary...* (New York, 1867), pp. 14–15; Henry M. Field, "The Continued Fever of New York City," *Trans. Med. Soc. State of New York*, 1867, p. 322.

provided concerned New Yorkers with much of their knowledge of such intolerable conditions. Many of the physicians participating in the careful sanitary survey sponsored by New York's Citizens' Association in 1865 were, or had been, dispensary physicians. And despite the comparatively low social status generally afforded physicians who engaged in public health work,[28] the task of the dispensary physician had its compensations: the few hundred dollars a year paid visiting physicians was a welcome addition to a beginning physician's slender income. Perhaps more importantly, it was an excellent way in which to sharpen clinical skills.

The larger dispensaries undertook a staggering amount of work. One of the largest, for example, was the Demilt at Twenty-third Street and Second Avenue. Its "district" was the East Side of Manhattan Island, from Fourteenth Street on the south to Fortieth on the north and from Sixth Avenue on the west to the East River. Some 110,000 New Yorkers lived in this area, 75,000 in tenement houses. The dispensary treated 29,070 new cases in 1866, 4,625 in their homes, while the apothecary prepared 58,520 prescriptions. The dispensary thus treated an average of some eighty new cases a day and filled daily about 160 prescriptions.[29] Though the Demilt published no statistics on this point, the great majority of its patients must have been immigrants or their children. This was clearly the case with other dispensaries publishing such records and established in similar areas. Of 20,301 patients treated by the Northern Dispensary during 1866, 11,184 had been born in Ireland. At the North-Western Dispensary, one district physician reported that of 684 patients he had visited, 311 were Irish by birth; less than half were born in the United States and of these, two-thirds were of foreign parentage.[30]

When such disadvantaged New Yorkers became gravely ill they entered a hospital. Without exception, these were purely eleemosynary institutions. Bellevue and Charity Hospitals, the city's two great hospitals, dwarfed all others. Bellevue, with a thousand beds, treated 7,725 patients during the year, while another 7,574 were ministered to at Charity Hospital on Blackwell's Island. No other hospital approached these figures, although the New York Ophthalmic Hospital and the New York Eye and Ear Infirmary treated impressive numbers of cases for special hospitals.[31]

28 Smith, *Doctor in Medicine*, p. 152; Cathell, *The Physician Himself*, p. 20; B. Howard Rand, *Valedictory Address to the Graduates of the Jefferson Medical College...* (Philadelphia, 1868), p. 11.

29 These statistics are drawn from: The Demilt Dispensary in the City of New York, *16th Annual Report...for...1866* (New York, 1867).

30 North-Western Dispensary..., *14th Annual Report*, p. 7; Northern Dispensary, *40th Annual Report* (New York, 1867), p. 17.

31 New York Commissioners of Charities and Correction, *Annual Report, 1866*, "Annual Report of the Warden of Bellevue Hospital," p. 4. The New York Ophthalmic

A stay in one of New York's hospitals in 1866 could not have been too pleasant. Patients were regarded with condescension and still expected to work in the wards as soon as they had recovered sufficiently. Convalescent women helped everywhere to care for others still sicker; in Bellevue and Charity Hospitals women were set to work sewing, the men at carpentry and cleaning. A few formed the crew of the rowboat which plied twice daily between Bellevue and Blackwell's Island. A pervasive moralism and – in the best hospitals – a species of heavy-handed paternalism burdened the patients as well. The Infant's Hospital, for example, charged seven dollars a month for children able to walk but ten dollars for the illegitimate. Even St. Luke's, probably the most liberally administered of New York's hospitals, which allowed visitors on weekdays, forbade them on the Sabbath. Patients might, in addition, be expelled for blasphemy, indeed for any insubordination.[32] Many of the desperately ill, moreover, could not be admitted to the city's hospitals. Patients with ailments judged incurable, cancer for example, were forbidden admittance by all of New York's hospitals; they could turn only to the Almshouse or to their own families' resources.[33]

Nursing was casual, hygiene inadvertent. Some years earlier, for example, a young New York physician advocating hospital reform had hopefully urged the installation of a spittoon in each ward and the thorough airing of beds and bedding. Nurses, he suggested, should have some badge of their station, and be "compelled to dress in clean garments, and not be allowed to wander over the building looking like the off-scouring of the city."[34] Though many of the city's leading physicians held attending and consulting posts, the lack of thorough clinical training in contemporary

Dispensary treated some 1,119 patients, and the Eye and Ear Infirmary noted that it had "prescribed for" 8,033 patients, 313 of whom were indoor cases.

32 *8th Annual Report of St. Luke's Hospital for the Year Ending... Oct. 18, 1866* (St. Johnland, 1867), pp. 30–31. The rules of the Nursery and Child's Hospital and Infant's Home are printed in *Medical Register for 1866*, p. 136. The *7th Annual Report* of the Commissioners of Charity (pp. 8–9) prints a list of items made by patients and notes the use of convalescents as oarsmen (p. 83).

33 See the remarks of William Muhlenberg, founder of St. Luke's Hospital, on the tragic circumstances of the "incurables" denied treatment. *8th Annual Report of St. Luke's Hospital*, pp. 8–9. Thomas Addis Emmett waged a bitter struggle with his board of managers when he sought to treat cancer patients in the Woman's Hospital. Emmett, *Incidents in My Life* (New York: Putnam, 1911), pp. 195–196. In 1866, however, the Protestant Episcopal Church did establish the city's first private "Home for Incurables" at West Farms, an act applauded by the medical profession. *New York Med. J.* 3 (1866): 318.

34 Valentine Mott Francis, *A Thesis on Hospital Hygiene for the Degree of Doctor of Medicine in the University of New York. Session 1858–59* (New York, 1859), pp. 194, 203. Since nurses at Bellevue and Charity Hospitals were paid $120 a year, it does not seem likely that the more able and ambitious served in these positions. Commissioners of Charity and Correction, *7th Annual Report*, p. 19.

medical schools must inevitably have meant a house staff inadequate in many instances – even by the standards of the day. And the young men of the house staff, of course, provided the bulk of medical care. Death rates for the several hospitals averaged in the vicinity of 10 percent, almost none lower and a few a bit higher. The highest death rate, one not included in this average, was among the foundlings brought to the Almshouse. Of the 771 admitted during the year, 644 died.[35] Hospitals were, finally, administered by lay boards, a fact which most physicians regarded with consistent hostility, and to which they attributed many of the hospital's inadequacies.[36]

Though perhaps not immediately apparent to the patients, these hospitals had already come to play a significant role in New York's medical growth. The elite among medical school graduates could compete for positions on the house staff and, increasingly, the medical schools themselves offered instruction utilizing the city's abundant "clinical material." By 1866, some physicians at least were able to state that the principal function of the city's hospitals lay not in the alleviation of individual suffering but in the teaching of medicine.[37] A few attending physicians had even begun to use their hospital facilities for the conduction of clinical investigations.

III

Diagnosis and therapy had in 1866 changed in some ways very little since the eighteenth century. Despite brave talk of reliance on hygiene, despite

35 J. Bayley Done, "Report of Department of Infants; Charity Hospital Report," Commissioners of Charity and Correction, *7th Annual Report*, p. 98. The poor condition of abandoned children when received and the consequent difficulties of trying to raise them on an artificial diet were, of course, the principal element in creating this mortality. The children were, as well, nursed by the Almshouse's elderly female inhabitants, who cared little for extra duties and saw that they were as transitory as possible.

36 D. B. S. John Roosa, *The Old Hospital and Other Papers* (New York, 1889), p. 232 and *passim*; Emmett, *Incidents in My Life*, pp. 199–201. Particularly illuminating is the story of Abraham Jacobi's bitter squabble with the Board of Lady Managers of the Nursery and Child's Hospital. Jacobi, "In re the Nursery and Child's Hospital. Letter to Mrs. R. H. Lemist, Secretary Board of Managers Nursery and Child's Hospital, New York, October 1870," *Collectanea Jacobi*, vol. VII (New York, 1909), pp. 11–42.

37 Society of the New York Hospital, *The Financial Condition and Restricted Charitable Operations of the Society of the New York Hospital. Majority and Minority Reports... Presented April 17, 1866* (New York, 1866), p. 8. The Ophthalmic Hospital was incorporated on April 21, 1865, "for the purpose of affording facilities for the instruction of medical students in the treatment of all diseases of the eye." James J. Walsh, *History of Medicine in New York* (New York: National Americana Society, 1919), vol. III, p. 855. Existing hospitals were, moreover, gradually being reorganized in terms of special services and clinics. In the spring of 1866, for example, the Charity Hospital was thus reorganized. "The Island Hospital," *Medical Record* 1 (1866): 63.

an invigorating skepticism in some circles toward the bulky materia medica, medicine was still in practical terms just that – the administration of medicine. "Prescribing for" a patient was still a synonym for seeing him. Diagnostic procedures too shifted slowly and with them the physician's prognostic ability. Inadequacies in therapeutics helped, of course, maintain the traditional importance of prognostic skills in determining a physician's success. "People in general," as Austin Flint put it, "are apt to estimate [the physician's] knowledge and ability by the correctness of his judgment in this regard."[38] In the hands of most practitioners, diagnosis was in all probability still based on asking questions, observing the patient's appearance, taking his pulse, and examining – and sometimes tasting – his urine.[39] Physical diagnosis was not employed routinely by the ordinary practitioner, but only by the better-trained and then, apparently, only when the case seemed a severe one.

It is extremely difficult, of course, to discover precisely how many physicians practiced physical diagnosis in New York a century ago and how expert they were. Some useful hints can be found, however, in the manuals prepared by the various insurance companies to guide their medical examiners. Insurance examiners were well-established physicians, certainly more skillful than the average practitioner; clearly, as well, their examination would be as thorough as the company's advisors could design. One learns from these manuals, for example, that auscultation and percussion were normally performed through underclothing.[40] The very detailed and explicit quality of the instructions indicates, moreover, that too much could not be assumed as to the physician's consistency in diagnosis. In 1866, physical diagnosis was not taught on an individual basis in medical schools; it was something which one had to learn either in practice, in the apprentice relationship (though this ancient mode of clinical instruction was falling increasingly into disuse), or more commonly in one of the small, semiformal tutoring classes attached to the city's medical schools. It would be safe, I think, to conclude that physical diagnosis was not an ordinary procedure in routine house visits; it had still the aura of high-level practice. The lag between the general academic acceptance of auscultation and percussion and their introduction in routine practice demonstrates quite

---

38 Flint, *A Treatise on the Principles and Practice of Medicine*, p. 102.
39 On the persistence of tasting urine to detect sugar, see: Edward L. Keyes, "Early History of Urology in New York," in Bransford Lewis, ed., *History of Urology* (Baltimore: Williams & Wilkins, 1933), vol. I, p. 77.
40 *Instructions to the Medical Examiners of the Security Life Assurance and Annuity Company of New York* (New York, 1868); Mutual Life Insurance Company of New York, *Instructions to Medical Examiners*, p. 6. Each year the *Medical Register* listed the medical examiners of the various insurance companies in New York, and the list always included a number of the city's more prominent physicians.

well the gap which existed in this period between the "best" practice and the day-to-day round of the average practitioner.

At the same time, of course, other newer modes of diagnosis were being introduced. Thermometry was known from the literature but was hardly considered by the general practitioner an appropriate part of his normal routine. In the fall of 1865, and then in 1866, clinical thermometry was introduced to New York City on an experimental basis, first at New York Hospital, then at Bellevue; it is clear, however, even in enthusiastic pleas for their use that thermometers were considered unnecessary, indeed wildly impractical by the average practitioner.[41] Other aids to diagnosis, the ophthalmoscope and laryngoscope especially, were well known but, of course, were used routinely only by those who specialized in ailments of the eye and ear and nose and throat.[42] The vaginal speculum was certainly used by many nonspecialists; it is doubtful, however, that its employment could have been routine if only because of contemporary standards of propriety. The analysis of blood, despite the influence in theoretical matters of hematological pathologies, was still an experimental procedure – and most often a postmortem one at that.

Therapy, as we have noted, was still heavily dependent upon the administration of drugs, less heroic than in an earlier generation perhaps, but still strenuous enough. It is, of course, difficult to quantify, but a pattern of multiple prescriptions was seemingly universal. Dispensary apothecaries compounded an average of almost exactly two prescriptions per case.[43] Certainly the average would have been higher in private practice.

It cannot be denied that a certain critical skepticism in matters therapeutic had been present and even increasing in the quarter-century before

41 E. C. Seguin, "The use of the thermometer in clinical medicine," *Chicago Medical Journal* 23 (1866): 193–201; Seguin, "Clinical thermometry," *Medical Record* 1 (1867): 516–519. Seguin reported that W. H. Draper and Austin Flint at New York and Bellevue Hospitals were the physicians sponsoring the experimental use of the thermometer in their services. Both, it should be noted, were members of the Medical and Surgical Society, which held a meeting in November 1866, at which the thermometer was discussed. Van Ingen, *A Brief Account of the First One Hundred Years of the New York Medical and Surgical Society*, p. 73. Austin Flint's *Practice*, which did not discuss thermometry in the first edition of 1866, added three pages (pp. 106–108) on the subject in its 1867 second edition. James J. Walsh noted, however, that: "It was well on toward the eighties before the thermometer was generally used by city physicians; it was nearly the nineties before it was generally employed in country practice." *History of Medicine in New York*, vol. 1, p. 258.

42 The very existence of such aids to diagnosis helped, of course, to create specialties. See also Louis Elsberg, 'Laryngology in America...," *Trans. Am. Laryngological Assn.* 1 (1879): 33–35.

43 This is based on the statistics of seven dispensaries which provided totals of the number of prescriptions administered during the year. For 160,156 cases, 305,731 prescriptions were provided.

1866. Beginning most clearly with Jacob Bigelow, a respectable number of American medical leaders had warned against the routine and uncritical use of severe drugs and bleeding. The logic of Bigelow's position and that assumed by like-thinking physicians was based on the assumption that most diseases were self-limited, their natural tendency even if untreated being to recovery not death. The physician should therefore, the argument followed, be cautious in his therapy, attempting simply to strengthen the body's vital powers in their struggle with disease. For ills that were not self-limited, on the other hand, there was usually little that could be done. Reliance should, therefore, be placed upon good food, favorable hygienic conditions, and stimulants such as alcohol or relaxing anodynes such as opium – as opposed to so-called depleting remedies, the traditional arsenal of cathartics and bleeding.

By the 1860s, the position of Austin Flint was probably representative of the best therapeutic thinking in American medicine.[44] Flint called his therapeutic stance "conservative medicine." The term had in reality two separate but complementary meanings, conservative in the sense of conserving the body's natural powers and conservative in the sense of abjuring harsh and unproven modes of therapy. Flint, for example, was famous in this generation for his emphasis in the treatment of tuberculosis upon fresh air – and enormous quantities of whiskey.[45] The emphasis of fashionable clinicians in the late 1860s upon the administration of alcohol and other stimulants was not altogether popular. Temperance writers were bitterly hostile and more than a few older practitioners considered this new practice a rather naively self-confident Neo-Brunonianism.[46] It is apparent,

44 Austin Flint, *Essays on Conservative Medicine and Kindred Topics* (Philadelphia, 1874). See also Jacob Bigelow, *Brief Expositions of Rational Medicine...* (Boston, 1858). Flint's conservative medicine was not unlike Bigelow's "rational medicine." A full bibliography of Americans adopting this more skeptical position would include scores of names in addition to the well-known ones of Bigelow and Oliver Wendell Holmes. Particularly influential in the mid-1860s was the English clinician Robert Bentley Todd and his emphasis on "stimulating therapy." *Clinical Lectures on Certain Acute Diseases* (Philadelphia, 1860).

45 The alcohol purchases of Bellevue Hospital in 1866 were staggering, including 1,637 gallons of best whiskey, 161 gallons of common whiskey, 40 gallons of brandy, 260 gallons of sherry, 68 gallons of port, 20 gallons of gin, 134 barrels of ale, and 85 cases of tarragona wine. On the other hand, Bellevue, significantly enough, ordered no calomel and only five pounds of jalap. Much of the alcohol listed must have found its way into the stomachs of attendants and Tammany politicians – but still the enormous quantities are of significance. "Report of Apothecary, Schedule of Liquors, Wines and Ales, Purchased and Expended," Commissioners of Charities, *7th Annual Report*, p. 25. Medicines are listed on pages 26–29. Despite some historical skepticism as to how routinely anesthetics were employed at this time, it is worth noting that Bellevue purchased 375 pounds of sulfuric ether and 20 gallons of chloroform during the year.

46 S. D. Gross was particularly acid. "Young Physic," he wrote in 1867, "boasts that he has never seen a lancet, and expresses surprise that such a weapon should ever have

however, from a survey of medicine and materia medica textbooks (including Austin Flint's *Practice*) that a rather elaborate drug therapy was assumed and suggested in the great majority of conditions.

Certainly, the casual employment of severe bloodletting and the almost automatic prescribing of harsh emetics and cathartics had decreased, though again the gap between the more sophisticated academic or quasi-academic practitioners and their less pretentious colleagues is difficult to evaluate.[47] Nor should the problem of generations be ignored: older men must have found it difficult to change accustomed practices, to abandon faith in the calomel and phlebotomy which had, apparently, served them so well. Cupping and leeches were still used routinely, and while venesection was in intellectual disfavor, texts still pointed out that in children under three, blood might be drawn from the jugular if other veins were difficult to locate.[48] Blisters and setons were still a part of the therapeutic armory. Most importantly, however, the therapeutic implications of a logically severe emphasis on the self-limited nature of most ills were still heresy to most physicians. Both characteristic and revealing is the frequency with which physicians could write on one page of the evils of traditional therapeutics and the self-limited quality of most ailments and on the next emphasize their contempt for expectant therapy. Certainly there was virtue in drugs, as T. Gaillard Thomas, a vigorous advocate of the self-limited nature of most ills, put it: "There was a vantage ground between the two extremes, neither verging toward meddlesome interference on the one hand, nor imbecile neglect on the other."[49]

been in universal use.... He looks with disgust at the conduct of his predecessors, loudly proclaiming against their want of judgment, and like the Pharisees in the Bible, devoutly thanks God that he is not like other men. Scrupulously abstaining from the spilling of blood, he entrenches himself behind his wine, his whiskey, his brandy, his milk-punch, and his beef essence, bids defiance to disease...." Gross, *Then and Now: A Discourse* ... , p. 23. Gross does note as well that emetics of any kind were now rarely given and "drastic cathartics" administered less frequently. See also Richard D. Arnold to Henry M. Fuller, March 28, 1868, Richard Shryock, ed., *Letters of Richard D. Arnold, M.D. 1808–1876* ... (Papers of the Trinity College Historical Society, XVIII–XIX) (Durham, N.C.: Duke University Press, 1929), pp. 135–137.

47 This statement is based on a survey of a number of contemporary guides to prescribing and collections of prescriptions, as well as textbooks of materia medica. I have, unfortunately, been unable to find the prescription records of any New York pharmacy or established practitioner in 1866. There does seem to have been some truth in the homeopathic charge that their influence had been important in turning allopaths toward less severe doses – even toward the coating of their own pills with sugar. William Todd Helmuth, "Annual address," *Proc. Am. Inst. Homoeopathy*, 1866, p. 53.

48 See also, among others, Charles West, *Lectures on the Diseases of Infancy and Childhood* (Philadelphia, 1866), p. 27. West's text was probably the most popular of the period, the edition cited being the fourth American, from the fifth English edition.

49 *Introductory Address Delivered at the College of Physicians and Surgeons, New York, October 17th, 1864* (New York, 1864), p. 31. See also Bigelow, *Brief Expositions of Rational*

And the patients themselves were a sturdy bulwark against any nihilism in therapeutics. People seemed to want medicines, and when the physician left, wished to be in the comforting possession of a prescription. (To support this view, one need simply mention the routine use of placebos by practitioners in this period and their general conviction that placebos played a significant, possibly even genuinely therapeutic, role in comforting patients and their families.) Devotees of homeopathy too quaffed countless doses – even if they had little physiological effect. Most of the drugs imbibed, moreover, were not prescribed by physicians. In addition to the omnipresent patent mixtures, drugs such as calomel, laudanum, even strychnine, were everywhere available at pharmacy counters.[50] Parents routinely administered cathartics to helpless children when they appeared a bit peaked; many others followed the dictates of traditional wisdom and administered purges every spring. Popular wisdom still held that infections in the blood would have to be driven out through the skin, resulting in the administration of countless doses of medicine, mustard plasters, and the like. And many Americans, of course, still felt comfortable with the calomel that had played so prominent a role in their own childhood.

With drug-taking so important in therapeutics, a central aspect of medical practice a century ago was the relationship between physician and pharmacist. A "course of treatment" was, as we have noted, essentially a series of prescriptions. It was the pharmacist's duty to fill these as carefully and accurately as possible; this was as far as his authority extended, at least in theory. In practice, apothecaries felt no hesitation in acting as medical advisors, suggesting particular patent medicines and, more importantly, casually refilling prescriptions at the patient's request. (In 1867, New York City's East River Medical Association voted to boycott local pharmacies which did not agree to forego this practice.) There was, not surprisingly, a good deal of chronic ill feeling between physicians and druggists. Apothecaries criticized physicians for occasionally extortionate demands for percentages of each prescription;[51] physicians, on the other hand, criticized

---

Medicine..., pp. iv., 29; Field, "The Continued Fever of New York City," *Trans. Med. Soc. State of New York*, pp. 338–339, 341; A. P. Merrill, "Homoeopathy and cholera," *Medical Record* 1 (1866): 275.

50 Druggists were also expected to have available their own compounds of traditional panaceas. Even the forward-looking Edward Parrish's textbook of pharmacy provided recipes for Dalby's Carminative, Bateman's Pectoral Drops, Opodeldoc, Hooper's Female Pills, Turlington's Balsam of Life, No. 6 Hot Drops (Thomsonian), and Composition Powders (Thomsonian). *A Treatise on Pharmacy. Designed as a Text-Book for the Student, and as a Guide for the Physician and Pharmaceutist...*, 3d ed. (Philadelphia, 1867), pp. 824–828.

51 Such covert financial arrangements were particularly embarrassing to ethical relationships between physician and pharmacist. A few physicians went so far as to refuse to visit patients unless they agreed to have their prescriptions filled at a

pharmacists for carelessness and for selling everything but drugs in their stores.[52] Essentially, of course, the problem rested in the embryonic state of professionalism within the guild of pharmacists, exacerbated by the state's failure to exert any control over the druggist's training, licensing, or operations. With a similar laissez-faire prevailing in regard to physicians, this state of things was inevitable.

IV

We have tended, thus far, in discussing medicine in New York a century ago, to emphasize factors which made for continuity. I should like, finally, to suggest a number of "unstable" areas within the profession itself that offered the possibility of change. These aspects of medicine are education, specialization, and values.

In each of these areas, moreover, the city itself played a significant role; effects of scale and organization helped make New York medicine a century ago foreshadow in a number of ways the shape of American medicine generally in generations to come.[53] Some of the influences exerted by the city are obvious, some more subtle. Most apparent are the simple effects of scale, the availability of abundant clinical material, for example, or the presence of large numbers of wealthy prospective patients; both attracted ambitious physicians and intensified specialization. And all such effects are, of course, cumulative, each building upon and magnifying the next. The metropolis served as well as a node for the gathering and distribution of knowledge. New York, the nation's largest city, was also its

particular pharmacy – the physician receiving, of course, a percentage of the prescription's cost for such devotion. Physicians charged druggists with carelessness in filling prescriptions, druggists physicians with carelessness in writing them (usually in pencil and many on scraps of newspaper). "Medicus," "Physician's prescriptions," *Druggist's Circular* 10 (1866): 106; [William Proctor, Jr.], "Percentages on prescriptions," *Am. J. Pharm.* 15 (1867): 89–90; Edward Dixon, *Back-Bone* (New York, c. 1866), pp. 355–358; J. C. Young, *Druggist's Circular* 10 (1866): 129. More ethically oriented pharmacists approved of the East River Medical Association's action. [John H. Maisch], "Prescriptions – whose property are they?," *Am. J. Pharm.* 15 (1867): 472–473.

52 Smith, *Doctor in Medicine*, p. 17; F. Stearns, "The pharmaceutical business . . . ," *Proc. Am. Pharm. Assn.*, 1866, pp. 202–203.

53 By the 1870s, it was becoming apparent that New York medicine was beginning to overtake the traditional leadership exerted by Philadelphians. "Is not Philadelphia paling before New York?," Richard Arnold wrote in 1871. "What one of us takes a Boston Journal, high in intellect and medical culture as Boston is?" *Letters of Richard D. Arnold*, p. 151. For an extremely perceptive analysis of the role of New York in fostering specialization – one paralleling many of the points made in the following passages – see George Rosen, *The Specialization of Medicine with Particular Reference to Ophthalmology* (New York: Froben Press, 1944), pp. 34–38.

leading port of entry. Inevitably, New York and other great cities provided a peculiarly stimulating context for the profession's institutional and intellectual growth.

Specialism was still a term of derision in the vocabulary of many physicians. General practitioners feared the specialist's competition and attacked any professed limitation of practice to specific classes of ailments as a symptom of quackery – which in the not-too-distant past it had usually been. (And which, it should be recalled, it still was in the case of numberless pox-doctors, cancer specialists, and the like proliferating at this time in American cities.) In 1866, coincidentally, the American Medical Association's Committee on Medical Ethics took a skeptical view of what the committee's majority termed exclusive specialism. Indeed, many forward-looking physicians of goodwill were critical of exclusive and seemingly premature specialism, feeling that it should develop only out of the broad opportunities for observation enjoyed by the general practitioner.[54] Despite this not entirely friendly climate, on the other hand, specialism was by 1866 clearly well-established in New York.[55] Busy and intelligent practitioners gradually concentrated upon certain classes of ailments, seeking them out in hospitals and dispensary work, finally having colleagues refer such cases when they appeared in private practice. In a city, with its great numbers of people and its complex social structure, there was obviously room for specialists; in rural areas there could be little opportunity for them either to earn a living or to perfect clinical skills.

In the intense competition, moreover, specialism was clearly a road to reputation and status. How else, indeed, was distinction to be won in a day of rapidly accumulating knowledge and before a purely academic career provided a realistic aspiration for American physicians? The majority, as we have noted, of the Medical and Surgical Society's members were specialists.[56] Even outside the Society's socially impeccable membership,

54 The logic behind this position was, of course, based upon the emphasis in contemporary etiological thought upon the need to understand the "whole man" and his environment. See also [George Shrady], "Specialties and specialists," *Medical Record* 1 (1867): 525–526; "Report of the Committee on Medical Ethics," *Trans. A.M.A.* 17 (1866): esp. pp. 504–506. Compare, however, the completely different orientation exhibited in Henry Bowditch's minority report, *Trans. A.M.A.* 17 (1866): 511–512.

55 In January 1864, for example, the New York Obstetrical Society was organized; in March, the New York Ophthalmological Society. The New York Medico-Legal Society was organized early in 1866 and the New York Dermatological Society in 1869. Walsh, *History of Medicine in New York*, vol. I, pp. 213–214, vol. III, pp. 688, 692. Other specialties, as in diseases of the chest or orthopedic surgery, were generally recognized by other physicians.

56 They also played prominent roles in both the Ophthalmological and Obstetrical Societies. Their influence was even more predominant in hospital appointments.

specialism was intricately related to the acquisition of status. Men like Louis Elsberg, Abraham Jacobi, Emil Noeggerath, Ernst Krackowizer, and a few years later Herman Knapp – to mention only a few distinguished German physicians active in New York a century ago – made reputations as specialists, eventually overlapping and merging with the establishment of "hospital men" seen in so concentrated a form in the membership of the Medical and Surgical Society. Not surprisingly, New York physicians played an extraordinarily prominent role in the founding of the first national specialty societies in this period.[57]

The new specialities were recognized not only in such informal terms, moreover, but institutionally as well in the creation of chairs in the city's medical schools and special clinics and services in the city's hospitals and dispensaries. Such institutional provisions are particularly significant, for they provide an opportunity for the ordered transmission of knowledge – while the availability of a sufficient number of cases made such institutional provisions feasible. And, once created, it is the tendency of all such arrangements to grow and consolidate themselves. With the increasing accumulation of knowledge and technique generally in medicine, with the trend within European clinical medicine quite clearly toward specialization, it was inevitable that similar and parallel developments should take place in this country. Certainly this was the case after the wedding – already achieved in New York by 1866 – of such intellectual influences with institutional contexts appropriate for their transmission and elaboration.

By 1866, in any case, the elite among New York's medical men were in large degree specialists – or surgeons, and even surgeons were beginning to show signs of specialization, with men like Lewis A. Sayre limiting themselves largely to orthopedic cases or Thomas Addis Emmett to gynecological surgery.[58] But this emphasis upon the emergence of specialism is easily exaggerated. Specialists in this period almost always acted to some extent also as general practitioners. Exclusive specialism, despite the anxieties of its critics, was still essentially in the future.

Medical education at once mirrored and fostered this growing differentiation within an as yet comparatively homogeneous group. For most

---

57 In medical education and medical publishing, however, Philadelphia was still ahead of New York. The larger city's dominance in the production of specialists would seem to have been a result of the larger "substrate" it offered, both in hospital patients and, perhaps more importantly, in prospective paying clients.

58 Emmett recalled his being atypically exclusive in his specialization, giving up all routine obstetrical practice. He remembered as well the hostility with which he was rewarded by other physicians; see Emmett, *Incidents in My Life*, p. 203. The best contemporary defense of specialism which I have seen was composed by New York ophthalmologist Henry D. Noyes, "Specialties in medicine," *Trans. Am. Ophth. Soc.* 1865, pp. 59–74.

would-be physicians, medical education had probably not changed for generations. Though somewhat longer, the regular session from October to March was filled with didactic, factual, and routinely pedantic lectures. The great majority of students graduating after such a two-year course must have been indeed ill-prepared to begin practice.[59]

For the better student, on the other hand, more highly motivated, more intelligent, wealthier perhaps, the possibilities of medical education within New York a century ago could be surprisingly broad. In an age of vigorous competition among medical schools, the availability of great clinical resources was an obvious inducement to be held out by the New York City schools to prospective students.[60] The city's three regular medical schools offered clinical instruction, both in hospital wards (open to students of all medical schools) and dispensary clinics. All three schools had as well by 1866 instituted special fall preliminary courses, optional but free of charge. Some offered summer courses as well. Both these innovations in the curriculum promised an emphasis upon clinical teaching greater than that possible in the constricted winter course. Many of the city's eminent teachers offered private instruction in diagnosis, or, more traditionally, quizzes in test-passing. Senior students were beginning to be entrusted with obstetric cases in the city's tenements. After graduation, there were desirable house-staff positions to be competed for; these posts, unlike senior consulting appointments, were often awarded on the basis of a competitive examination, not simply through influence. Then, of course, there were the dispensaries and the possibility of perfecting one's skills, perhaps even developing a specialty in their clinics.[61]

Most students, of course, never took advantage of these opportunities. Many failed even to attend regularly scheduled clinics, for they were never

59 Traditional preceptorial responsibilities had, moreover, come to be regarded as a mere formality. [George F. Shrady], "Medical preceptorship," *Medical Record* 1 (1866): 429–430.

60 The following remarks are based largely on the annual announcements for 1865–1866 and 1866–1867 of New York's three medical schools, the Medical Department of the University of New York, the Bellevue Hospital Medical College, and the College of Physicians and Surgeons. Writers on medical education, it might be noted, unanimously urged the need for combining clinical instruction with traditional didactic methods. A certain defensive tone was also to be found in writers discussing the opportunities of small-town and rural practice; cf. Theophilus Parvin, *The Subjective Utility of Medicine. Introductory Address Delivered before the Class of the Medical College of Ohio... Oct. 6, 1868* (Cincinnati, [1868]), pp. 18–19.

61 The volunteer clinic physicians were younger men, unlike the established practitioners who occupied the dispensaries' consulting positions. On the importance of the dispensaries in providing opportunities for clinical training, see William Ludlum, *Dispensaries. Their Origin, Progress and Efficiency* (New York, 1876), p. 26; Abraham Jacobi, "Address at the twenty-fifth jubilee of the German Dispensary of New York," *Collectanea Jacobi*, vol. VIII (New York, 1909), pp. 62–63.

specifically tested on such practical knowledge.[62] The better students, however, and especially those with adequate funds, were exposed to the possibility at least of a far more elaborate, if informal, medical education than one might have thought at first glance possible. Ordinary practitioners, perhaps, did not take advantage of these opportunities, but the leaders-to-be of New York medicine certainly did. The New York medical education of William Henry Welch, for example, clearly illustrates this pattern. Welch competed and studied throughout the city, seeking out the best teachers and the most desirable positions in which to develop his skills.[63] Just as we have seen in the beginning of specialization a gradual elaboration of structure within the medical profession, so we have in medical education the simultaneous creation of institutional mechanisms through which an elite, still small in numbers perhaps, might be trained in the values and techniques of the new clinical medicine.

It might be argued, of course, that Welch and many others like him completed their studies in Europe. Such foreign study, however, is not an act of arbitrary impulse. Although clinical and laboratory teaching may have been far more advanced in the Old World, the values which accepted this superiority and chafed against American inadequacies were already being formed in the New World. A spirit of urgent, and in some cases aggressive, positivism was widely disseminated among younger intellectuals in the profession.[64] Book reviews in both of New York's medical journals, the *Medical Record* and the *New York Medical Journal*, tended in the mid-1860s to exhibit a fine scorn for the subtleties of mere speculation; closet philosophy was no substitute for solid laboratory or clinical investigation. Certainly such a rationalistic spirit influenced the contemporary debate over therapeutics. American physicians were as well beginning to acknowledge their awareness of German knowledge and acumen, of the emergence of a new leader in world medicine. The New York Medical Journal Club,

62 [George H. Shrady], "Clinical instruction," *Medical Record* 1 (1866): 261–262; [Shrady], "The extension of the lecture term," *Medical Record* 1 (1866): 213–214; R. Cresson Stiles, *An Introductory Lecture to a Course of Demonstrative Instruction in Histology and Pathological Anatomy* (New York, 1866), p. 4. Stiles urged that students offer proof before graduation of having attended a "demonstrative" course in auscultation and percussion. The quality of formal clinical instruction did not improve for some time. E. C. Seguin, "Higher medical education in New York. III. The system of clinical teaching in colleges," *Arch. Med.* 6 (1881): 57–64.

63 Simon Flexner and James Thomas Flexner, *William Henry Welch and the Heroic Age of American Medicine* (New York: Viking Press, 1941), pp. 58–71.

64 The younger Seguin was probably the most self-conscious and vocal. See, for example, his articles cited in note 41 on the use of clinical thermometry and his "The aesthesiometer and aesthesiometry," *Medical Record* 1 (1867): 510–511, in which he called for the general adoption of the "new instruments of positivism" in clinical medicine and noted at the same time the fall of the French and the rise of the German school of medicine in the preceding twenty years.

for example, which, like the New York Pathological Society, included in its membership the great majority of New York's scientifically oriented physicians, subscribed in 1866 to more German journals than it did to French, English – or even American.[65]

A significant role in the transfer of knowledge and values was played, moreover, by European physician émigrés, by the Seguins, for example, and Abraham Jacobi. All sought to spread the gospel of scholarship and investigation in a nation which must have seemed to them lamentably shoddy in the standards it demanded of its medical practitioners.[66] Such men would naturally choose to practice in New York or some similar eastern city; in addition to the other advantages of metropolitan life, its large immigrant population offered the possibility of conviviality and financial security. American physicians too flocked to New York City; in medicine as in business it promised boundless opportunity. The great majority of New York medicine's intellectual leaders in the latter part of the nineteenth century were born outside the city.[67]

The values of world science were, of course, still a minor, if somewhat disturbing, current in the total life of New York medicine. The acquisition of "business" was still the physician's primary concern. It was still possible for medical men to more or less casually abet malpractice suits, to squabble in private and public. Puffing, the planting of one's name in news columns, and the signing of endorsements for anything from patent medicines to galoshes were still favorite means of acquiring publicity. Most importantly, of course, it did not seem to most New York physicians that one could be a success in any full sense of the word without the attainment of financial independence.[68]

65 *The Medical Register for 1866*, pp. 67–68, provides a list of journals. The large number of German physicians, many of them comparatively recent arrivals, probably explains this fact; however, their very presence was part of the process in which knowledge and values were transmitted.

66 William Welch, for example, attributed the awakening of his interest in German medicine to the influence of Jacobi. Flexner and Flexner, *William Henry Welch and the Heroic Age of American Medicine*, p. 70. The need to foster research and raise standards in American medicine was a pervasive theme in Jacobi's own addresses. For the reactions of two other German physicians, see Ernst P. Boas, "A refugee doctor of 1850," *J. Hist. Med. & Allied Sc.* 3 (1948): 79–84; and "Aerztliche Zustände in Amerika. Aus New-York," *Wien. med. Presse* 7 (1866): 358–359.

67 Among obstetricians and gynecologists in the 1860s, for example, it is difficult to find any prominent teacher and practitioner born in the city. T. Gaillard Thomas, E. R. Peaslee, A. K. Gardner, J. Marion Sims, Thomas Addis Emmett, Emil Noeggerath, Fordyce Barker, J. Lewis Smith, and Abraham Jacobi were all born and raised outside New York. A study comparing medical leadership in New York, Philadelphia, and Boston in this period would be of value.

68 For a particularly illuminating view of the casual ethical standards of the time, see the details of the malpractice suit launched by a Mrs. Walsh against Lewis A. Sayre several years later. Willard Parker and J. W. Carnochan, well-established and successful

It is my hope in these pages to have suggested something of the texture of American medical practice a hundred years ago. Conclusions of any dogmatic sort are certainly premature, but this cross-sectional survey does, I think, indicate a number of general points. One is the interdependence of ideas and the institutional contexts in which they are elaborated. Another is the interrelation of status and learning, the existence of an already well-articulated pattern in which knowledge, practical success, and status were distributed within the profession.

American medicine was, a century ago, disturbed by a number of labile elements. The practitioner's status was uncertain, protected neither by state sanctions nor by the universal trust and admiration of laypersons, certainly not by the transcendent faith accorded medical science today. Many aspects of the physician's practice and ideas have thus to be seen in terms of a need to secure his financial and social status. At the same time, a number of the more ambitious, academically successful practitioners, men atypically secure by contemporary standards, were disturbed by the challenge and availability of new ideas, new techniques, and – most important-antly – new aspirations. From the hindsight of a century, it seems clear enough that these contrasting and coexisting instabilities of status and values were ultimately to cancel each other. The progress of the scientific disciplines within medicine was eventually to raise the level of objective – and to the layperson increasingly visible – achievement, thus insuring the ultimate willingness of society to control both medical education and access to the profession. This limitation of access coupled with better and more specialized medical training in a society increasingly prosperous was in the twentieth century to largely banish these anxieties of status.

physicians, thought nothing of endorsing the patient's claim – without apparently even bothering to make a thorough examination. *The Alleged Malpractice Suit of Walsh vs. Sayre* (New York, 1870); *Comments of the Medical Press on the Alleged Malpractice Suit of Walsh vs. Sayre* (New York, 1871); Lewis A. Sayre, *Introductory Lecture of 1868–69, at Bellevue Hospital Medical College* (New York, 1869), p. 11. The possibility of science forming the basis of a new system of values, one opposed implicitly to the morally compromising conditions of America's commercially centered medicine, was clear enough to at least some contemporaries. Stiles, *An Introductory Lecture to a Course of Demonstrative Instruction in Histology and Pathological Anatomy*, p. 9; Smith, *Doctor in Medicine*, pp. 130–131.

8

Social class and medical care in nineteenth-century America: The rise and fall of the dispensary

❧ Like many of these chapters, this one was conceived in a moment of celebratory inadvertence – as a contribution for a symposium honoring Richard H. Shryock, pioneer historian of American medicine. I used the occasion to explore the rise and fall of the outpatient dispensary, an institution that had been central to the delivery of health care in America's growing cities – but which had been largely ignored by historians of medicine. I had first become aware of the dispensary's centrality – both to the medical profession and to urban working people – when completing research for Chapter 7, on mid-nineteenth-century New York. That essay emphasizes the pivotal interdependence between the internal history of the medical profession and the development of urban social institutions. But my interest remained latent as I worked on a variety of unrelated topics in the late 1960s and early 1970s. The focus of the Shryock symposium on social history provided an ideal incentive – and occasion – to pursue this relationship in another context. ☙

To most mid-twentieth-century physicians, the term *dispensary* evokes the image of a hectic hospital pharmacy. To their mid-nineteenth-century counterparts, it was both the primary means for providing the urban poor with medical care and a vital link in the prevailing system of medical education. These institutions had an effective life span of roughly a hundred years. Founded in the closing decades of the eighteenth century, American dispensaries increased in scale and number throughout the nine-teenth century and remained significant providers of health care well into the twentieth century. By the 1920s, however, the dispensaries were on the road to extinction, increasingly submerged in the outpatient departments of urban hospitals. Historians have found the dispensary of little interest; even those contemporary medical activists seeking a usable past for experiments in the delivery of medical care are hardly aware of their existence.[1] Yet a study of the dispensary illustrates an important aspect of medicine and philanthropy in the nineteenth-century city, and the social logic implicit in the rise and fall of the dispensary underlines permanently significant relationships between general social needs and values and the narrower world of medical practice and ideas.

The dispensary was invented in late eighteenth-century England; it was an autonomous, free-standing institution, created in the hope of establishing an alternative to the hospital in providing medical care for the urban poor. Like most such benevolent innovations, it was soon copied by socially conscious Americans; dispensaries were established in 1786 at Philadelphia, 1791 at New York, 1796 at Boston, and 1800 at Baltimore. Their growth was at first very slow. No additional dispensaries were established until 1816, when the managers of the Philadelphia Dispensary helped established two new dispensaries, the Northern and Southern, to serve their city's rapidly developing fringes.[2] New Yorkers established the Northern Dispensary in 1827, the Eastern in 1832, the DeMilt in 1851, and the Northwestern in 1852. By 1874 there were twenty-nine dispensaries in New York, and by 1877, thirty-three in Philadelphia. Their growth was equally impressive in terms of the number of patients treated; in New York, for example, the city's dispensaries treated 134,069 patients in 1860, roughly 180,000 in 1866, 213,000 in 1874, and 876,000 in 1900.[3]

The dispensaries shared certain organizational characteristics. Almost all had a central building – with the prominent exception of Boston which had none until the 1850s – and usually employed one full-time employee, an apothecary or house physician who acted as steward, performed minor surgery, often vaccinated and pulled teeth, and prescribed for some

---

1 The most valuable study of the dispensary is still that by Michael M. Davis, Jr., and Andrew R. Warner, *Dispensaries: Their Management and Development* (New York, 1918). The most useful account of the early years of any single dispensary is: [William Lawrence], *A History of the Boston Dispensary* (Boston, 1859). For an example of contemporary interest, see George Rosen, "The First Neighborhood Health Center Movement – Its Rise and Fall," *American Journal of Public Health* 61 (1971): 1620–1637.

2 Philadelphia Dispensary, Minutebook 18, June 25, 1816, Archives of the Pennsylvania Hospital, Philadelphia (hereafter APH). See also "Brief History of the Southern Dispensary," Southern Dispensary, *Eighty-first Annual Report* (Philadelphia, 1898), pp. 6–10.

3 See Chapter 7 of this volume; and F. B. Kirkbride, *The Dispensary Problem in Philadelphia. A Report made to the Hospital Association of Philadelphia, October 28, 1903* (Philadelphia, 1903). By 1900, Davis and Warner (*Dispensaries*, p. 10) estimated that there were roughly one hundred dispensaries in the United States, seventy-five general and twenty-five special.

patients. (Though most dispensaries limited their aid to prescriptions written by their own staff physicians, a few would fill prescriptions for the indigent patients of any regular physician.)[4] By mid-century the house physicianship had in the larger dispensaries evolved into two separate positions, resident physician and druggist-apothecary. Most dispensaries also appointed younger physicians who visited patients too ill to attend the dispensary. Such "district visiting" was the principal task of the Philadelphia Dispensary when founded in 1786, remained the sole activity of the Boston Dispensary until 1856, and was continued by almost all urban dispensaries until the end of the nineteenth century, though the treatment of ambulatory patients grew proportionately more prominent in all. The dispensaries also appointed attending and consulting staffs from among their community's established practitioners, the attending staff treating patients well enough to visit the dispensary, the consulting staff serving a largely honorary role.

The dispensaries were shoestring operations. Most, with the exception of those in New York which enjoyed state and city subventions, were supported by private contributions and the often-voluntary services of local physicians.[5] As late as the 1870s and 1880s − when a dispensary might treat over 25,000 patients a year − budgets of four or five thousand dollars were still common and annual reports vied in reporting how little had been spent for prescriptions − an average of under five cents per prescription was common. The Boston Dispensary and Philadelphia Dispensary gradually accumulated some endowment funds, though most others remained financially marginal. All, however, were sensitive to cyclical economic shifts, for contributions declined in periods of depression while patient pressure increased proportionately. As a result of the economic downturn in 1857, for example, New York's Eastern Dispensary reported an increase in cases of 22 percent over 1858 and 42 percent over 1856.[6] A useful index to the shaky financial condition of many of the dispensaries was their frequent practice of renting a portion of their building to commercial tenants; such income often constituted a substantial portion of the insti-

4 As late as 1899, the city of Baltimore still compensated the Baltimore Dispensary when it filled prescriptions for the indigent patients of any legal practitioner. Baltimore General Dispensary, *Charter, By-Laws, &c. . . . Revised 1899* (Baltimore, 1899), p. 14.
5 New York's Eastern Dispensary reported in 1857 that the city's donation to the New York Dispensary had been set at $1,000 in 1827. As other dispensaries were founded, these too received the same subvention. Eastern Dispensary, *23rd Annual Report, 1856* (New York, 1857), p. 19.
6 Eastern Dispensary, *25th Annual Report, 1858* (New York, 1859), pp. 16–17. The panics of 1857, 1873, and 1893, as well as the Civil War years, all represented such periods of stress for the dispensaries. New York's Northeastern Dispensary, for example, was so pressed by the Panic of 1873 that it could not even publish annual reports in 1874 and 1875. Northeastern Dispensary, *15th Annual Report, 1876* (New York, 1877), p. 6.

tution's budget and could not be given up even when the dispensary needed room for expansion.[7]

Some of the dispensaries published detailed statistics of the numbers and kinds of ailments treated by their physicians; thus we can begin to reconstruct their everyday responsibilities. Most cases were, of course, relatively minor – for example, bronchitis, colds, and dyspepsia – and rarely were the numbers of deaths equal to more than 2 or 3 percent of the patients treated. Consistently enough, the number of female patients was always greater than that of males, in some instances as much as twice as great; working men, that is, had necessarily to tolerate disease symptoms of far greater intensity before feeling able to consult a physician. In those cases serious enough to be treated at home by visiting physicians sex ratios tended to be more nearly equal. (It was not until the end of the century that dispensaries began to consider evening hours for workers.) Although the general level of mortality among all dispensary patients was low, mortality among patients treated in their homes approached the 10 or 11 percent normal for hospitals at the beginning of the century. Such death rates were particularly discouraging, for the district physician never treated many intractable cases. Chronic and degenerative ailments brought incapacity and eventual almshouse incarceration; these cases never found their way into the dispensary's mortality statistics. The dispensaries also performed minor surgery, treating fractures, contusions, and lacerations – as well as casual if frequent dentistry, essentially the "indiscriminate extirpation" of offending teeth.[8]

The dispensaries also played an important public health role in providing vaccination for the poor and vaccine matter for the use of private practitioners. From a purely demographic point of view, indeed, vaccination was the most important function performed by the dispensaries. The dispensaries not only made vaccination available without cost, but some mounted door-to-door vaccination programs in their citys' tenement dis-

7 As late as 1891, Philadelphia's Northern Dispensary bemoaned the fact that it could still not afford to stop renting their second floor, despite the establishment of five new specialty clinics and consequent need for space. Northern Dispensary, *74th Annual Report, 1891* (Philadelphia, 1892), p. 9. As early as 1803, the Philadelphia Dispensary was happy to rent its basement to a commercial tenant. Minutes, December 12, 1803. The typical pattern was illustrated clearly by the New York Dispensary's decision in 1868 to build a four-story building, the basement, first, third, and fourth levels to be rented, and only the second to be used by the Dispensary itself. New York Dispensary, *77th Annual Report, 1868* (New York, 1869), p. 12.

8 Eastern Dispensary [New York], *23rd Annual Report, 1856* (New York, 1857), p. 22. S. L. Abbott to G. F. Thayer, April 6, 1844, Chronological File, Boston Dispensary Archives, New England Medical Center, Boston (hereafter BDA). The phrase describing the dispensary's casual dentistry is from New York Dispensary, *81st Annual Report, 1870* (New York, 1871), p. 17.

tricts. In periods of intense demand, most frequently at the outset or threat of a smallpox epidemic, the dispensaries were able to supply large amounts of vaccine matter at short notice. In the opening months of the Civil War for example, the New York Dispensary provided vaccine matter for all the state's recruits.[9]

Despite ventures into surgery, dentistry, and vaccination, dispensary therapeutics generally consisted of the writing of prescriptions; dispensaries dispensed. Throughout the first three-quarters of the nineteenth century, the phrase *prescribing for* was generally synonymous with seeing a patient; busy dispensary physicians could hardly be expected to do more than compose hasty and routine prescriptions. (Dispensary managers tended by mid-century to demand the use of formularies limited in both cost and variety; later in the century some dispensaries were charged with filling prescriptions by number, the dispensing physician being constrained by an abbreviated list of numbered and preformulated prescriptions.)[10] In this routine and exclusive dependence on drug therapy lay the principal difference between the care provided the urban poor and that paid for by the middle class. Physicians in private practice relied consistently in their therapeutics upon adjusting the regimen of their patients, especially in chronic ills; such injunctions were hardly appropriate in dispensary practice. The city poor could not well vary their diet, take up horseback riding, visit the seaside, or sail to the West Indies.

Not surprisingly, the dispensaries tended to develop both formal and

9 For a convenient summary of early vaccination work by the dispensaries, see: DeMilt Dispensary [New York], *25th Annual Report, 1875* (New York, 1876), pp. 20–22. For the role of the dispensaries in the Civil War, see New York Dispensary, *72nd Annual Report, 1862* (New York, 1863), pp. 9–10. Eastern Dispensary [New York], *25th Annual Report, 1861* (New York, 1862), pp. 23–25. Though the poor were normally uninterested in vaccination, the threat of epidemics often created a sudden upsurge of interest; in one case, indeed, the New York Dispensary could refer to a "vaccination riot" on their premises. New York Dispensary, *76th Annual Report, 1865* (New York, 1865), p. 20. Some of the dispensaries were financially dependent on their sale of vaccine matter.

10 George Gould, "Abuse of a Great Charity," *Medical News, N.Y.* 57 (1890): 6; Medical College of the Pacific, Faculty Minutes, January 29, 1878, July 22, 1881, Lane Medical Library, Stanford University. New York's Eastern Dispensary was so lacking in funds that its patients were given neither bottles nor printed instructions: "The patients universally bring a bottle or tea-cup to receive and hold the medicine." Eastern Dispensary, *25th Annual Report, 1861* (New York, 1862), p. 14. There were only occasional conflicts between physicians and lay managers in regard to such cutting of corners. A revealing incident of this kind shook the Boston Dispensary in 1844 when the managers sought to compel their visiting physicians to employ scarification and bleeding instead of the far more expensive leeches. The physicians argued not only that the leeches had a different physiological effect, but that they had well-nigh banished more painful modes of bloodletting from private practice. G. T. Thayer to Visiting Physicians, February 8, 1844; S. L. Abbot et al. to Thayer, April 6, 1844; S. L. Abbott et al. to President and Managers [February 1844], BDA.

informal ties with other urban charities – in New York, for example, with the Commissioners on Emigration, the Association for Improving the Condition of the Poor, and the Children's Aid Society; in Philadelphia with the Board of Guardians for the Poor.[11] Dispensary physicians were in this sense *de facto* social workers. In New York, for example, a note from the dispensary physician was necessary for the commissioners to issue a ration of coal; thus a mid-century whimsy referred to "coal fever," an illness which struck suddenly during cold weather in the city's tenements.[12] In the post–Civil War decades, efforts to provide such physical amenities became somewhat more organized; dispensary physicians continued to work with existing philanthropic agencies and began as well to establish their own auxiliaries in hopes of providing food and nursing in deserving cases. In Philadelphia, the Lying-in and Nurse Charity and the Lying-in Department of the Northern Dispensary had provided some nursing service since the 1830s, while others had paid occasionally for nursing in selected cases since the opening years of the century. In a more contemporary idiom, the Instructive Visiting Nurse Service of the Boston Dispensary began in the 1880s to aid the dispensary's district physicians in their work, not only nursing, but educating the poor in hygiene and diet. In Boston and New York, diet kitchen associations provided nourishing food for patients bearing a dispensary physician's requisition. By 1883, the New York Diet Kitchen Association was operating three kitchens in cooperation with the dispensaries and fed 7,699 patients, filling 53,893 separate requisitions from dispensary physicians during the year.[13]

Another trend marking the nineteenth-century evolution of the dispensaries, reflecting and paralleling a more general development within the medical profession, was their internal reorganization along specialty lines. As early as 1826, the New York Dispensary reorganized itself, dividing patients treated at the Dispensary into "classes" according to the nature of their ailment. Pioneering dispensaries for diseases of the eye and ear had come into being as early as the 1820s. By mid-century, the need for specialty differentiation was unquestioned. When the Brooklyn Dispensary opened in 1847, for example, it announced that patients would be distributed among the following classes; women and children, heart, lungs and throat, skin and vaccination, head and digestive organs, eye and ear,

---

11 For an example of such ties in a particular dispensary, see DeMilt Dispensary, *2nd Annual Report, 1852–53* (New York, 1853), p. 12; *4th Annual Report, 1855* (New York, 1856), pp. 10–11.
12 Eastern Dispensary [New York], *32nd Annual Report, 1865* (New York, 1866), p. 14.
13 New York Diet Kitchen Association, *11th Annual Report, 1883* (New York, 1884), p. 5. On nursing, see, for example, Philadelphia Dispensary, Minutes, February 15, 1853, October, 17, 1854, APH.

surgery, and unclassified diseases. In the second half of the century, specialty designations became increasingly narrow and gradually closer to modern categories; nervous and genito-urinary diseases, for example, were among the most frequently created of such departments in the late 1870s and early 1880s. By 1905, the forward-looking Boston Dispensary boasted these impressively varied outpatient clinics: surgical, general medical, children, skin, nervous system, nose and throat, women, eye and ear, genito-urinary, and x-ray.[14] An important related late nineteenth-century trend was the increasingly frequent establishment of specialized dispensaries, institutions that treated only particular ailments or ailments of particular organs.

These in brief outline were the chief characteristics that marked the growth of the dispensaries between the end of the eighteenth century and the last decades of the nineteenth century. Why did the founders and managers of our pioneer dispensaries find them so plausible a response to social need? What factors led to their initial adoption and subsequent growth?

In their appeals for public support, dispensary founders and supporters left abundant records of their conscious motives. Most prominent in the last years of the eighteenth and opening decades of the nineteenth century was a traditional sense of stewardship. "It is enough for us," as one physician-philanthropist put it, "to be assured that the poor are always with us, and that they are exposed to disease."

> Benevolence [he continued] is not that passive feeling which can be satisfied with doing no injury to our neighbor, or rest contented with mere good wishes for his well-being when he needs our assistance.

The poor, as a prominent New York clergyman explained the need for supporting the dispensary's work, "have feelings as well as we; they are bone of our bone and flesh of our flesh; men of like passions with ourselves."[15] Such sentiments remained deeply felt and were explicitly articulated throughout the first half of the century.

Other, more mundane motives always coexisted with such humanitarian appeals. One was the familiar mercantilist contention that maintaining

14 Brooklyn Dispensary, *Trustee's Report, April, 1847* (New York, 1847), p. 8; *Boston Dispensary, 108th Annual Report* (Boston, 1905), pp. 10–12. For the crediting of the New York Dispensary with this particular first, see DeMilt Dispensary, *25th Annual Report, 1875* (New York, 1876), p. 19n.

15 John G. Coffin, *An Address delivered before the Contributors of the Boston Dispensary, ... October 21, 1813* (Boston, 1813), pp. 6, 15; John B. Romeyn, *The Good Samaritan: A Sermon, delivered in the Presbyterian Church, in Cedar-street, New York, ... for the Benefit of the New York Dispensary* (New York, 1810), p. 16.

the health of the poor would not only save the tax dollars spent on the almshouse or hospital care of chronically ill workers, but would aid the economy more generally by helping to maintain the labor force at optimum efficiency. (These appeals assumed, of course, the ability of the dispensary physicians to diagnose ills at a stage when they might still respond to available treatment.) A related argument urged the dispensaries' function as first line of defense against epidemic disease; though such ills ordinarily began and reached epidemic proportions among the poor, once established they might attack even the comfortable and well-to-do. No household could feel immune when servants and artisans moved easily from the world of their betters to that of tenement-dwelling friends and families.[16] These arguments soon hardened into rhetorical formulas and were ritually intoned throughout the first two-thirds of the century. Thus, for example, a mid-century dispensary spokesman could, in appealing for support, argue that

> the political economist will find here cheapness and utility combined. The statesman will discover the greatest good of the greatest number combined promoted. The city official will find his sanitary police materially assisted. The heads of families will soon find how much the lives and health of their household are cared for and secured. The tax-payer will see his burdens diminished. The benevolent will have opened to his view in the Dispensary and its kindred and associated charities the widest field for the exercise of good will towards man; and the Christian will find a new proof of the truth that they do not love God less who love mankind more.[17]

Finally, and matter-of-factly, their advocates always contended that dispensaries would serve as much-needed schools of clinical medicine.

But to catalogue the arguments of managers and fund-raisers is not precisely to explain the logic of their commitment. Why did the dispensaries grow so rapidly? Obviously because they worked – worked, that is, in terms of particular social realities and expectations. At least four such factors help explain the evolution of the dispensary in nineteenth-century America. First, they were entirely functional in terms of the internal organization of the medical profession. Second, they were entirely consistent with available therapeutic modalities. Third, they were effectively scaled to the needs of a small and comparatively homogeneous community; once established they became indispensable as urban growth dramatically increased their client

---

16 "Servants," one board of managers argued at mid-century, "who have relations and friends in the lower walks of life, and who are in the habit of visiting them, often in company with the children of their employers, would be subject to more danger than they are now exposed." DeMilt Dispensary, *3rd Annual Report, 1853–54* (New York, 1854), p. 10.

17 DeMilt Dispensary, *5th Annual Report, 1855–56* (New York, 1856), p. 11.

constituency. Fourth, the dispensaries made sense in terms of their founders' expectations of the roles to be played both by government and by private citizens.

Most fundamental was the relationship between the dispensary and the world of medical education and status. Without the initiative and voluntary support of the medical profession dispensaries would not have been created nor could they have survived. Physicians formed the core group in the formation of almost every American dispensary from the end of the eighteenth to the beginning of the twentieth century.[18]

In the first third of the nineteenth century, when formal clinical training could not be said to exist outside that presumed in the preceptorial relationship, the dispensary helped fill an important pedagogical void. Not only could visiting and attending physicians themselves accumulate experience and reputation while more firmly establishing their private practice, but they could use their dispensary appointment as a means of providing case materials for their apprentices. Thus Benjamin Rush could recommend Drs. Wistar and Griffitts as preceptors since both held dispensary positions, "where a young man will see more practice in a month than with most private physicians in a year." Almost from the first years of the dispensaries, indeed, critics often charged that students and apprentices were allowed to treat the poor. (In Philadelphia, for example, such complaints found their way into newspapers as early as 1791.)[19] In the second quarter of the nineteenth century, as the preceptorial system grew less significant, the role of the dispensaries in clinical training grew even more prominent; mid-century medical schools vied actively in establishing dispensaries for the benefit of their students.

Most significantly, dispensary physicianships served as a step in the careers of elite physicians. Despite the complaints of articulate mid-century critics as to the wretched state of medical education and practice, even a cursory analysis of the profession's structure indicates the existence of a well-defined elite, largely urban, often European-trained, and almost always enjoying the benefits of hospital and dispensary experience. It was

18 For typical examples later in the century, see Central Dispensary and Emergency Hospital of the District of Columbia, *24th Annual Report... Including an Historical Sketch of the Institution* (Washington, 1894), pp. 8–10; Camden City Dispensary, *26th Annual Report, 1892–93* (Camden, N. J., 1893), pp. 6–9.

19 Rush to John Dickinson, October 4, 1791, *Letters of Benjamin Rush*, ed. by L. H. Butterfield (Princeton, N. J., 1951), I, 610; Philadelphia *Dunlap's American Daily Advertiser*, August 16, 18, 179; Minutes, Philadelphia Dispensary, August 26, 1791. See also [William Lawrence], *History of Boston Dispensary*, pp. 90–91, 98–99. Another dispensary noted at mid-century that they had "often been accused, as being rather the schools, where the young and inexperienced might find patients to their hands, than benevolent institutions where sufferings might be allayed and diseases cured." DeMilt Dispensary, *2nd Annual Report, 1852–53* (New York, 1853), p. 8.

just such ambitious young practitioners who served as dispensary visiting and attending physicians while they accumulated experience and gradually made the contacts so important to later success – contacts, it should be emphasized, with older, established physicians at least as much as with prospective patients.[20] (Prestigious and largely honorary consulting physicianships were normally reserved, in dispensaries as in hospitals, for a community's most influential and respected physicians.) Contemporaries never questioned the dispensary's teaching function. The trustees of the New York Dispensary admitted, for example, in 1854 that their institution served as "a practical school for physicians," but, they contended, it was a perfectly defensible policy: "for, by this system, these Physicians must become accomplished practitioners, by the time the growth of their private practice shall oblige them to resign their posts at the Dispensary."[21] With the growing importance of specialization as a prerequisite to intellectual status and economic success after mid-century, the increasingly specialized dispensaries served as *de facto* residency programs, allowing ambitious – and often well-connected – young men to accumulate experience and reputation. Though formal statements by medical spokesmen uniformly disowned "exclusive" specialism until long after the Civil War, devotion to a pragmatic specialism was established much earlier in America's cities. In 1839, for example, the editor of the *Boston Medical & Surgical Journal* remarked, in commenting on the specialty organization of New York's Northern Dispensary, that "such is manifestly the tendency in our times, in the great cities, and it is the only way of becoming eminently qualified for rendering the best professional services – to learn to do one thing as well as it can be done."[22]

If the dispensary made excellent sense in terms of the institutional needs of American medicine, it was equally consistent with the technological means available – both at the end of the eighteenth century, and through the first half of the nineteenth. Beyond the stethoscope – not routinely

---

20 Surviving archives of the Boston Dispensary, for example, indicate in letters of recommendation for district physicians the pattern we have suggested: The Bigelows, James Jackson, and Oliver Wendell Holmes recommend and are recommended. Successful candidates had frequently studied in Europe and the Tremont Medical School or served as house physicians at the Massachusetts General Hospital. See also James Jackson to Board of Managers, August 3, 1831; O. W. Holmes to William Gray, September 3, 1845; and letters in 1836 file from John Collins Warren, Jacob Bigelow, and George Hayward recommending O. W. Holmes as a visiting physician. BDA.

21 New York Dispensary, *Annual Report, 1854* (New York, 1855), p. 9. A year later, the same Dispensary contended that their staff members "in a few years, hope to be the eminent physicians of New York, and it is their right to expect, and of the community to require, that the unequaled advantages to be found here, should be freely offered them." New York Dispensary, *Annual Report, 1855* (New York, 1856), p. 10.

22 *Boston Medical & Surgical Journal* 20 (1839): 351.

applied before mid-century – no special aids to diagnosis were available to any physician, and no therapeutics beyond bleeding, cupping, and administration of drugs. Surgery was ordinarily limited, for rich and poor alike, to the treatment of lacerations and fractures, the reduction of occasional dislocations, and the lancing of boils and abscesses. Dispensaries seemed, for many decades into the nineteenth century, fully able to provide both adequate care for the poor and adequate training for their attendants.

The dispensaries seemed equally appropriate to the needs of a small and relatively homogeneous community. The world of the late eighteenth century assumed – even if it did not necessarily practice – face-to-face interaction between members of different social classes, interactions structured by customary relations of deference and stewardship. This social world-view is concretely illustrated in the acceptance by the dispensaries' founding generation of the contributor recommendation as basis for patient referrals. A certificate of recommendation was necessary, that is, before the dispensary would undertake treatment of a particular patient. This followed English hospital and dispensary practice. As the century progressed, however, the dispensaries which maintained the practice sometimes found it a cause of conflict between medical staff and lay managers. By-laws specified the privileges of recommendation accompanying each contributing membership; a typical arrangement was that in which a five-dollar annual subscription brought with it the right to recommend two patients at any one time during the year. A fifty-dollar subscription typically bought the same privilege for life. Similarly, early dispensary by-laws indicate that members of boards of managers were expected to play an active and often personal role; the New York Dispensary, for example, created a trustees' committee to accompany visiting physicians on their rounds once a month.[23]

Equally revelatory of the world-view shared by the pious and benevolent Americans who founded the dispensaries was their assumption that a crucial difference separated the dispensary from the hospital patient; the dispensary patients would be drawn from among the worthy poor, hard-working and able to support themselves except in periods of sickness or general unemployment. Such worthy poor might also include widows,

23 New York Dispensary, *Charter and By-Laws*... (New York, 1814), p. 8. Another indication of the social assumptions of the generation which created the dispensaries was their concern over whether servants and apprentices were appropriate patients. John Bard argued in New York that servants should indeed be treated, but not at their place of work – which would have compelled "gentlemen to visit the servants to families in which they had no acquaintance with the Masters or Mistresses." *A Letter from Dr. John Bard... to the Author of Thoughts on the Dispensary*... (New York, 1791), p. 20. See the entry for July 17, 1786, in the Minutes of the Philadelphia Dispensary for the question of the treating apprentices.

orphans, and the handicapped. The lying-in department of Philadelphia's Northern Dispensary declared in 1835, for example, that it could aid only married women of respectable character, "such as require no aid when in health." Financial support for the dispensary would, the argument followed, keep such honest folk from almshouse residence and from morally contaminating contact with those abandoned souls who were its natural inmates. Dispensary spokesmen tirelessly repeated these stylized categories by way of argument even as experience indicated that this neat and comforting ideological distinction failed to reflect reality. In 1830, a physician of the Boston Dispensary could complain indignantly that persons of the "most depraved and abandoned character frequently apply who think they have a right of choice between the Alms-House and the Dispensary." As late as 1869, the Philadelphia Dispensary could still explain that

> the principal object of this institution is to afford medical relief to the worthy (not the lowest class of) poor, in those cases where removal to a hospital would for any approved reason be ineligible. . . . In a thrifty population like our own, it is the exception . . . where removal to a hospital should be considered eligible.[24]

The dispensaries were founded and grew, finally, because they were entirely consistent with the assumptions of most Americans in regard to the responsibilities of government and the appropriate forms and functions of the public institutions which embodied such responsibilities. The prostitute, the drunkard, the lunatic, and the cripple were the city's responsibility – social subject matter for the almshouse or city physician. The dispensary, on the other hand, represented an appropriate response of humane and thoughtful Americans to the needs of hard-working fellow citizens, a response demanded both by Christian benevolence and community-oriented prudence; it was a form of social intervention, limited, conservative, and spiritually rewarding. In the second third of the nineteenth century, as demographic realities shifted inexorably, this traditional view still served to justify the now-expanded work of the dispensaries – and at the same time to avoid systematic analysis of the changing nature and social condition of the constituency they served. It was only very slowly, and only in the minds

---

24 Philadelphia Northern Dispensary, Philadelphia Lying-In Hospital, "Rules and Regulations, Adopted November 4, 1835," Historical Collections, College of Physicians of Philadelphia; [?] to Board of Managers, October 1, 1830, BDA; *Rules of the Philadelphia Dispensary with the Annual Report for 1869* (Philadelphia, 1870), p. 10. As late as 1879, the organizers of a specialized New York dispensary contended that they appealed to those patients able to pay a small fee and thus "saved the necessary associations of a public, free dispensary." *Report of the East Side Infirmary for Fistula and other Diseases of the Rectum* (New York, 1879), p. 5. See also Pitttsburgh Free Dispensary, *3rd Annual Report, 1875* (Pittsburgh, 1876), p. 9.

of a minority of those associated with dispensary work, that it became clear that many of their city's honest and industrious laboring men were unable to pay for medical care even in times of prosperity.

Dispensaries continued to change throughout the second half of the nineteenth century. We have already referred to their increase in numbers and degree of specialization. Equally significant was expansion of the dispensary form under new kinds of auspices. First, most urban – and even some small-town – medical schools anxious to compete for students established their own dispensaries so as to offer "clinical material" for their embryo physicians. Second, hospitals not only increased in number in the last third of the century, they also began to provide more outpatient care, in some localities duplicating services already offered by dispensaries. In Philadelphia with its flourishing medical schools the rivalry between hospitals and dispensaries emerged as early as 1845.[25] In certain areas outpatient facilities competed for patients, medical school clinics in particular advertising in newspapers and posting handbills. All these events were correlated, of course, with a growing demand within the medical profession for clinical training at every level, for the possession of attending and consulting physicianships, and for the accumulation of specialty credentials. At the end of the century, finally, a growing public health movement used the by now familiar dispensary form to shape and deliver medical care and would-be prophylactic measures in slum areas – most conspicuously in the identification and treatment of tuberculosis.

Underlying these developments were a series of parallel changes, first in the scale of the human problems the dispensaries faced, second in the intellectual tools and social organization of the medical profession. First in time came an absolute increase in the numbers and shift in the social origins of those urban Americans calling upon the dispensary. Second, in terms of chronology if not significance, were shifts within the world of medicine which made the dispensary increasingly marginal in the priorities of medical men. One need hardly demonstrate the significance to medical practice of increasing specialization, the germ theory and antisepsis, the development of modern surgery, x-ray, and clinical laboratory methods, and the increasing centrality of the hospital; the way in which demographic and social changes reshaped the dispensaries is perhaps less familiar.

Whatever degree of reality there had been in the original vision of a community bound by common ties of assumption and identity, this unifying vision corresponded less and less to reality as the nineteenth century progressed. The accustomed social distance between physician and charity patient seemed increasingly unbridgeable. A practical measure of this

25 Philadelphia Dispensary, Minutes, December 26, 1845, APH.

increasing social distance – and one which correlates with population and immigration statistics – was the growing disquietude of dispensary physicians in contemplating their patients. As early as 1828, New York's Northern Dispensary asked contributors to sympathize with their staff physicians'

> great sacrifices of feeling and comfort, which they must necessarily make, by being forced into daily and hourly association with the miserable and degraded of our species, loathsome from disease, and often still more so by those disgusting habits which go to the utter extinction of decency in all its forms.

The traditional system, in which would-be dispensary patients or their messengers, in seeking a recommendation, called first upon contributors and then upon visiting physicians at their regular homes or offices, also showed signs of strain. In Boston, where the dispensary's lay managers had long opposed the establishment of a "central office," a major factor helping to overcome this reluctance in the 1850s was the unwillingness of district physicians to have their offices used by so "ignorant and degraded a class." "It is undesirable," as Henry J. Bigelow explained it, "for most physicians to receive at their own apartments the class of applicants who now form the mass of dispensary patients."[26]

The patients who seemed most familiar, closest to the physicians' own experience, were those most capable of evoking sympathy and understanding. Thus the plight of those fallen in fortune, of the genteel widow, of the orphaned child of good parents, were those which touched visiting physicians most deeply.

> It is not infrequently that we witness much feeling manifested by those who have been able to employ their own physicians and purchase their own medicines, when through reverses of fortune they have for the first time applied for assistance from the Institution; such constitute the most interesting portion of our patients.[27]

26 Northern Dispensary [New York], *1st Annual Report, 1828* (New York, 1828), p. 10; DeMilt Dispensary, *2nd Annual Report, 1853* (New York, 1853), p. 12; Bigelow to D. D. Slade, August 22, 1855, BDA. Cf. D. D. Slade to My Dear Sir [William Lawrence], September, 3, 1855, BDA; [Lawrence], *History of the Boston Dispensary*, pp. 178–80.

27 Northern Dispensary [Philadelphia], *Annual Report, 1847* (Philadelphia, 1848), p. 10. Such sentiments were familiar ones. A "Contributor" to the Boston Dispensary explained in 1819 that its appropriate clients were those "many persons … who have been reduced from a state of competence to one little short of poverty, who while blessed with health, can, by industry, support themselves, but when attacked by sickness, and laid upon a bed of illness, find it imposible to pay the physician and apothecary." *New-England Palladium and Commerical Advertiser*, January 12, 1819. The earliest rules of both Philadelphia and Boston dispensaries emphasized their wish to comfort "those who have seen better days … without being humiliated." Boston Dispensary, *Institution of … 1817* (Boston, 1817), p. 7.

Other patients were far less interesting.

There were, of course, the venereal and alcoholic; but these had always existed and their existence had always implied a certain conflict between morals and medical care. Far more unsettling by the 1840s were the new immigrants who streamed into America's cities and soon constituted a disproportionate part of the dispensary's clientele. By the early 1850s it was not uncommon for an absolute majority of a particular institution's patients to have been born in Ireland; in the districts of individual visiting physicians over 90 percent of those treated might be foreign-born. Not surprisingly, the 1840s and 1850s saw dispensary administrators and trustees pointing again and again to the immigrant as they sought to explain the difficulties of their work and their ever-increasing financial need.[28]

It was not only the numbers and poverty, but the alienness of the immigrants which intensified the differences between them and their would-be medical attendants. It must be recalled that the desirability of dispensary appointments guaranteed their being filled by young physicians of at least middle-class background – thus insuring as well a maximum social distance between physician and patient. As early as 1831, for example, Boston Dispensary visiting physicians, dismayed by the conditions they encountered, elected to survey the economic and moral status of their patients. In that age of temperance and pietism, it was only to have been expected that the district physicians found intemperance to be the most important single cause of disease in their patients – and intemperance to be most common among the foreign-born. The Irish seemed particularly undesirable, filthy, drunken, generally inhospitable to middle-class standards of behavior. "Upon their habits – their mode of life," a dispensary physician explained in 1850, "depend the frequency and violence of disease. This I am fearful will continue to be the case, since no form of legislation can reach them, or force them to change their habits for those more conducive to cleanliness and health." "Deserving American poor," another Boston Dispensary physician complained, were "often deterred from seeking aid because they shrink from seeming to place themselves on a level with the degraded classes among the Irish."[29] The unfamiliar

28 In the New York Dispensary, for example, in 1853, of 7,188 patients treated, 1,582 were born in the United States and 4,886 in Ireland. At the Philadelphia Dispensary in 1857, 1,906 were born in the United States, 3,649 in Ireland. New York Dispensary, *64th Annual Report, 1853* (New York, 1854), p. 12; Philadelphia Dispensary, *Rules... with Annual Report for 1857* (Philadelphia, 1858), p. 14. Some dispensaries would not allow venereal cases to be treated, some imposed a special fee, while still others allowed individual physicians to decide whether they would treat such errant souls.

29 Luther Parks, Jr. to Board of Managers, June 10, 1850, Boston Dispensary Archives. On the temperance question, see, for example, J. B. S. Jackson to Board of Managers, October 8, 1853, BDA.

attitudes and habits of these patients often added to their troublesomeness; they ignored hygienic advice and often defied the physician's simplest requests. The Irish, for example, considered it dangerous to have lymph removed from the lesion of an individual vaccinated for smallpox; thus they refused to return to the dispensary after the required week to have the lesion checked (and to supply the lymph so useful in helping balance the dispensary's budget).[30] Later immigrant groups brought their peculiar beliefs and problems of communication; Jews and Italians replaced the Irish as objects of the dispensary physician's frustration and disdain.

A good many dispensary physicians were, of course, sympathetic to their patients, and in some cases not only sympathetic but convinced that environmental causes contributed to their clients' chronic ill health. Yet even those individual physicians whose personal convictions made them most sensitive to the deprivation of their city's slum dwellers shared the ambivalence and even hostility of their peers. The same mid-century physicians, that is, who denounced basement dwellings, exploitative landlords, rotting meat, and adulterated milk, shared a distaste for the intemperance, imprudence, filth, and apparent sexual immorality of those victimized by such conditions. One of the harsher dispensary critics of mid-century tenement conditions could, for example, contend that

> there is much squalor and other evidences of poverty which might be remedied had the patients more pride in cleanliness and more ambition to be doing well in the world.

As another mid-century physician explained, his patients' degradation and ignorance called "not for pity alone, but for the greatest exercise of patience and forbearance."[31]

A concern with social realities was, moreover, supported by and consistent with mid-nineteenth-century etiological assumptions. Both acute and constitutional ills were seen as related closely to an individual's powers of resistance – itself a product of interaction between constitution and environment. And the conditions encountered by dispensary physicians were exactly those which seemed to lower resistance and hence increase the incidence and virulence of disease. Thus a dispensary physician could

---

30 New York Dispensary, *64th Annual Report, 1853* (New York, 1854), p. 10; New York Dispensary, *72nd Annual Report, 1862* (1863), p. 20. When, in an effort to solve this problem, New York's dispensaries initiated a small deposit to be refunded when the patient returned to have the vaccination checked, these intractable – and seemingly ungrateful – patients chose to regard it as a payment absolving them of any responsibility to the institution.

31 J. Trenor, Jr., physician to middle district, Eastern Dispensary [New York], *25th Annual Report, 1858* (New York, 1859), p. 32; New York Dispensary, *Annual Report, 1837* (New York, 1838), p. 7.

note casually that scarlet fever was particularly virulent one year, since it proved as fatal to the rich as to the poor. Similarly, a pioneer ophthalmologist could urge the need for ophthalmological dispensaries because of the relationship between poverty and diseases of the eye:

> The sickly hue, and the toil worn features of these poor people are but the results of constitutional derangements . . . and as clearly reveal the inseparable union between the health of the body and the health of the eye, as between poverty and disease.

Throughout the century articulate dispensary spokesmen were aware of the need to provide food and clothing for their patients, convinced that medicines could be of only marginal help when patients had to return to work before their complete recovery, while their homes had no adequate heat, their tables only impure and decaying food. "No persons can more readily appreciate than we," as one put it, "the utter uselessness of drugs, if there is no possibility of nourishing and warming the patient."[32]

The attitudes of mid- and late nineteenth-century physicians can best be described in terms not of hostility, but of ambivalence – and perhaps most importantly an ambivalence characterized by a world-view which related disease and morals alike to general social conditions. Both morality and morbidity were seen as resultants of the interactions between environmental circumstance and culpable moral decisions. This mixture of social concern, moralism, meliorism, and deep-seated antipathy was clearly apparent by mid-century and marked the writings of most dispensary spokesmen until the end of the century; it could not prove the basis of a long-lived commitment to the dispensary and the necessity of its peculiar social function.

Nevertheless, a handful of articulate spokesmen for the dispensary did elaborate a characteristic point of view by the century's end, in which disease was seen not only as related inextricably to environment, but which emphasized the dispensary's capacity to reach out into the homes of the sick poor, so as to deal with problems more fundamental than the symptoms which brought the patient to their attention. The ability of the dispensary to relate to the community surrounding it became in the arguments of such dispensary defenders an indispensable aspect of a socially adequate medical care system. Visiting physicians and nurses could not be replaced by a hospital outpatient department. Advocates of this higher

---

32 Edward Reynolds, *An Address at the Dedication of the New Building of the Massachusetts Eye and Ear Infirmary, July 3, 1850* (Boston, 1850), p. 15; Mission Hospital and Dispensary for Women and Children, *2nd Annual Report, 1876* (Philadelphia, 1877), p. 10. The scarlet fever reference was by William Bibbins, DeMilt Dispensary, *6th Annual Report, 1856–57* (New York, 1857), p. 17.

dispensary calling argued again and again that one could not simply treat a patient's symptoms and do nothing about an environment which had much to do with causing those very symptoms. Such ideas were implemented perhaps most fully in the tuberculosis dispensaries established so widely in the first decade of the twentieth century.[33]

Such would-be rationalizers of American medicine as Edward Corwin, S. S. Goldwater, Richard Cabot, and Michael Davis contended that the dispensary could, in addition to supplying primary treatment for the indigent, supplement the necessarily unfinished work of the general practitioner in those numerous cases where the patient could not afford a specialist's consultation or expensive x-rays and laboratory tests. The dispensary could, that is, serve a vast urban constituency able perhaps to afford the services of a general practitioner but unable to manage the cost of more extended or elaborate medical care. And such occasions increased steadily as the profession's ability to understand and even cure increased. Yet even as they urged such prudent considerations, these advocates of social medicine were well aware of the threat posed to the independence and ultimately to the existence of the dispensary by rapid changes in medical ideas, techniques, and institutional forms.

These arguments were consistent as well with the motivations and social assumptions of the contemporary settlement house movement and other pioneer social welfare advocates. The settlement houses were often involved in dispensarylike programs themselves. But in a precisely timed irony, the dispensary as a viable independent institution was dying just as its most self-conscious advocates were formulating these brave contentions.

How did this come about? The dispensaries could hardly be said to have lost their social function; we have become quite conscious in recent years that their function is still not being adequately fulfilled. In retrospect, however, their dissolution was inevitable. By the 1920s, most significantly, the dispensary had become as marginal to the needs of the medical profession as it had been central in the first two-thirds of the nineteenth

33 For useful descriptions of the tuberculosis clinics, see, for example, F. Elisabeth Crowell, *The Work of New York's Tuberculosis Clinics*... (New York, 1910); Louis Hamman, "A Brief Report of the First Two Years' Work in the Phipps Dispensary for Tuberculosis of the Johns Hopkins Hospital," *Bull. Johns Hopkins Hosp.* 18 (1907): 293–297. For samples of the more positive defense of the dispensary and its appropriate role, see S. S. Goldwater, "Dispensary Ideals: With a Plan for Dispensary Reform...," *Am. J. Med. Sci.* n.s. 134 (1907): 313–335; Richard Cabot, "Why Should Hospitals Neglect the Care of Chronic Curable Disease in Out-Patients?" *St. Paul Med. J.* 10 (1908): 110–120; Cabot "Out-Patient Work. The Most Important and Most Neglected Part of Medical Service," *J. Am. Med. Assn.* 59 (1912): 1688–1689; Good Samaritan Dispensary [New York], *29th Annual Report, 1919* (New York, 1920), p. 8. The most complete statement of a positive dispensary program is to be found in Davis and Warner, *Dispensaries*.

century. A century of work in the city's slums, a growing – if always somewhat ambiguous – awareness of the relationship between health and environment, the conscious commitment of a small leadership group to the need for working in that human environment, all proved ultimately of little importance.

As hospital-centered intern and residency programs became a normal part of medical education – following inclusion of clinical training in the undergraduate years – it was inevitable that those elite physicians who would in earlier generations have been anxious to receive a dispensary appointment would now prefer hospital posts. Not only had hospitals increased greatly in number, but they contained beds, laboratory and x-ray facilities, and a cluster of appropriately trained specialists. The hospital's increasingly exclusive claims to practice the best, indeed the only adequate medicine, seemed to grow more and more plausible. When, for example, the Managers of the Philadelphia Dispensary decided in 1922 to merge with the Pennsylvania Hospital, they explained that they had "found it practically impossible for an independent dispensary, unassociated with the facilities and specialists of a large modern hospital, to render the public adequate service."[34]

As the intellectual and institutional aspects of medicine changed, economic pressures also pointed toward the centralized and capital-intensive logic of the hospital. Expensive laboratory facilities, x-ray units, modern operating rooms all demanded the investment of unprecedently large sums of money. The routine low-budget dosing which characterized the independent nineteenth-century dispensary seemed no longer a real option; dispensary boards had to face a growing and embarrassing asymmetry between their limited resources and the demands of high-quality medical care. The hospital outpatient department seemed to many medical men a substantial and inevitable improvement over its predecessor institution. The growing tendency in the twentieth century for medical schools to forge strong hospital ties only increased the centrality of the hospital.

Shorn of its relevance to the career needs of aspiring physicians, the dispensary was left with the clearly residual function of providing public health – charity – medical care, in itself a low-status occupation throughout

34 Philadelphia Dispensary, Minutes, January 8, 1923, APH. At the end of the nineteenth century, for example, the Boston Dispensary began a search for beds; it seemed a necessity if bright young men were to be kept on the staff. *Report of the Dinner given to the Board of Managers of the Boston Dispensary by the Staff of Physicians ... January 25th, 1909* (Boston, 1909), p. 13. Once allied with a hospital, the dispensary had invariably a lower status. Francis R. Packard charged in 1903 that hospitals would casually spend two or three hundred dollars for new surgical instruments yet balk at ten or fifteen for the dispensary. F. B. Kirkbride, *Dispensary Problem in Philadelphia*, p. 21.

the nineteenth century. Dispensary appointments had brought prestige and clinical opportunities in generations during which there were few other badges of status or roads to the acquisition of clinical skills; by the end of the century, there were other, more prestigious options for the ambitious young physician. Positions as municipal "outdoor physicians" had a comparatively low status throughout the nineteenth century. The dominion of fee-for-service medicine remained essentially unchallenged by the liberal critics of the Progressive generation. Those ambitious young men incapable of remaining content with the mere accumulation of fees were – as the twentieth century advanced – ordinarily attracted not by social medicine but increasingly by the "higher" and certainly less ambiguous demands of research; and even clinical investigation seemed in its most demanding forms to have little place in the dispensary.

If the dispensary had lost much of its appeal for the medical elite by the end of the nineteenth century, it had lost whatever goodwill it had had in the mind of the average practitioner decades earlier. There had always been occasional complaints in regard to the dispensaries intervening unfairly to compete with private physicians for a limited supply of paying patients. From the earliest years of their operation, American dispensaries had warned that their services were only for "such as are really necessitous." None however chose to investigate systematically the means of their patients until after the Civil War. Until the 1870s, criticism was comparatively muted; throughout the last third of the century, however, and into the twentieth, the dispensaries were widely attacked as purveyors of ill-considered charity to the unworthy. The more constructive critics sought to find alternatives, the most popular – besides simply demanding a small fee – being the provident dispensary, a species of prepaid health plan which had proven workable in some areas in England. In city after city, local practitioners called meetings and commissioned reports predictably concluding that a goodly portion of those using dispensary services were quite capable of paying a private physician's fees.[35] Americans found it difficult to understand the social configuration of the society in which they lived; only abuse by those in fact capable of paying medical bills could possibly

35 Probably most significant is the tone of this debate. It was the ordinary practitioner who generally resented the way in which dispensaries with their elite house staffs attracted cases which might otherwise have remained in the hands of private practitioners. Discussions of "dispensary abuse" also served to express the resentment of many practitioners against the monopolization of hospital and dispensary posts by a minority of well-connected physicians. In its report on charity abuse, for example, the Medical Association of the District of Columbia also urged limited tenure in hospital staff appointments and access to hospital privileges for all "reputable members of the profession." *Report of the Special Committee ... on the Hospital and Dispensary Abuse in the City of Washington* (Washington, 1896), pp. 15–16.

explain the vast numbers who utilized dispensary services. To doubt this was to assume that large numbers of worthy and hard-working Americans were indeed too poor to pay for even minimally adequate medical care.[36]

Physicians were often unwilling to refer their paying patients – even if the payment were only twenty-five or fifty cents – to the more specialized facilities of neighboring dispensaries. As late as 1914 the director of Pennsylvania's tuberculosis program charged that local practitioners refused to refer patients in the early stages of the disease, unwilling to relinquish treatment until such working people were too deteriorated to work – and pay. Attacks on the dispensary system were generally supported as well by the charity organization movement which, in city after city, attacked dispensary medicine as an excellent example of that undiscriminating alms-giving which served only to demoralize its recipients. (It should be noted that the majority of empirical studies of dispensary patients completed between the 1870s and the First World War indicated that most dispensary patients were not in fact able to pay for medical care.)[37]

By the last quarter of the nineteenth century the dispensary patient no longer fit into that same vision of an ordered social universe which had guided and inspired the efforts of those benevolent Americans who had founded the first dispensaries a century earlier. Those older views of community and stewardship implied in the contributor-sponsorship system had faded by mid-century, paralleling changes in the scale and social composition of America's older cities. Similarly, it would have been hardly plausible to argue that New York or Boston tenement dwellers should be visited in their homes so as to spare them the indignity of hospitalization. The constituency of both hospital and dispensary had changed. By the closing years of the nineteenth century, the dispensary had very clearly become the provider of charity medicine for a class who – if indeed worthy of such charity – were sharply differentiated from paying patients and who ordinarily lived in a section of the city removed physically from that of contributors, physicians, and private patients. Before mid-century and especially in the first quarter of the nineteenth century, dispensary managers still sought to enforce requirements that visiting physicians actually reside in the district they served – a natural enough sentiment in the eighteenth century but impracticable in postbellum America.[38] The arguments em-

---

36 [William Lawrence], *Medical Relief of the Poor. September, 1877* (Boston, 1877), pp. 3–4; James Keiser, "The Abuses in Hospital and Dispensary Practice in Reading," *National Hospital Record,* 1899.

37 Albert P. Francine, "The State Tuberculosis Dispensaries," *Penn. Med. Journ.* 17 (1914): 940. See Davis and Warner, *Dispensaries,* pp. 42–58 for a brief discussion of patient eligibility.

38 G. F. Thayer to William Gray, April 12, 1838, BDA.

ployed by the end of the century to attract contributions had become almost exclusively prudential, appealing little either to explicitly religious convictions or to a feeling of identity with those at risk. Fund-raising circulars emphasized instead the need to avert crime, pauperism, and prostitution.

Positive support for the dispensaries was, on the other hand, shaky indeed; aside from the support implicit in the inertia developed by all institutions, only a small group of socially active physicians and proto-social-welfare activists defended the dispensaries as a positive good. Many social workers, as we have indicated, evinced little affection for an institution which seemed to embody so casual and unscientific an approach to philanthropy. Even the oldest dispensaries did not survive as independent institutions past the early 1920s.

Historians have devoted little attention to the dispensary. Yet as our contemporaries begin to concern themselves with the delivery of medical care this neglect may end; for the dispensary provides such would-be reformers with a potentially usable past. The dispensary did at first provide a flexible, informal, and locally oriented framework for the delivery of public medicine. But the analogy to contemporary problems is limited; the flexibility and informality of the dispensary were a result of medicine's still primitive tools, its local orientation a consequence of the contributors being in some sense – or assuming themselves to be – part of the community served by the dispensary. Such conditions ceased to exist well before the end of the nineteenth century. And even within its own frame of reference, the nineteenth-century dispensary provided second-class, routine, episodic medicine, was a victim of shabby budgets, and even in its earliest decades was marked by unquestioned distance between physician and patient. (A distance *perhaps* made tolerable by traditional attitudes of hierarchy and deference.)

Yet despite these imperfections, the death of the dispensary and the transfer of its functions and client constituency to general hospitals have not been an unqualified success. And though the history of the rise and fall of the dispensary provides no explicit program for contemporary medicine, it does have a simple moral: any plan for the reordering of medical care must be based on the accommodation of at least three different factors. The first is felt social need, felt, that is, by those with power to change social policy. A second factor is general social values and assumptions as they shape the world-view and thus help define the options available to such decision-makers. Third, there are the needs of the medical profession, needs expressed in the career decisions of particular physicians and needs defined by medicine's intellectual tools and institutional forms. Without a strong commitment to government intervention in health matters – a commitment impossible without an appropriate change in general social values – factors internal to the world of medicine have determined most forcefully the specific forms in which medical care has been provided for the American people. Thus the rise and fall of the dispensary; it was doomed neither by policy nor by conspiracy but by a steadily shifting configuration of medical perceptions and priorities.

9

From almshouse to hospital: The shaping of Philadelphia General Hospital

❧ The distinction between public and private philanthropy, means tested and universal aid, stigmatizing as opposed to nonstigmatizing government expenditure is as old as the history of social welfare itself in North America. And it characterizes the gratuitous provision of medical care just as it does any other aspect of public welfare. We see it at the end of the twentieth century in the distinction between medicare and medicaid; in an earlier period Americans experienced it in the distinction between almshouse (later municipal hospital) and voluntary hospital care. The problems that created the need for our earliest hospitals – poverty, trauma, and chronic disease – have not gone away and our modes of responding to them are still marked by traditional attitudes and assumptions, most significantly, the distinction between "worthy" and "unworthy" recipients of public benevolence. In American welfare policy at least, the more things change the more they seem to stay the same.

This continuity is demonstrated with unmistakable clarity in the following case study of Philadelphia's now-deceased public hospital. In formal terms, the Philadelphia General Hospital evolved from its beginnings as one aspect of the aid provided in an almshouse – an undifferentiated facility in which all those Philadelphians unable to provide for themselves received minimum care. In the course of the nineteenth-century, the almshouse's medical wards gradually evolved into a hospital in name and bureaucratic identity. But not even in the twentieth century has Philadelphia General ever been precisely the same sort of institution as its not-for-profit peers. The seeming victory of medicine in redefining the almshouse's hospital function only masked its continued, and stigmatizing, identity as a welfare institution. The burden of poverty and chronic illness that had always constituted its defining social burden remained to distinguish it from the great majority of the city's private hospitals. ❧

In 1932, the Philadelphia General Hospital proudly celebrated its bicentennial. David Riesman, chairman of the hospital's medical board and a principal speaker on this occasion, was certain that despite the Depression and its threat to traditional medical care patterns,

> in the coming realignment of all the forces making for better health the public hospital will occupy a central position, a position of far greater importance than in the past. The New Philadelphia General Hospital aided by a progressive staff and a liberal municipality will take its rightful place in the coming era.[1]

This was no mere effusion of parochial loyalty. The Philadelphia General was not simply a very old institution, it could make a strong claim to being America's first hospital, and by the 1930s had attained an international reputation for clinical teaching and research. Nevertheless, its history after the Second World War – like that of many other municipal hospitals – grew increasingly bleak; and in 1976 Philadelphia announced plans to close its municipal hospital. It succumbed with surprisingly little public protest. To many observers, the hospital's demise seemed only a particularly dramatic but entirely representative symptom of a more general decay in the quality of public medicine in America's older cities.

The story of Philadelphia General is, in some ways, a bit atypical – it was larger than most municipal hospitals, more prestigious clinically, and founded earlier than almost all – but in other ways it was characteristic. Our older municipal hospitals all developed as welfare institutions, many, like Philadelphia General or New York's Bellevue, out of one aspect of a city's almshouse. The gradual differentiation of such municipal welfare mechanisms into a half-dozen successor functions and agencies was a complex and ambiguous process; the municipal hospital cannot be understood without a more general understanding of that elusive and in some ways still incomplete evolution.

By the first decades of the nineteenth century, every American city had established an almshouse; the larger the city, the greater the number of rootless and dependent who were its natural clients. "I visited the almshouse today," a young Bostonian reported from Philadelphia in 1806, "where I saw more collective misery than ever before met my eye."[2] The internal makeup of the almshouse inevitably reflected the diversity of misfortunes afflicting its clients. One set of wards housed the chronic unemployed (and often unemployable), another "old men" and "old

---

1 D. Riesman, "How the New Blockley Came into Being," *Medical Life* 40 (1933): 137–148.
2 G. C. Shattuck to R. Shirtleff, November 10, 1806. Shattuck Family Papers, Massachusetts Historical Society.

women," and others the sick, the delinquent, the minor dependent, the crippled and blind, and the mentally incompetent. During the eighteenth century, in the larger cities such as New York or Philadelphia, special wards were assigned to the sick and physicians engaged to care for these unfortunates; by the 1820s, almshouse populations were in practice selected more by sickness than by any other single factor – other than dependence itself.[3]

Doctors, of course, were anxious to enlarge their opportunities to teach and learn – and thus eager to staff these institutions. In Boston, for example, such almshouse beds provided the only institutional medicine in the years before the Massachusetts General Hospital accepted its first patients in 1821; in Charleston, the almshouse served the same function until the 1850s, when the city's Roper Hospital opened its doors.[4] Even in smaller communities such as Salem, Massachusetts, or Richmond, Virginia, aspiring physicians were happy to serve as almshouse visitors. At no time was public medicine not related to medical careers – and at no time was it easily distinguishable from the more pervasive problem of dependency and the values associated with it.

In the following pages I have chosen to emphasize the history of Philadelphia's municipal hospital, partly because its records are uniquely complete, partly because it was important and influential, and most importantly because its problems were representative. Each of our older cities constituted a somewhat different social environment and elaborated a similarly distinct history of policy decisions. Boston, New York, Baltimore, Philadelphia, and Chicago, for example, were all to arrive at somewhat different institutional solutions to their need for a municipal hospital; yet just as many of the older British workhouse hospitals are still identifiable in the National Health Service, none of America's older city hospitals could entirely erase the marks of their almshouse ancestry.

An old institution in a New World

As early as the first years of the nineteenth century, the sick wards in Philadelphia's almshouse were the city's most important hospital facility; this reality did not change throughout the century. As late as 1894, the

3 J. K. Alexander, "Philadelphia's 'Other Half': Attitudes toward Poverty and the Meaning of Poverty in Philadelphia, 1760–1800" (unpublished Ph.D. diss., University of Chicago, 1973); S. E. Wiberley, "Four Cities: Public Poor Relief in Urban America, 1700–1775" (unpublished Ph.D. diss., Yale University, 1975).
4 N. I. Bowditch, *A History of the Massachusetts General Hospital*, 2d ed. (Boston: Trustees of the Massachusetts General Hospital, 1872); J. I. Waring, *A History of Medicine in South Carolina, 1825–1900* (Charleston: South Carolina Medical Association, 1967).

Philadelphia General Hospital treated as many patients at one time as all the city's other flourishing hospitals put together.[5] In the first decade of the century, the almshouse averaged some 200 occupied "sick" beds, while the Pennsylvania Hospital cared for no more than thirty to sixty at any one time. In the years between 1804 and 1811, the almshouse admitted some 1,300 to 2,100 hospital patients each year – and its lay administrators were understandably resentful that their more socially elevated competitor continued to receive state aid, while the almshouse was ignored. Although its hospital function was somewhat obscured by other responsibilities, Philadelphia's almshouse was by the 1820s very largely a hospital. In 1821 the institution had fifteen wards for adult females; this had increased to eighteen by 1826. Three were for women well enough to work and two were for vagrants; the rest were all medical wards. There were nineteen wards for adult men in 1826 – and of these, only three were for inmates well enough to work regularly.[6]

The almshouse not only treated what were for the time enormous numbers of patients, but these patients were also drawn overwhelmingly from among those Philadelphians without roots in the community and from groups sharply divergent from the Quakers and Episcopalians who dominated so much of the city's business and philanthropic life. In an 1807 census of the almshouse, more than half of its inmates were immigrants (71 percent of the male and 58 percent of the female patients).[7] This was typical of almshouse inmates; in 1796 only 102 of New York City's 622 almshouse residents were American-born.[8] The Philadelphia almshouse population remained overwhelmingly poor and disproportionately alien; a census of 1821 showed that 43 percent of the inmates were foreign-born; in 1840–1841 the figure was 46 percent and a decade later it had risen to 68 percent.[9]

Even by contemporary standards, almshouse conditions were brutal and

5 Philadelphia General Hospital, *Annual Report for 1894* (1895), p. 70. The *Annual Report* is hereafter cited as *AR* followed by the year covered in the report; the reports were always published in the following calendar year.

6 P. S. Clement, "The Response to Need: Welfare and Poverty in Philadelphia, 1800–1850" (unpublished Ph.D. diss., University of Pennsylvania, 1977); W. H. Williams, *America's First Hospital: The Pennsylvania Hospital, 1751–1841* (Wayne, Pa.: Haverford House, 1976).

7 *Philadelphia Almshouse Census for 1807*, Philadelphia City Archives. Archival materials from this repository are hereafter cited in brief form. For a complete description of materials relating to Philadelphia General Hospital, see the appropriate sections in John Daley, *Descriptive Inventory of the Archives of the City and County of Philadelphia* (Philadelphia: City of Philadelphia, 1970).

8 R. J. Carlisle, *An Account of Bellevue Hospital with a Catalogue of the Medical and Surgical Staff from 1736 to 1894* (New York: Society of the Alumni of Bellevue Hospital, 1893).

9 P. S. Clement, "The Response to Need."

the distance between patients and their physicians was vast. The minutes of Philadelphia's late-eighteenth-century Overseers of the Poor underline these particular realities. On January 20, 1797, the Overseers noted that a patient had been sent to the Pennsylvania Hospital "at the charge of this Institution with a broken jaw occasioned by a stroke from Dr. C." The costs implied a dilemma. "Quere? Ought Dr. C not be prosecuted as it is thought he is liable for all damages?" Some months earlier, the Overseers could reflect with some whimsy on the fate of "John R.*** noted dirty worthless customer, noted as a tender or waiter among the Fish sellers, etc. etc. and also among the dirty hussies by the name of 'Cock Robin' and they have now cooked him up indeed or fully and fowly done him over, he being highly venereal."[10] This was indeed a personal stewardship exerted by the Overseers of the Poor, but one rather less pious than that exerted by the Quaker Board of Managers at the Pennsylvania Hospital; "Cock Robin" would never have been admitted to the board and care provided at that private institution.

Admission to an almshouse ward – even for unavoidable illness or injury – was a confession of failure. For both the institution's internal order and its process of recruitment mirrored closely the values and relationships that reigned outside its walls. Most significant was the unavoidable blurring of the distinction between sickness and dependence, for in fact the primary requirement for admission to an almshouse ward was dependence, not some particular diagnosis. Those Philadelphians who could be treated at home obviously preferred such outpatient care to the stigmatization of becoming an "inmate" (the term was used into the present century) in an almshouse. It was at once refuge and punishment for the morally and physically incapacitated, for the alcoholic and the diseased prostitute or sailor, as well as for the longshoreman or teamster who might have been injured at work.

In the categories of popular social understanding, hard-working and churchgoing citizens did not belong in the company of paupers, prostitutes, alcoholics, and the dependent generally; indeed, a significant motivation in the founding of private hospitals and dispensaries was that very desire to maintain a distinction between the hard-working worthy poor and the almshouse's appropriate pauper residents.[11] Philadelphia's Overseers of the Poor supported the work of "outdoor physicians" partially at least in the hope that their home-visiting would serve to keep their patients outside the morally debilitating walls of the almshouse. In practice, of

10 R. J. Hunter, *The Origin of the Philadelphia General Hospital. Blockley Division* (Philadelphia: Rittenhouse Press, 1955).
11 C. E. Rosenberg, "Social Class and Medical Care in Nineteenth-Century America: The Rise and Fall of the Dispensary," Chapter 8 of this volume.

course, there was often nowhere else for them to go. Private hospital beds were limited in number throughout the antebellum years and hedged in by admission rules that excluded many potential patients – the chronic and incurable, children, sufferers from contagious ills. And in the first half of the century especially, private hospitals in effect excluded those without a place in the community's structure of deference. It was no more than fair for the city's Guardians of the Poor to characterize the Pennsylvania Hospital in 1804 as "shut against the poor."[12]

The difficulty of distinguishing the dependent from the sick, the unworthy from the worthy recipient of public assistance, remained as ill-defined within the almshouse itself as it was in shaping admission to it. Were the occupants of the "old ladies" ward dependent or sick? Should they be considered a part of the hospital or of the *outwards*, the term used to describe that portion of the institution assigned to paupers well enough to work? The decision was determined as much by the accident of circumstances as by the application of clear and universal criteria. If hospital beds were crowded, the sicker among the old people would of necessity be treated in the outwards; if beds became available, the same people might be removed to the hospital. As medical men were all too aware throughout the century, no neat distinction could be made between such cases. Late in 1884, for example, the Board of Guardians Hospital Committee resolved that all persons occupying beds in the hospital who no longer needed care be removed if they were not serving as nurses; a month later, the crowding had not abated and the hospital's resident was instructed to move certain chronic and semichronic patients (such as those suffering from superficial ulcers) to the outwards. It was only natural that house officers should have protested against the recurring need to treat acute cases in the outwards.[13] Chronic illness and geriatric debility remained the peculiar burden of the municipal hospital; it was a reality that no increase in medical sophistication and autonomy could solve. Indeed, as the voluntary hospitals came to define themselves in terms of acute illness and timely therapeutic intervention, the role of chronic ailments grew only the more prominent in municipal hospitals.

Another characteristic difficulty for the municipal hospital lay in the distribution of authority. What were to be the respective roles of layperson and physician? Were physicians or public officials to dominate the hospital's internal order? The relationship between a politically appointed governing board and the physicians who did their bidding was almost certain to be a

---

12 Williams, *America's First Hospital.*
13 Minutes of the Hospital Committee of the Board of Guardians, December 12, 1884; January 16, 1885.

stormier one than that between the trustees of voluntary hospitals and their appointed medical staffs. The social ties between lay board and medical board were more likely to be close at the voluntary hospitals. Lay members of municipal hospital governing boards were – from early in the century – men of a rather different sort. Though the mechanisms through which such positions were filled varied, board members tended to have much closer ties to Philadelphia's political process and to be men of lower social status than those who served the Pennsylvania or Episcopal or later the University Hospital. As we shall emphasize, the last third of the nineteenth century was a period that saw a steadily increasing role for medical men and medical needs in the municipal hospital; nevertheless, the values and priorities of the medical world were never entirely to shape the wards of a Philadelphia General or a Bellevue Hospital. The almshouse heritage and the very magnitude of the need that filled their wards guaranteed that an enormous gap should separate private and public hospitals in our older cities.

The almshouse heritage: A society writ small

Like any social institution, the Philadelphia almshouse-hospital was obviously a microcosm of the social values, structures, and careers which characterized the larger society outside it. Perhaps the most important and unavoidable reality was the public image enjoyed by the institution; despite the fact that it had been in function and fact essentially a hospital throughout the century, it never occupied that morally neutral niche in the public mind. The hospital's resident physician made precisely that argument in 1856 when he emphasized that the so-called almshouse included within itself a smallpox hospital, a lunatic asylum, a children's asylum, a lying-in department, a nursery, a hospital for medical and surgical cases, and wards for venereal and alcoholic cases "besides the Almshouse properly so called which is in reality an infirmary for the blind, the lame, the superannuated, and other incurables so decrepit as not to be able to earn for themselves a livelihood." The number of able-bodied, he continued, was in reality quite small and consisted largely of the casual criminal and vagrant who alternated between prison, almshouse, and "low dens of vice"; it was their presence, he concluded, that brought a stigma upon the sick and unfortunate, "which would not attach to them if this place was in name, and, in the opinion of many in the community, what it is in reality, a hospital."[14]

Though the almshouse did not formally subscribe to the principle of less eligibility – a widely accepted policy which dictated that conditions within

14 C. Lawrence, *History of the Philadelphia Almshouses and Hospitals* (Philadelphia, 1905).

the almshouse for the well pauper always be less desirable than those he or she might find outside – its governors were still committed to the need for providing, and demanding, work from those able to perform it. Thus surgical patients were expected to pick oakum as soon as they were well enough to walk to the "Manufactory."[15] The most frequent form of work, however, was as nurse, or "assistant" in the hospital and asylum. In 1849, the Board of Guardians stated that of 756 male paupers in the house, 449 were hospital patients and 67 were employed as nurses; it left comparatively few of the "able-bodied" for whom "useful employment" had to be found.[16] And, in fact, several years earlier the board had closed their "House of Employment," sold the machinery on which inmates had worked, and converted the building into more hospital space. And, as we shall emphasize, even those inmates capable of some small amount of work were in many cases able-bodied only by the kindest of definitions.

Patient population

Not surprisingly, average lengths of stay were always longer in Blockley (as the almshouse came to be called after it moved in 1834 to a then rural area in West Philadelphia bearing that name) than in its private peers. Similarly, death rates continued to be high throughout the nineteenth century and into the twentieth; the municipal hospital was always the recipient of those cases for which neither recovery nor remission could be hoped. Similarly a far greater number of male than female patients filled its wards – and among the males a disproportionate number were single or widowers. A man with a place in the community would not ordinarily have found his way into the almshouse unless the victim of a lengthy and debilitating illness or old age itself. Such considerations applied even more strongly to women; it was disgraceful to allow a mother or sister, or even a domestic servant, to enter a hospital or almshouse. As late as 1879, a house officer noted that "nearly all the fracture cases in the house at the present time are old maids, no doubt due to the fact that when one of these unfortunate beings meets with such an accident her kin are anxious to get rid of her, while if a mother or wife is so unfortunate, her husband or child will take care of her at home."[17]

15 Minutes of the Hospital Committee, June 29, 1842.
16 Philadelphia Guardians for the Relief and Employment of the Poor, *The Reply of the Guardians of the Relief and Employment of the Poor...*, *to Certain Remarks made in their Presentments by the Grand Inquests Inquiring for the County of Philadelphia for February and April Sessions 1849* (Philadelphia: Crissy & Markley, 1849).
17 E. M. Flick, *Beloved Crusader: Lawrence F. Flick, Physician* (Philadelphia: Dorrance, 1944).

Long convalescences and a large proportion of "old men and women" increased the difficulty of distinguishing in practice between the recipients of care in the hospital and alms in the institution's outwards. The hospital's clerk noted in 1864, for example, that a good many patients had actually been treated in the outwards, "especially upon the female side, where many of the old women are so comfortable, that it is with great difficulty that they can be prevailed upon to go to the hospital." Such practices, the same officer noted four years later, were almost unavoidable for there was often an inadequate number of acute beds in the hospital. And the distinction between acute and chronic was sometimes as difficult to apply in practice as that between the sick and the simply debilitated; a decade later, the Board of Guardians' Hospital Committee was warning its medical staff not to treat acute diseases in the outwards for longer than thirty-six hours.[18]

Many almshouse patients were "regulars," readmitted again and again before ending their days in its wards. John Miller, for example, a Scottish-born fifty-year-old blacksmith died and was autopsied in the almshouse in 1864. Miller was described as intemperate. His health had been good until mid-1862 when he was admitted with cramps in his legs which he attributed to a "debauch" and sleeping outdoors. Four months after that he was admitted again as a drunkard and sent this time to the drunkards' ward instead of to male medical. He was then transferred to medical to be treated for a cough that hinted at incipient tuberculosis. In the spring he was sent to the male outwards where he assisted in making iron bedsteads. In August he left the house "on liberty," but returned in early October complaining of a severe pain in his leg. The limb became livid and Miller died a few weeks later.[19] Only the comparative rapidity of Miller's physical deterioration set him apart; otherwise his life was typical of that of the working men who filled so large a proportion of Blockley's beds.

Admissions, significantly, had to be certified by an agent of the Board of Guardians; only when the patient entered the almshouse did its medical staff play a role in assigning him or her to an available (and if possible appropriate) ward. Discharge perhaps even more than admissions incorporated social as well as biological dimensions. In mid-century, for example, hospital patients who were not natives of Philadelphia were often discharged with fare sufficient to return them to their place of birth or previous residence; prostitutes were ideally discharged into the hands of an employer or a society for the reform of "fallen women". Illegitimate children and their mothers might not be discharged until an effort had been made to find the financially responsible father.

18 *AR for 1864*, p. 42; *AR for 1868*, p. 52; Minutes of the Hospital Committee, March 1, 1878.
19 Casebook, Male Medical, 1864–1869, p. 5.

Such realities changed only in detail during the course of the century. In 1883, for example, the obstetric staff recommended that women be allowed to stay only three months after confinement. The children treated at the children's asylum were in practice the residue of orphans and chronic cases who could not be placed in an appropriate home; they were, in the words of the "children's visitor" in 1884, "deformed, crippled, diseased eyes, nervous, etc. These children are not acceptable or desired as boarders at private homes, nor, indeed, could they get, in private homes, the constant nursing and medical care which they receive in the Children's Asylum."[20] Were these children a medical or a welfare problem? To phrase the question is to admit its meaninglessness. Such problems could not easily be solved. As late as 1898, for example, one duty of the nurse in the venereal ward was to make sure that discharged patients were issued shoes.[21] It was difficult indeed to apply strictly medical criteria to any stage of the patient's experience – admission, care, or discharge.

Within Blockley, of course, factors other than the biological or the narrowly economic also helped shape an inmate's experience. The deviant and the low in status – prostitutes, alcoholics, blacks, and the aged – fared particularly badly even in an institutional context in which no one fared particularly well. And all inmates, including nurses, servants, assistant nurses, and house officers, were subjected to a paternalistic discipline throughout the century, one that mirrored more general assumptions about the appropriate responsibilities of the several social classes.

Female venereal cases were a particular thorn in the sides of generations of administrators and physicians. Almost all, of course, were prostitutes and their incarceration was as much penal as therapeutic. They were made to work whenever possible, and the resident physicians were given special powers to discipline these bawdy and unremorseful objects of municipal benevolence. Their diet was almost invariably worse than that of other medical patients; in the 1820s, indeed, it was explicitly ordered that they be fed the same diet as that offered healthy paupers, one designed explicitly to discourage extended almshouse stays. This double standard continued throughout the century. In dress, in freedom of movement, even in the right to borrow library books, venereal patients found themselves treated very differently from their fellow patients with less stigmatizing ills. Visitors were always carefully limited – in part as an aspect of the ward's punitive character, in part because of the fear that prostitutes might seek to ply their trade on a retail basis within the hospital's walls. Venereal patients at the end of the century were assigned blue bedspreads while all the other

20 *AR for 1884*, p. 20.
21 C. G. Dalbey to G. O. Meigs, July 11, 1898, chief resident's letterpress copybook, p. 438.

patients were issued white spreads. Employees working in the venereal wards were asked, moreover, to change their clothes before eating in the staff dining room.[22]

Even within the venereal wards, physicians worried constantly about the need to maintain moral distinctions. One of the great problems, as contemporaries saw it, in both venereal and lying-in wards was the danger of contaminating erring but still salvageable females. In 1865, Blockley's clerk recommended that the female venereal ward be divided into two,

> one for abandoned characters, the other for those admitted the first time, many of whom show a willingness to reform; and if the immoral and debasing influence of those who are almost continual residents of the ward could be prevented, a small proportion, at least, might become useful members of society.[23]

A decade later, a prominent physician demanded a similar division in the lying-in wards. "Lying-in hospitals," he conceded, "are never schools of virtue, but if their inmates leave them morally worse than when they entered, we are bound to ask whether this sad result could not be prevented by some practicable change."[24]

At Blockley one of the amenities offered even the most humble was racial segregation; even paupers, it was assumed, deserved to be segregated by race and sex. (Revealingly, this was true for all but venereal patients.) Black patients were always present in nineteenth-century Blockley (and often in numbers greater than their proportion in the population), and routinely occupied the least desirable wards. In 1846, for example, when the hospital needed more bed space for "lunatics," patients were removed from the black male medical ward to the attic.[25] The attics were, of course, the most unpleasant part of the institution, cold in the winter and stiflingly hot in the summer. A generation later, the "colored wards" were still in the attic. "Those wards are unfit for the care of any sick people," a reformist member of the Board of Guardians charged in 1873,

> but they are used solely for the reason that there is no other room for them; every other available spot being occupied. . . . The house was not built with the intention of having the attics used for wards, conse-

22 Minutes of the Hospital Committee, August 12, 1859, and January 22, 1886; Memorandum, acting chief resident, October 27, 1902, chief resident's memorandum book, p. 93.

23 *AR for 1865*, p. 50.

24 I. Ray, *Social Science Association of Philadelphia. Papers of 1873. What Shall Philadelphia do for its Paupers? Read March 27, 1873* (Philadelphia: The Association, 1873; also in *Pennsylvania Magazine*, April, 1873).

25 Minutes of the Hospital Committee, January 28, 1846; Clement, "The Response to Need."

quently they were not furnished with flues for the admission of hot air from the furnaces.

A medical man added that the ward was not over twenty feet wide and the ceiling no more than eight feet in height, the beds were crowded closely together, and inadequate ventilation was provided by several windows two feet long and eighteen inches high.[26] But given the social assumptions of most nineteenth-century Americans (even in Quaker-influenced Philadelphia) such segregation was only to have been expected.

The treatment of alcoholics needs even more explanation, for they occupied a gray area between that of the legitimately (morally neutral) sick and that occupied by the culpable offender. True, the alcoholic might not be immediately responsible for his actions – even for the delirium tremens so dangerous to himself and destructive to hospital routine – but he was ultimately responsible for the decision to drink, which over time brought about his addiction. And alcoholics were ordinarily brought in by the police or committed by magistrates; in an administrative sense they were inmates indeed. Most of the inhabitants of the "men's drunkards ward" (as it was called in official reports) were diagnosed simply as "debauch"; in 1873, 530 of 585 were so diagnosed, and a year later 440 of 457. Only the handful of patients diagnosed as suffering from delirium tremens were actively treated. Within the hospital, they were at first placed in cells with a keeper, not a nurse. Only in 1848 did the Board of Guardians' Hospital Committee vote to change the name of drunkards' "cells" to "wards"; a year later they resolved that these wards were now part of the hospital and no longer part of the outwards, and the keeper's duties were to be performed by a nurse and an assistant nurse.[27] The location of these wards and the activities that went on in them had not changed, but had begun to be viewed in a new framework of perception. The alcoholic's dilemma was physiological as well as moral; no medical man doubted, no matter what the drinker's original responsibility, that delirium tremens could and often did kill, and was especially dangerous to inmates thrown untreated and unattended into cells to sober up.

In Blockley, and in every other nineteenth-century municipal hospital, discipline was tenaciously sought. As late as 1896, an editorialist reminded readers that "a difficult and discontented class in the community is being cared for" in public institutions, and "discipline is so absolutely necessary to the success of management."[28] In antebellum Blockley, patients con-

---

26 Ray, *Social Science Association of Philadelphia.*

27 *AR for 1873*, p. 69; *AR for 1874*, p. 57; Minutes of the Hospital Committee, September 29, 1848; April 20, 1849.

28 "Boston Public Institutions" (editorial), *Boston Medical & Surgical Journal* 135 (1896): 422.

fronted a wide variety of rules and punishments. The *Rules* of 1822 specified, for example, that paupers who failed to work or who acted in a disorderly or disrespectful manner could be placed in the lunatic cells and fed on bread and water. Through the middle third of the century, unruly inmates could be placed in punishment cells, be given forcible cold showers, and have their normal diet curtailed. In December of 1846, for example, the Hospital Committee of the board ruled that Caleb Butler

> be kept in the cells on Bread and Water for 48 hours, and soon as the Physician in Chief says his health will permit, he is to receive one shower bath per day for one week, and two Shower Baths per day for two weeks – Making 3 weeks – Subject to the Order of the Physician in Chief.[29]

The Hospital Committee had to be careful indeed in seeking to oversee such punishments, for house officers seem often to have preferred a casual blow. Many of the hospital patients were ambulatory and their movements had to be carefully controlled; passes had to be obtained before a patient or nurse could go on "liberty" and harsh punishments awaited those late in returning. Patient mobility within the institution had to be carefully constrained as well. The separation of male and female patients was a particularly difficult problem; gates between the male and female wards tended not to stay closed and blinds had to be placed on the windows of the men's wards to keep patients from conversing with their female counterparts.

Perhaps the most fundamental aspect of discipline was the work – often meaningless and repetitive – that all but the most debilitated were expected to perform. As Blockley's steward explained it in 1875, the work was not only valuable to the institutions in a period of lean budgets, but was "beneficial" to the patients, "and has enabled me more easily to preserve proper order and discipline in the management of the institution."[30] To find refuge or work in an almshouse was to surrender a citizen's normal autonomy. Paternalistic rules applied to nurses, house officers, and minor functionaries as well. Enforcement was often erratic, but the institution's right, indeed duty, to demand strict discipline was unquestioned.

Impressionistic evidence indicates, however, that the Blockley reality was a good deal less ordered than such rules might have implied. Throughout the century, for example, there seems to have been an irrepressible black market in alcohol and a brisk trade in pilfered food and drugs. If the steward placed blinds on the patients' windows, the men persistently removed them and used the windows for the disposal of trash, bottles, and

29 Minutes of the Hospital Committee, December 11, 1846.
30 *AR for 1875*, p. 27.

other "offensive matter."[31] The mixture of prostitutes among the inmates and political appointees on the staff made for a chronic occasion of sin. And discipline implied an orderly chain of command and predictable patterns of punishment; here again order was elusive. House physicians, for example, were a difficult and often unruly lot, resentful both of their senior attending physicians and of the laypersons who in theory administered the institution. They formed a weak link in any chain of disciplinary command.

Public and private hospitals

A good many of the same social values and relationships of status and deference were present in voluntary hospitals, but the differences between public and private hospitals was always marked in nineteenth-century America. In fact, that very difference was a fundamental aspect of the municipal hospitals. First, as we have seen, the almshouse-hospital was always a last resort; patients were unwilling to apply for admission until driven to desperation. The creation of private outpatient dispensaries and the ministrations of municipalities' own "outdoor physicians" were not simply humanitarian gestures, but were seen consciously as a rational (and economical) means of saving the worthy poor from the degraded status of almshouse inmate. The ability of the voluntary hospitals to pick and choose among their cases – and the corresponding need for the almshouse-hospital to serve as the refuge of last resort for the tubercular, the chronic, the alcoholic, and the moribund – meant that Blockley inevitably served as a dumping ground for such cases. Indeed, patients were often transferred there when they proved disruptive, did not respond to treatment, or, even more scandalously, were in extremis.

Within the medical profession, as well, municipal hospital appointments tended to be a bit less desirable than the corresponding appointments at private hospitals; the rough social environment as well as the prevalence of chronic and "uninteresting" cases could discourage the youthful practitioner. "The diseases are not of a very varied character," one wrote in 1840 as he began his Blockley apprenticeship.

> The indolent ulcer is by far the most common presenting few or no varieties and generally the result [sic] accidental injuries inflicted upon broken down or vicious constitutions, a few fractures & a tolerable

31 Minutes of the Hospital Committee, January 23 and June 26, 1863.

display of hernias, contusions, and diseases of the spine completing the list.[32]

The lay steward and political appointees who dominated the almshouse were also less congenial than their counterparts in the city's more prestigious private institutions. Only the scarcity of hospital appointments and the sheer volume of "clinical material" allowed Blockley to compete effectively for the services of young house officers.

Not surprisingly, conditions at municipal hospitals generally and at Blockley in particular were often far below the standards tolerated at private institutions. Throughout the century, well-meaning Philadelphians found conditions at Blockley a scandal. Diet, accommodations, and washing facilities were chronically inadequate and prompted recurrent demands for reform. Nurses in 1859 were charged with seeing that the straw in the beds was changed "at least once in each month during the summer season, and see that the beds are preserved free from vermin." They were also to see that patients changed their linen at least once a week. How closely these worthy injunctions were followed remains unclear. Penury and corruption inevitably lowered hospital standards. In 1844 nurses were warned against tearing up shirts to provide needed bandages. Two years later a request for a bathtub in the "operated ward" was rejected because of the expense. Doctors found themselves without lancets – still considered a necessity – in the 1850s, while the eminent surgeon Samuel D. Gross complained in 1862 that scurvy was endemic in the hospital.[33] (And physicians had known for well over a century that fresh fruits and vegetables were preventive.) But conditions did improve – if at a somewhat glacial pace. In 1870, Blockley's steward could report that the bathtub in the women's bathhouse had been enlarged by almost a half – and could now accommodate about a dozen patients at one time! A year later, it was suggested that the lying-in department be furnished with a water closet, hot water, and wash basins. Nurses had complained the previous year that the roof leaked so badly that a good many patients had to be moved during every rain storm. A few months later – in December – a prominent attending physician could complain that ward temperatures were dangerously low and the supply of blankets inadequate.[34] Until the end of the century, conditions were crowded and patients were stowed in rooms never designed for human

32 E. K. Kane, "Hospital Notes." Manuscript Division, American Philosophical Society, 1840–1841.
33 Board of Guardians, Rules, 1859, p. 61; Minutes of the Board of Physicians, September 9, 1840; Minutes of the Hospital Committee, October 23, 1844; April 15, 1853; January 26, 1855; March 14, 1862.
34 Minutes of the Hospital Committee, February 25 and March 4, 1846; September 6 and December 27, 1872; AR for 1870, p. 28; AR for 1873, pp. 31–32.

occupancy. Convalescents as well as blacks were isolated in attic rooms, for example, and as late as 1887, the Department of Charities (the new-model title of the Board of Guardians of the Poor) could complain of

> the fearfully overcrowded condition of the Hospital attics appropriated to the so-called convalescents from the men's medical and surgical wards. . . . When the beds are prepared for the night there is barely room enough left to enable one to walk from one of the rooms to the other. Many of the patients are compelled to sleep two in a bed.[35]

The details shifted, but the fundamental reality changed only in degree throughout the century; conditions at Blockley were always forbidding and always worse than those that prevailed at Philadelphia's private hospitals.

It is hardly surprising that working men and women, even the most helpless, showed little willingness to enter the almshouse. A spokesman for Pennsylvania Hospital put the distinction between public and private with unavoidable clarity. The Pennsylvania Hospital, he explained in 1867,

> is the house for the better class of our poor, when sick or wounded; the abject poor finding a refuge in the Blockley Hospital of the almshouse.
>
> Now, I think no person comes in here thinking to carry away spot or blemish connected with the fact of a sojourn made in our house; for no man nor woman is forced in by the mandate of a magistrate or the constraint of a policeman.[36]

When a group of mid-century philanthropists sought to establish a hospital in Philadelphia they had only to cite the almshouse as motivation for the creation of such an institution – not a reason to make it unnecessary. The almshouse, they emphasized,

> is necessary, but, while it is the legal receptacle for all whose destitution is the result of idleness, profligacy, and licentiousness, it communicates a character to its inmates which causes those who have any remaining feeling of respect for their own reputation, or that of their children, or connections, to be willing to endure, to the utmost limit of possibility, all the evils of sickness and poverty rather than submit to the stigma which attaches to those who enter its walls.[37]

Such assumptions did not easily change; thirty-five years later, Philadelphians employed remarkably similar arguments when a group of

---

35 *AR for 1887*, pp. 10–11; *AR for 1888*, p. 6.
36 Pennsylvania Hospital, *Proceedings of a Meeting held First Month (January) 15th, 1867* (Philadelphia: Collins, 1867), pp. 19–20.
37 Episcopal Hospital of Philadelphia, *Appeal on Behalf of the Sick* (Philadelphia: Lindsay & Blakiston, 1851), pp. 18–19.

Methodist laypersons sought funds to establish a Methodist Episcopal hospital. Blockley, a prominent medical man argued, "is not worthy to be called a hospital. It is nothing but a part of the Almshouse; its inmates are stigmatized as paupers; it is in improper buildings and the pure and impure are mingled indiscriminately together." There was not a voluntary hospital bed, Dr. Wood emphasized, in the entire city, "in which a poor man or woman, without influence, can feel sure of being cared for in the hour of trouble."[38]

Chronic disease

The problem was not sickness alone, but chronic illness, for it was such cases that private hospitals felt unwilling or unable to admit and which filled large numbers of long-term beds at Blockley. As late as 1887, for example, the census at Blockley was 1,200, while the Pennsylvania Hospital was treating only 164 patients. "We have of classes that the Pennsylvania Hospital cannot receive for want of means," the Blockley authorities emphasized, "568 chronic or incurable cases, such as consumptives, paralytics, epileptics, and patients with cancer."[39] The problem of chronic disease was apparent throughout the century. It was one of the motives in the founding of Philadelphia's Episcopal Hospital (and New York's St. Luke's as well). "It is a well known fact," a committee of the new Episcopal Hospital's medical board reported in 1858,

> that there exists in Philadelphia no place excepting the Almshouse to which the poor afflicted with chronic incurable diseases are admitted. To the Almshouse the more respectable class of them entertain an intense aversion & unless compelled by the direct necessity never resort. Everyone who has mixed among the poor has noticed this, and it cannot be doubted.[40]

But if the pious low-church Episcopalians who staffed and administered Episcopal Hospital could not help feeling concern for the chronically ill, most of their medical contemporaries were anxious to keep such long-term sufferers out of hospital wards. In Boston, for example, the Boston City Hospital was in theory to be established as a separate hospital so as to allow the poor to be treated outside the stigmatizing walls of the almshouse. Yet as one strong advocate of the new city hospital argued, it was necessary that

38 *Philadelphia Public Ledger*, December 17, 1886, p. 1.
39 *AR for 1887*, p. 10.
40 Minutes of the Medical Board, Archives of Episcopal Hospital, Philadelphia, April 23, 1858.

it only admit patients suffering from acute ailments. The costs, added to the problem of overcrowding, "imperatively forbid the admission, into a hospital, of patients who can be equally well cared for in an almshouse. The object of hospitals is to treat disease, not to afford an asylum for the idle or decrepit."[41] The stigma of charity and the burden of age and chronic disease were never to be solved; even within the almshouse itself, the aged and helpless were the least desirable. Just as the city's private hospitals sent their chronic patients to Blockley, so the aged and particularly feeble within the city hospital were transferred to the "insane department."[42]

World within the walls

The municipal hospitals were in many ways a world unto themselves. With much of its labor recruited from onetime inmates, the hospital was not only a reflection of the larger society's values and priorities, but also a distinct and self-contained work culture, centering on a "job ladder" and dominated by the influence of long-time employees. Throughout the century, administrators had bewailed the problems created by the use of inmate labor – alcoholism, pilferage, incompetence. As early as 1825, the almshouse medical board had asked that a "regularly trained" nurse of good reputation be assigned to each ward, but warned that this could not be done without an increase in salary. A decade later, the Board of Guardians bravely resolved to hire no more nurses from among the pauper inmates and replace those presently employed with "persons of known integrity and steady and temperate habits." Significantly, the original resolution had included the phrase "and assistant nurses"; but even in a reform mood, the board realized that it was unrealistic to hope that they could find sufficient funds to hire assistant nurses. The reference to assistants was stricken from the minutes.[43] It was not until the last decades of the century that such goals could be considered more than well-meaning rhetoric. And of course much of the common labor – cooking, butchering, laundering, carpentry, even the compounding of prescriptions – was performed by inmates. Nursing was little differentiated from other inmate tasks.

Or at least assistant nursing. For one can discern traces of a career line at Blockley, one in which patients might first work as they recovered, then stay and work for board and room as assistants, then gradually be paid, first

41 John Green, *City Hospitals* (Boston: Little, Brown, 1861).
42 *AR for 1868*, p. 49.
43 Minutes of the Board of Physicians, March 7, 1825; Minutes of the Board of Guardians, September 7, 1835.

with plugs of tobacco and alcohol, then clothing, then a small monthly salary. Finally, through skill and reliability (and possibly political connections), he or she might be promoted to ward nurse. A few workers could rise even higher in the hospital hierarchy. John Miller was not only a ward nurse, but a cupper and leecher (for which he received extra pay). Frank Johnson, another ward nurse, achieved even more authority. He was put in charge of Blockley's surgical instruments and physicians had to request them from him; Johnson also supervised the cleaning of the grounds and was subsequently given charge of issuing all the hospital's alcohol.[44]

It was only to have been expected that these positions, and especially the supervisory ones, would become enmeshed in a web of political patronage. One mid-century nurse who killed two patients by giving them the wrong drug – while he was drunk – was only suspended for a week. Even more egregiously, a Mr. Lane who was in charge of the receiving ward was brought up on charges ranging from disobedience toward the steward to "ungentlemanly" conduct toward a lady; at one hearing he insolently repeated his inappropriate language in front of the Board of Guardians' Hospital Committee itself. Still, it was not until more than four years after this incident that Lane was replaced; and by a man to be paid less than half Lane's $18.00-a-month salary. Lane must certainly have had influential friends and protectors.[45] Such mundane ties only strengthened the hospital's localistic and antiprofessional ethos. It was a community of like-thinking fellow workers who fought back aggressively when in the 1880s the Board of Guardians engaged a Nightingale-trained superintendent for their nursing school; her administrative control over graduate and student nurses recruited from outside the institution represented an immediate threat to Blockley's well-established social order.

It was only natural that the young physicians who served as house officers should often have walked Blockley's grim wards like officers of an occupying power. "The doctor must be wary," one resident wrote in 1877, "if he wants to have control of his wards, for the vicious and often criminal elements therein will stop short of nothing to circumvent him."[46] The resident's impressions were only typical. The Blockley experience could be traumatic for such protected young men. And, unlike their patients and aides, these educated and self-conscious practitioners sometimes recorded their impressions. Fortunately, two such young men kept journals in the

---

44 Minutes of the Hospital Committee, December 6 and 27, 1861; March 8 and May 24, 1872; August 29, 1873; February 27, 1874.
45 Minutes of the Hospital Committee, October 1, 1852; August 16, 1850; January 10, 1851; October 14, 1853; January 27 and February 3, 1854; May 4, 1855.
46 J. B. Roberts, "Notes of Life in a Hospital by a Resident Physician, 1877," Historical Collections, College of Physicians of Philadelphia.

early 1880s; their experiences are both illuminating and significantly parallel. Most striking is the ambivalence they felt toward their charges, who seemed of a different breed from the people the young men had grown up with. A. A. Bliss, for example, one of these physicians, described the patients in his obstetrics ward as

> women with their first children, young, ignorant, without any self-control, sometimes with instincts and manners like savages. Of course very few of them were married. In rare instances, the mothers manifested a real and lasting interest in their children, but usually the feeling was an evanescent, physiological, maternal instinct, not as deep or as serious as a cat would feel for its kittens, or a cow for its calf.[47]

The same young man was astonished while on ambulance duty to see the kindness and helpfulness shown by his patients' tenement neighbors. "I was among the lowest of the low," he reflected, among

> people so wretchedly poor, that, in Philadelphia, the city of cheap homes, they housed, or rather kenneled, in this rotting tenement. I don't suppose they knew much of the fine distinctions between right and wrong.... I strongly suspect that, like beasts, they lived in promiscuous intercourse, but a wave of emotionalism or, perhaps, divine pity, swept over them.[48]

It was a structured relationship that degraded in their different ways both physician and patient. "After living in such circumstances for several months," Dr. Bliss confessed, "we became naturally overbearing, dogmatic, and it must be confessed, more or less brutal."[49]

Material conditions within the hospital only mirrored such emotional brutality. Resident Lawrence Flick noted in January of 1880 that it was no wonder his patients were infested with lice, since they had no change of clothes and no adequate bathing facilities. For three months they had been short of linen; if a woman's nightshirt needed to be washed they would have to send the clothing out to be washed and keep the woman in bed until it was returned. Food was consistently poor in quality: eggs were rotten, the cold meat was doled out in infinitesimal portions, and the sugar used in the nursery "looked like sawdust soaked in some brown fluid." And patients were, of course, expected to work as soon as they could; Flick spoke with uncharacteristic warmth of an uncharacteristically respectable young girl who had given birth one evening at ten, been thrown out of her

47 Arthur A. Bliss, *Blockley Days. Memories and Impressions of a Resident Physician* ([Philadelphia]: Privately Printed, 1916), p. 49.
48 Bliss, p. 35.
49 Bliss, p. 89.

stepfather's home − and who was at work on a Blockley sewing machine the next day.[50]

Though many of the patients seemed unsympathetic − paupers who failed to show a humility appropriate to their station − others seemed victims of a system that demanded a poor man's dignity in payment for a hospital stay. The presence of the almshouse, as young Dr. Bliss noted, made any poor but respectable Philadelphian unwilling to apply for hospital admission, except as a last resort. And when they were driven to apply, he learned gradually, medicine and medical men were perhaps less understanding than the political functionaries who represented the city's Board of Guardians of the Poor. As Bliss recalled, the Guardians owned a small house on Seventh Street (in central Philadelphia, several miles from Blockley) where applicants for hospital or outward admission were examined by a hospital resident in conjunction with a lay official of the board. "It must be confessed," Bliss concluded, "that the young medical man was often too disposed to be sarcastic, cynical, suspicious, and anxious to drive away every applicant who did not bear in his or her body the symptoms of being an interesting medical or surgical case."[51] The city's political appointees, on the other hand, were sympathetic, never spoke harshly to the supplicants who appeared before them, and often admitted them, even when the resident decided that they were not sick enough. The categories of medical diagnosis might seem intellectually, and in a sense morally, superior to the imperatives of sordid patronage; they did not always transcend them in humanity.

Doctors and guardians: The medicalization of Blockley

Almost from the beginning of the nineteenth century, Blockley's physicians had sought to distinguish the hospital in which they worked from the almshouse. But they were never entirely to succeed. Blockley was becoming more and more a hospital − yet a hospital that could not escape the almshouse aura that had surrounded it since the eighteenth century.

At first the medical presence in Blockley was comparatively small. Senior attending physicians appeared only on "regular prescribing days," and even then might send students or substitutes. But this did not discourage the medical staff from seeking to control medical practice in the hospital. In 1825, they asked to examine all candidates for house physician, although the power of appointments still lay in the hands of the Board of Guardians.

50 Ella M. Flick, *Beloved Crusader. Lawrence F. Flick* (Philadelphia: Dorrance & Co., 1944), pp. 70 and 68−112.
51 Bliss, p. 14.

Even earlier they had sought to increase the opportunities for postmortems and dissection.[52]

But in 1834, with the transfer of the almshouse to West Philadelphia – then a green and pleasant area of small farms and quiet settlements – the problems of differentiation emerged in sharper form. A year later, the medical board suggested that the name "Philadelphia Hospital" be used as a proper designation for the building that housed the almshouse sick. At almost the same time, significantly, the medical staff resolved to admit no one to the medical and surgical wards without an examination, and protested against the continued necessity of treating severely ill paupers in the outwards. (Nevertheless, admissions could still take place only upon a written order of the Board of Guardians agent.) In return for a continued hold on the hospital's medical administration, the medical board promised to make daily visits and generally place the institution "on a footing with some of the best hospitals in London and Paris."[53]

Such estimable goals could hardly be attained while the hospital was administered as an almshouse. It was inequitable, the medical argument followed, to both patients and physicians. An almshouse and a hospital should and must be separate institutions. The arguments were reiterated again and again in succeeding decades. In 1873, for example, Isaac Ray, a prominent expert on psychiatry, addressed the self-consciously reformist Philadelphia Social Science Association and affirmed the need to differentiate the two institutions as a preliminary step in providing the city's worthy poor with adequate medical care. Minor improvements, he emphasized,

> will fall short of the end in view, if the hospital is to be managed in the spirit of a pauper establishment. The paramount consideration must be, not how cheaply the patients can be kept, but how speedily they can be cured, and how far their sufferings can be alleviated.

Those in the almshouse were the city's legitimate concern, Ray continued, and few of the city's respectable understood the reality of Blockley: "In a continuous pile of buildings, just across the Schuylkill, it has gathered them together, from 3,600 to 4,000 in number, varying with the season, and constituting one seething mass of infirmity, disease, vice and insanity."[54]

What underlay the physicians' appeals was an unmistakable social consensus that assumed the reality and usefulness of the distinction between the worthy and unworthy poor, between the demoralized pauper and

52 Minutes of the Board of Physicians, March 7, 1825.
53 Minutes of the Board of Guardians, August 19 and November 2, 1835.
54 Ray, *Social Science Association of Philadelphia.*

the hard-working but unfortunately ailing worker. "I conceive," Dr. Horatio C. Wood added in endorsing Ray's argument, "that there can be no plainer and more sacred duty of a community than that of taking care of its destitute, sick and poor; no greater mistake than that of confounding vicious idleness with the need that sickness may bring any day to the poor." Yet the only way a poor man could guarantee himself medical care was to have himself labeled a pauper. "The city must have a municipal hospital," Wood contended, "unconnected with and uncontaminated by association with the workhouse – a hospital maintained purely and solely as such, where the poor man, or woman, or child, can always go, knowing that poverty and sickness are the only needful passports for admission."

The issue did not redefine itself, even as the hospital grew ever more prominent and self-contained. In 1900, for example, Blockley's medical staff again formulated the now commonplace demand. The hospital, they charged,

> being a part of the Almshouse, there is strenuous objection on the part of many people to take advantage of the treatment therein accorded patients, because of the stigma of pauperism which they believe is attached to an inmate of the institution.
>
> In order to overcome this feeling your Board desires to separate the two institutions, removing the Almshouse to a suitable location, where the inmates may be properly cared for and yet have some light duties to perform so as to help sustain themselves and to make of the present location a hospital in every sense of the term, one from which the stigma is removed, and that no citizen would hesitate to enter when in need of treatment.

Significantly, this plea was made as part of an effort to "promote, encourage and enlarge the clinical teaching at the Philadelphia Hospital" so as to "make it one of the best medical and dental schools in the world."[55] Yet it was not until the 1920s, as we shall see, that the physical separation of the almshouse, hospital, and lunatic asylum became a reality.

Every aspect of the patient's experience reflected the dual system into which he or she entered; sickness and dependency were not easily distinguished. Admission, as we have seen, was certified by a physician and a lay agent of the Board of Guardians acting together (if not precisely in concert) into the 1890s. In addition, as late as 1853, visitors to the poor – a kind of proto–social worker – could send patients into Blockley's hospital wards. It was not until 1848 that a smokehouse was converted into the institution's first receiving ward. And this ward was more an adminis-

---

55 *AR for 1900*, pp. 8, 10 (contemporaries were particularly concerned at the plight of the aged forced to enter an almshouse); *AR for 1887*, pp. 16–17.

trative than a medically oriented facility; patients were bathed and their clothes were stored, but they were not necessarily examined and evaluated clinically. As late as 1880 there was no thermometer in the receiving ward and in 1899 the assistant resident physician could still complain that he kept being called to the front gate to examine patients (presumably emergencies) presenting themselves for admission.[56]

Once admitted, however, the patient was affected by a medical presence that grew steadily throughout the century. Paralleling physician demands for an explicit distinction between almshouse and hospital were staff requests for more liberal teaching privileges and an increasing differentiation among cases, one reflecting a more general growth of interest in the specialties. Like many other nineteenth-century hospitals, Blockley responded grudgingly, yet inexorably, to medical demands for the creation of specialized services and wards. As early as the 1820s, the almshouse had had a ward for "eye cases," and an accepted distinction between male and female, medical and surgical cases. Venereal patients had, for a number of reasons, always been treated separately. In 1840, the medical staff had urged the creation of a ward for "uterine" disease as useful both to patients and to "medical science." Thirty-five years later, in 1875, staff physicians called for a separate tuberculosis pavilion (though it was a quarter of a century before their request was granted); and in 1897 they outlined the need for a pediatric department. Dermatology and neurology had been recognized in 1877.[57]

As in most other hospitals, surgery grew increasingly important in the last quarter of the century – though contemporaries noted that it was never as significant in Blockley as it became in private hospitals; too large a proportion of its cases were the chronic, geriatric, and contagious ills unwelcome elsewhere. As late as 1900, Blockley's surgical wards housed comparatively few patients who had actually undergone major surgical procedures. The medical staff, nevertheless, worked steadily to keep pace with surgical facilities and procedures of sister institutions. In 1873, Blockley organized a ward for the preparation and recovery of surgical patients; the 1880s had brought "the Antiseptic process," although in a manner so gradual "that it is impossible to fix an exact date even to the year." In 1898 an "anaesthesizer of the Philadelphia Hospital" was appointed.[58]

56 Flick, p. 93; *AR for 1891*, p. 58; Sherman Gilpin, Diary, 1899–1901, Temple University Urban Archives; Philadelphia General Hospital, *Rules Governing Internes* (1903), p. 15.
57 Minutes of the Board of Physicians, December 4, 1826; September 9, 1840; *AR for 1897*, p. 62; J. W. Croskey, *History of Blockley: A History of the Philadelphia General Hospital from its Inception, 1731–1928* (Philadelphia: F. A. Davis, 1929).
58 *AR for 1873*, p. 31; *AR for 1890*, pp. 7–8; D. E. Hughes to C. Lawrence, March 18, 1898, chief resident physician's letterbooks.

Long-term neurological cases were a particularly difficult problem; they demanded a good deal of care and were unwelcome at all of the city's other hospitals. Blockley staff members made a virtue of necessity and their chronic neurological wards became a center of teaching and research. The evolution of this clinically prestigious situation was complex and instructive. As early as 1866, the superintendent of the hospital's insane department asked that the epileptics "not insane" be removed to the hospital proper (though it seems not to have been done until 1871). A year later, the Guardians' Hospital Committee, at the request of two of its prominent visiting physicians, moved "that the paralytic ward now embraced in the Out Wards be made a proper hospital ward, with suitable nurses and food." In 1883, members of the medical staff requested that the patients in the "paryletic" wards be removed "to some portion of the Hospital." Four years later, Blockley administrators could announce the erection of two "well-appointed" buildings for male nervous patients; the department had now four nationally prominent visiting physicians, C. K. Mills, Wharton Sinkler, F. X. Dercum, and J. H. Lloyd.[59] Blockley authorities were proud to emphasize that the insane department as well as the neurological work had

> become more truly than ever before an integral part of the Hospital and has been absolutely removed from the category of "asylums:" where restraint or confinement were the chief objects aimed at, – not treatment, improvement, and cure. The services of four eminent specialists in nervous and mental diseases are now given to the inmates of this department. . . . The enormous mass of valuable material which these wards contain is being classified, studied, and utilized, primarily for the benefit of the patients themselves, but also for the advancement of medical science and the good of the community.

Within the Blockley context, physicians and administrators never doubted that those patients who made up this "enormous mass of valuable materials" were far better off in a medically controlled and defined context than in the almshouse outwards in which they had previously vegetated.[60]

All of this seemed morally as well as administratively appropriate. It was consistent with efforts to allow medical patients to wear clothing different in color and style from that worn by the "paupers." And it was part of a more general movement toward the assimilation of Blockley's overly general and stigmatizing category of inmate into the seemingly more neutral role of patient. Numerically most important were the feeble outward inhabitants,

59 *AR for 1866*, p. 38; *AR for 1870*, p. 28; Minutes of the Hospital Committee, September 13, 1872; January 19 and August 3, 1883; *AR for 1888*, p. 45.
60 *AR for 1887*, p. 13.

the great majority of whom were in need of medical care. Almost 80 percent of the female inmates in the outwards, the medical staff contended in 1887,

> are affected by disease or insanity to such an extent as to make them fit subjects for hospital treatment and care. Many of these belong, as do so many of the hospital cases, to the chronic or incurable class. Most of the remaining twenty percent of these inmates are frequently the subjects of rheumatic, bronchitic, and other troubles, and almost constantly require medical attention. . . . The medical staff strongly urges the desirability of such a modification of the existing classification as would include the women's out-wards under the rules and regulations of the Hospital. This change would involve no additional expense.

Early the next year, this administrative change was put into effect; the matron was replaced by a graduate nurse and the night nursing undertaken by training school students instead of inmate assistants.[61]

In other areas, the authority of medicine seemed to increase with greater certainty. Blockley offered extraordinarily attractive opportunities for an ambitious and intellectually oriented physician. And from the Civil War to the end of the century, such practitioners lobbied steadily to raise the level of medicine taught and practiced in Philadelphia's almshouse hospital.

Pathology was the first area in which such values manifested themselves. "Morbid anatomy" had been the key to medical eminence in the middle third of the nineteenth century; and Blockley with its enormous numbers of patients represented, despite sporadic harassment from lay authorities, an excellent place to perform systematic autopsies. William Gerhard, for example, a Paris-trained clinician working at Blockley, was able to demonstrate the pathological distinction between typhus and typhoid fevers in 1836–1837. Similar opportunities at the Blockley deadhouse a half century later helped attract William Osler from Montreal to a post at the University of Pennsylvania.[62]

With the growing acceptance of the germ theory in the 1880s, and in particular the discovery of the causative organisms of tuberculosis, typhoid, and cholera, the assumed responsibility of the municipality to care for such cases created a demand for appropriate facilities to diagnose and isolate infectious disease. The community's responsibility for contagious ills had a

61 *AR for 1887*, p. 14; *AR for 1888*, pp. 45–46. For the attempt to differentiate clothing of "paupers" from patients, see Minutes of the Hospital Committee, January 2, 1874; May 9, 1884.

62 W. W. Gerhard, "On The Typhus Fever, which occurred at Philadelphia in the Spring and Summer of 1836 . . . ," *American Journal of the Medical Sciences* 19 (1837): 289–322; 20: 289–322; H. Cushing, *The Life of Sir William Osler* (Oxford: Clarendon, 1925), I: 250–253.

long history; in the eighteenth century, Philadelphia had supported a "pest house" and administered a sporadic quarantine.[63] But the era of bacteriology and immunology meant a new set of options. The possibilities of laboratory diagnosis and subsequent isolation of infectious ills led to the support of a new medical capacity – that of clinical pathology and especially bacteriological diagnosis. It led as well to a gradual integration of the clinical laboratory into the hospital's ward routine.

Blockley had appointed James Tyson as its "microscopist" as early as 1866; and he called immediately for more careful and systematic use of the microscope in evaluating tissues and fluids:

> In the present advanced and progressing state of Pathological Anatomy, a condition to which the use of the microscope (especially in its connection with medical chemistry), has contributed more than any other means of modern research, the history of few cases can be considered complete, while in a large number we can scarcely be considered as having performed our duty as physicians, without a microscopical and chemical examination of the blood and more important secretions and excretions of the body.

Brave words. But Tyson also noted that only seventeen pathological examinations had been ordered all year in a hospital with an average census of over 800 patients. By 1883, A. A. Bliss – the youthful house officer we have already quoted – described the pathological laboratory as including "glass pipettes of every size and shape, glass retorts and flasks, test tubes, and many strange and rusty machines long unused and the very use of which were forgotten."[64] The laboratory made slow progress in Blockley's penurious atmosphere.

Yet by the end of the century, the clinical laboratory was becoming a normal part of hospital routine; the seemingly boundless new opportunities offered by bacteriology had dramatized the need for integrating *all* the laboratory's results with the clinician's physical findings. A chief resident's memorandum of 1897 explained that the junior medical intern was responsible for ordering a chemical and microscopical examination of every patient on his service within twenty-four hours of admission. In 1903, the hospital reorganized and expanded its clinical laboratory. A year later the laboratory reported having examined 13,542 specimens; by 1906, the

63 R. Wolman, "Some Aspects of Community Health in Colonial Philadelphia" (unpublished Ph.D. diss., University of Pennsylvania, 1974).

64 *AR for 1868*, pp. 96–97; E. T. Morman, "The Development of Clinical Pathology in America, 1870–1920" (unpublished ms., University of Pennsylvania, 1979); J. H. Clark "The Development of a Pathological Laboratory at Blockley," *Medical Life* 40 (1933): 237–252; A. A. Bliss, *Blockley Days: Memories and Impressions of a Resident Physician, 1883–1884* (Philadelphia: privately printed, 1916).

number had risen to 22,627, an increase far more dramatic than that in admissions. Two years later, the hospital reported the appointment of a full-time resident in pathology, supplementing the three-month stints of regular medical and surgical residents. The laboratory's director could in 1904 record with satisfaction that it "has come to be indispensable to the institution." Research and instruction of house staff had been integrated into the overwhelming volume of routine clinical work. Blockley promised an unlimited field for clinical investigation: "The hospital, presenting as it does, unequalled and almost unlimited opportunity for research work of practical and scientific value, we look upon the present state of development of the laboratory as only the inception of the great work naturally expected in a modern municipal hospital."[65] This was rhetoric directed immediately toward the city council; it would be repeated again and again as staff members sought more adequate facilities.

Similarly, the x-ray was quickly incorporated into the hospital's clinical routine. The first formal radiology laboratory was equipped in 1900. In 1903, the laboratory was expanded and a director appointed; previously, radiographical work had been performed by an assistant resident in his evening hours. The hospital was soon providing therapeutic as well as diagnostic radiological services and by 1910 could boast that its x-ray laboratory's research results "have made the Department known throughout the country."[66]

By the First World War, at least a dozen specialties had established themselves in the hospital's wards and teaching routine; it was an institution that ever more self-consciously felt itself to be a hospital – and prided itself on the quality of its teaching and care. No physician could ignore the "professional advantages," as the Department of Charities put it as early as 1892, "resulting from official connection with a Hospital of size, importance and character we believe unsurpassed on this continent."[67] In 1890, *Philadelphia Hospital Reports* was begun as a vehicle for the publication of clinical studies conducted at Blockley; in 1904, the hospital's annual report included a bibliography of articles in which Blockley "materials" had been used. Philadelphia's municipal hospital was gradually being integrated into the world of medical status and intellect.

Teaching had grown steadily more prominent in postbellum Blockley, and, as it did so, it moved gradually from the lecture theater to the bedside. It had, of course, almost always been present. As early as the first years of

65 Philadelphia General Hospital, chief resident's memorandum book, [1897]; *Rules Governing Interns*, 1903, p. 11; *AR for 1903*, pp. 46–49; *AR for 1904*, p. 63; *AR for 1906*, pp. 273–276; *AR for 1908*, pp. 84–87.
66 *AR for 1910*, p. 46.
67 *AR for 1892*, p. 11–12.

the nineteenth century, the almshouse attending physicians had made it clear that their service at the hospital implied the right to use the wards for instructing their apprentices. In 1823 they had established a "clinical ward" in which patients for "demonstration" could be kept together; access to Blockley patients was a valuable asset in the antebellum competition for students that enlivened Philadelphia's medical world. The University of Pennsylvania and Jefferson Medical College were the principal contenders, but not the only applicants for student access to patients. As a result of hostility between the medical staff and lay board, there was a period of almost a decade at mid-century in which no formal teaching was undertaken, yet the trend was clear. Despite the handicap implied by the lay board's efforts to safeguard patient rights to refuse to be used in teaching, the presence of medical students in Blockley grew increasingly routine throughout the century. By 1891, hospital authorities could report with pride that their medical staff had been offering clinics through nine months of the year, to an average audience of 200. The clinics were held on Wednesdays and Saturdays from nine to noon. And that year, for the first time, a student clinic in "morbid anatomy" had been arranged with attendance averaging 150. The tension that had accompanied the provision of teaching facilities in antebellum years had gradually dissipated. By 1901 Blockley could boast that 13,547 medical students had attended at least some of their clinical lectures.[68]

But such amphitheater performances were no adequate substitute for the bedside teaching demanded by educational reformers; it was not until the first decade of the present century that such small-group clinical instruction became a reality at Blockley. But when it was finally introduced, there was little opposition. This increase in bedside instruction brought a decrease in attendance at the showpiece amphitheater lectures that had been such a source of pride (and advertisement) in a previous generation. "While each year shows a diminution in the number of students attending general clinics," the hospital reported in 1904, "continuous advance is made in bedside instruction and lectures to small classes." Over 27,000 had attended at least some clinical instruction that year, as opposed to roughly half that number in 1903. A year later the number had risen to almost 35,000 and the Wednesday amphitheater clinics had become obsolete; students would attend only the Saturday morning presentations. The new system seemed advantageous for both student and hospital:

68 *AR for 1891*, p. 84; *AR for 1900*, p. 44; *AR for 1901*, p. 32; D. H. Agnew, *Lecture on the Medical History of the Philadelphia Alms House. Delivered at the Opening of the Clinical Lectures, October 15th, 1862* (Philadelphia: Holland & Edgar, 1862); W. S. Middleton, "Clinical Teaching in the Philadelphia Almshouse and Hospital," *Medical Life* 40 (1933): 191–200, 207–225.

Bedside instruction and ward rounds by students accompanied by
members of the staff, have increased and become more thoroughly
organized. This method by which the student performs as nearly as
may be, the duties of a resident physician, seems to most effectually
hold the interest of the student and to have the greatest teaching value.

And the trend continued. In 1909, medical students paid almost exactly
50,000 visits to Blockley; 39,000 were for the purpose of small-group
bedside instruction.[69]

The fear of being used as "clinical material" obviously affected almost
every patient suffering from anything but the most routine ailment. But
teaching was only one way in which the increasing role of medicine
affected the patient and the hospital generally. Another was the development of a medical staff organization with a formal structure and influential
standing committees. Even more important was the day-to-day administrative authority of the chief resident physician. This post was created in
mid-century as an instrument for exerting the Board of Guardians' authority; by the end of the century the chief resident had become in effect a
chief executive officer. Beginning with authority to make emergency admissions or discharges, he gradually accumulated a measure of control over
house and visiting staff, medical care policies, and – in some measure –
even the nurse training school. A major obstacle to medical control,
however, was the continued authority of a politically appointed lay superintendent who enjoyed general oversight over all Blockley's divisions.
Conflict was inevitable, not only in Blockley, but in every American
municipal hospital. "The prostitution of the Goddess of Medicine," as one
administrator put it, "to the demons of politics is a plague spot on the face
of our liberty and republican government."[70] Partially in response to such
reformist sentiments, Philadelphia's welfare administration was reorganized
in 1903 (its title changed to Department of Public Health and Charities)
and an advisory board that numbered among its members some of the city's
most prominent and influential physicians was created to work with the
department's new director. Despite a lingering political influence, Blockley
was becoming administratively more and more a hospital like any other.

Imposing order

Within the hospital itself, no change was more important than the development of a nurse training school and the assumption of nursing duties by
women recruited from outside the hospital. But it was a gradual change

69 *AR for 1904*, p. 52; *AR for 1905*, p. 327; *AR for 1909*, p. 95.
70 A. Goldspohn, "Hospital Management," *National Hospital Record* 5 (1901): 15–17.

and one far more subtle than reformist histories of nursing might indicate. At the end of the Civil War, Blockley was still staffed by a traditional mixture of former patients and a handful of long-term employees. "The present system," the institution's clerk wrote in 1866,

> employs irresponsible persons whose only inducement to hold the position is the opportunity it affords to appropriate food and stimulants intended for the patients under their care. Those who are willing to remain as assistants belong to that dissolute class who are unable to keep out of the House, and from whom we can scarcely expect a conscientious discharge of duty.[71]

Poor pay and harsh discipline meant that assistants were not only unreliable as to the quality of their ward performance, but also were likely to leave those wards as soon as they could; only a small minority had the character, ambition, or connections to attain the position of ward nurse.

Nevertheless, it was not until the spring of 1883, a decade after the establishment of Bellevue's pioneer nurse training school, that the Board of Guardians began to investigate the establishment of a training school; it was not until the next year and with private support that the hospital engaged Alice Fisher, an experienced English nurse-administrator, to direct the training school and supervise the hospital's nursing. Gradually the new-model trained nurses made their way into the hospital's wards: first the female medical, and finally the male, insane, and venereal wards were brought under their control.[72] This change necessarily sharpened the line between patients and attendants; and far more important, it introduced a new source of workers, ones possessed of a carefully cultivated sense of vocational identity and recruited from a class different from the one that ordinarily provided almshouse patients and workers. And as they sought to impose a Nightingale-like order in Blockley – one incorporating moral as well as procedural elements – the trained and student nurses helped create a new atmosphere on the wards. Although the crust of order and professionalism they imposed was often thin, the nurses were in a cultural sense the foot soldiers of an occupying army – of middle-class values, ideas, and personnel in a population which seemed little amenable to such influences.

The nurses were only one element, if perhaps the most important, in a more general bureaucratization of the hospital. It manifested itself in a

71 *AR for 1866*, p. 59.
72 And not without persistent opposition from Blockley's existing staff; the indomitable Miss Fisher even had rotten eggs thrown through her window. J. McFarland, "The History of Nursing at the Blockley Hospital," *Medical Life* 40 (1933): 177–191; S. A. Stachniewicz and J. K. Axelrod, *The Double Frill. The History of the Philadelphia General Hospital School of Nursing* (Philadelphia: George F. Strickley, 1978).

number of ways, both essential and trivial, such as the centralization of cooking, laundry, and medical administration; the telephone's replacement of the previously omnipresent runners; and the provision of uniforms for all staff members visibly marking their function and status. As early as the 1870s, female nurses were required to wear a cap and apron; some time after that the male nurses were required to wear a uniform consisting of a blue blouse with ornaments according to rank. Nurses and assistants were to display a three-inch Maltese cross on their left sleeve midway between elbow and shoulder. Resident physicians were ordered to outfit themselves in an even more elaborate, military-style uniform: a dark blue cap, a coat with two gold bands on the sleeve and a star above it, buttons with the Pennsylvania coat of arms, and trousers with gold cord running down the seam.[73] Order and efficiency were gradually being imposed on Blockley's much older social system.

The almshouse enters a new century

Despite the brave words of reformers and the professional strivings of nurses and physicians, Blockley remained a hybrid of hospital and almshouse as it entered the new century. Almost half of its inmates were single white males, many "regular customers" who were admitted again and again. A large proportion were immigrants, almost 60 percent in 1892.[74] Roughly three times as many men as women filled Blockley's hospital wards, a ratio that changed little in the years before the First World War. (Significantly, the ratio was three to two among blacks, a measure of the more tenuous social and economic status of the black community and of the exclusionary policies of many of the city's private hospitals.) Death rates, of course, remained high, as they would be expected to in a hospital that could not exercise the option of turning away chronic, incurable, and even moribund patients.

Traditional vagueness of distinction between dependence, sickness, and delinquency remained characteristic of Blockley. A substantial proportion of admissions fell into the categories of venereal, alcoholic, and detention – roughly a third of the patient load in 1902. Even more revealing was the hospital's continuing difficulty in maintaining the line between hospital and outwards; in 1896, for example, 335 men and 124 women were transferred from the outwards to the hospital and 591 men and 146 women from the hospital to the outwards. "These figures clearly indicate," the hospital's

73 Minutes of the Hospital Committee, November 13, 1874; June 4, 1875; April 6, 1877; October 19, 1883; May 9, 1884; November 19, 1886.
74 *AR for 1892*, p. 34.

annual report had emphasized a year earlier, "the close relation existing between the hospital and the out-wards so-called." The fundamental
identity between many of the outward and hospital patients continued; in
1906, to cite another year, the hospital treated 10,057 adult patients, 2,339
were "transferred," and 1,567 died.[75] The great bulk of these transfers
were, of course, to the outwards – patients too old and sick to support
themselves, but no longer sufficiently ill to fill an acute bed.

Even within the hospital, categories of illness remained more discrete in
theory than they could become in practice. What, for example, was to be
done with "feeble-minded" children and adolescents? "It is hardly necessary to state that they should not be placed in a hospital ward surrounded by
the sick but mentally sound; or in the Department for the Indigent, where
corruption and demoralization would occur on the one hand, and injury
and maltreatment on the other." Venereal patients were still crammed in
suffocating attics and, like their deviant peers in the drunk and detention
wards, were not allowed to receive visitors without special permission.[76]
Not surprisingly, most Philadelphians remained as they had been for more
than a century, unwilling to pass behind the forbidding walls of Blockley.

And despite ever-increasing budgetary commitments, per capita costs at
Blockley remained far below those of most comparable institutions. In
1907, when the average per diem cost at Philadelphia's private hospitals
averaged $1.81, Blockley expended less than a third of that amount.[77] A
good deal of the work that would now be performed by aides was still being
done by convalescent or recovered patients. Ratios of graduates to student
nurses varied from year to year, but always remained low. Blockley authorities could complain in 1905 to the city's lawmakers that their greatest
handicap was a lack of trained employees: "The most liberal apportion-
ment of workers possible leaves the hospital with less than one-third the
number of trained salaried and unsalaried workers than is the rule in most
hospitals." A year later, they could thank the city council for underwriting
the cost of thirty-two additional orderlies and "cleaners"; but still the
shortage of nursing remained. Blockley had only fifteen graduate nurses
and ninety-two pupil nurses to care for nearly 1,500 patients – a number
that would demand 200 nurses in a properly staffed institution; as it was,

75 *AR for 1895*, p. 73; *AR for 1896*, p. 60; *AR for 1906*, p. 244–245. Rules for interns in this
   period indicate the difficulty in practice of distinguishing between the hospital and
   outward patients as well as the often moribund aspect of patients admitted.
   Philadelphia General Hospital, *Rules of Internes*, 1903, pp. 14, 16–17.
76 *AR for 1907*, p. 7; *AR for 1900*, p. 12; *AR for 1908*, p. 81; Middleton, "Blockley in the
   Changing World of Medicine," *General Magazine and Historical Chronicle* 42 (1940):
   431–447.
77 *AR for 1907*, p. 26.

"each head nurse has charge of a Department larger than the ordinary Hospital."[78] As we have seen, the title of Blockley's lay board had changed in a century from the Overseers of the Poor, to the Board of Guardians of the Poor, to the Department of Charities and Corrections, to the Department of Public Health and Charities. Realities could not be changed quite so neatly.

But statistics and administrative pleas for more generous support do not re-create the texture of that reality. No one knew the *fin de siècle* hospital better than Daniel Hughes, its chief resident physician. His letters, memoranda, and reports paint a picture of a grim and still intractable institution.

Discipline was perhaps his most difficult problem. Visiting physicians were often casual in their attendance and interns inattentive to clinical directives. House officers could be suspended for even chatting with a nurse in the wards. On one occasion a nurse had to be disciplined for striking a patient, on another an intern removed as "uncouth, boorish, and [unaware of] his shortcomings."[79] But Blockley's patients remained his most difficult disciplinary problem. Male venereal patients were, for example, a particularly truculent lot; they made trouble in the yards if let out for exercise and spent their evenings lounging and smoking in the bathrooms and water closets. And he could no longer use the threat of showers or cells; regulations did not allow even the chief resident to dismiss patients for disciplinary reasons.

Hughes's fundamental problem was, of course, the nature of Blockley's patient population, shaped by the unwillingness of most Philadelphians to enter unless forced by circumstance, and the parallel, if paradoxical, difficulty of finding a responsible home for patients ready to be discharged. Blockley served as the working man or woman's last resort. It was hardly surprising that so many should have been in extremis when admitted; as was, for example, Margaret Ashley, black, nineteen, single, domestic, who arrived in 1898

> in a state of collapse, with a history of having been in labor for past three days. The foetus was dead, the umbilical cord protruding from the vagina from which came a fetid discharge. Doctor Peck, Visiting Obstetrician, had the patient placed under ether and opened the abdomen as the only means of delivering the child. It was found that the uterus had ruptured and the child had dropped into the abdominal cavity. The patient died before the operation was completed.

78 *AR for 1905*, p. 329; *AR for 1906*, p. 271, 280.
79 Daniel Hughes to Alfred Moore, June 20, 1896, and Hughes to William Lambert, December 2, 1896, chief resident's letterbook.

It was only to be expected, Hughes noted, that Blockley should report a death rate of 13 percent.[80]

Overcrowding was another chronic difficulty, a result of the enormous numbers who were Blockley's natural constituency. Such overcrowding, Hughes warned his residents in July 1902,

> necessitates my calling your attention to the matter of discharging all patients who are capable of being treated by a district physician providing they have a home to go to when discharged.
> Kindly examine each of your patients with this object in view. Patients should not be required to sleep upon the floor at this season of the year; a time when the census of the hospital should be greatly reduced.

Eighty-nine patients had slept on the floor the previous night. The problem, of course, lay in the continued presence of patients who no longer needed attention, but could not be discharged because they were unable to care for themselves, "and if we send them away when they are unfit to care for themselves we open the way for adverse criticism." Many of those legitimately occupying beds were old and chronically ill, sufficiently ill to need some care but not so ill as to require active medical treatment:

> This group of patients crowd the hospital wards and interfere with the satisfactory treatment of those requiring more active medication. If space could be found for the establishment of special wards for these elderly and somewhat helpless patients, it would be of great advantage to the aged themselves, while giving a needed relief to the medical and surgical wards.

And the outwards remained an inappropriate place to treat anyone, filthy, overrun with vermin, and ill-suited to maintaining the shaky health of their feeble inhabitants. Chronic wards tended inevitably to be ignored and to sink into a custodial lethargy; when special tuberculosis wards were established at the end of the century, Hughes soon found that physicians were neglecting to make regular rounds among the consumptives.[81]

Hughes's picture, of course, is that of a harried administrator seeking to subdue a difficult reality. Sherman Gilpin, his assistant resident physician for almost three years, kept a diary that illustrates even more immediately both the professional attractions and the dismaying realities that Blockley presented to an ambitious young physician. "Blockley is an unhealthy,

80 Hughes to S. H. Ashbridge, [1898], chief resident's letterbook; *AR for 1899*, pp. 52–53.
81 Hughes to the Resident Staff, July 21, 1902, chief resident's memorandum book; Hughes to J. Musser, February 9, 1898, chief resident's letterbook; *AR for 1899*, p. 59; Hughes to Resident Staff, May 7, 1903, memorandum book.

miserable place to live," Gilpin confessed, "but it is very healthy for growth in medical knowledge."[82] Despite a crushing burden of routine work – he might admit more than thirty patients on busy days – Gilpin attended postmortems and tried to perfect his German. Politics and petty discipline made a difficult job even more frustrating. One Sunday he planned to attend church but couldn't because he was unable to find the chief resident to get permission. "This being a slave I don't like" (February 5, 1900). Even worse was the continued authority of political appointees, especially the superintendent. "If we had a man for Supt. and not a gruff, ignorant hypocrit [sic] of politician we might enjoy life a little even in Blockley." All the house staff ("medicals") detested the superintendent, Gilpin elaborated on another occasion:

> He is a politician, an ex-councilman, and sail-maker. He is everything but what a Dr. wants him to be. He is like the common run of Politicians, lazy, officious, small in brains, who cares for himself & his money. He has no use for medical science and hasn't the brains to appreciate it. We want a medical Supt. (February 25, 1900).

Even more dismaying was his enforced contact with a class of patients who seemed so different from himself. "So many destitute cases," he described one day's work, "lousy and dirty, just sick enough to need hospital care" (February 8, 1900). It was good, he complained wearily one Sunday, "going to church and realizing all the world are not paupers" (March 19, 1900). Another evening, spent with a lady friend, meant an evening lost to study; but he reassured himself that "I must meet a few people at least out of Blockley in order to round off the rough edges acquired by my contact with paupers" (January 5, 1899). The gap that separated doctors and patients in the antebellum almshouse hardly narrowed in the last third of the century.

By 1910, the year of the Flexner Report and its call for a closer integration of hospital, medical science, and medical education, the Philadelphia General had become in some ways a hospital like any of its large, metropolitan, voluntary sisters. Indeed, it was far larger than most and boasted an enviable reputation as a place to teach and study clinical medicine. Its 13,000 admissions demanded the attention of seventy-three visiting staff members – ten surgeons, twelve physicians, and eight each of obstetricians and neurologists. A majority held teaching positions in the city's medical schools (the largest number at the University of Pennsylvania). Fifty of the seventy-three lived in the fashionable square bounded by Broad and Twenty-second Streets on the east and west, Market on the north, and

---

82 Gilpin, Diary, entry for January 12, 1899. Quotations from Gilpin's Diary are hereafter cited in the text by the date of the entry.

Pine on the south. The hospital also boasted a house staff of twenty-seven interns directed by the chief resident, an assistant chief resident, and a resident pathologist.[83] Blockley had become an integrated part of the twentieth-century medical world, articulated into both its intellectual and social structure.

On the other hand, as we have emphasized, it was still an almshouse. The hospital's death rate remained at 12 percent, and a large proportion of its patients were chronically ill. In 1910, the average stay was thirty-five days at Blockley, and nineteen at Pennsylvania Hospital. The more things had changed, that is, the more they had remained the same. Blockley was still the residuary legatee for those cases desired least by Philadelphia's voluntary hospitals. And Blockley Hospital was still physically part of the almshouse complex – one known and feared by Philadelphia's working people. It was not until 1920 that the city opened a physically separate "Home for the Indigent," and not until the years between 1919 and 1926 that the "insane hospital" was moved to a separate location in the then still-rural northeastern part of the sprawling city. Several more generations of interns and residents had still to contend with the oversight of political appointees.

The city's social problems were not as amenable to a seeming technical solution – or even redefinition – as its medical ones. The chasm in social value between the public and the private sector remained. Class and social location still remained the primary determinant in deciding who would occupy Philadelphia's municipal hospital beds; and the problems of age, race, and chronic disease loomed if anything more prominently as the twentieth century progressed. With the retreat of the classic infectious diseases, the place of such problems only increased. For several years after the city of Philadelphia officially closed Philadelphia General Hospital in 1977, several hundred aged chronic patients remained in its depressing wards; the city had not yet remodeled a chronic disease hospital for them. These were patients that not even the promise of third-party payment could make palatable to other city hospitals and nursing homes. They were a fitting legacy for Blockley.

83 AR for 1910, pp. 121–127.

10

Making it in urban medicine: A career in the age of scientific medicine

• The three previous chapters, respectively on medicine in New York in 1866, the rise and fall of the dispensary, and Philadelphia's General Hospital, focus on the institutional fabric of urban medicine, one emphasizing interrelationships at a particular moment in time, the other two following institutions across time. This essay looks at the same urban setting, but employs a very different analytical strategy. It attempts to reconstruct that professional setting in terms of specific choices as perceived by a contemporary actor seeking to make his way among them. I wrote it partially because of an accident: my stumbling upon the extraordinary – and atypical – correspondence on which it is based; the letters were simply too rich and circumstantial to be ignored. But I also wrote it with the more general intent of demonstrating the relevance of biography to social and cultural history. I had heard too many comments from academic historians disparaging the conceptual deficiences of biography and the narrow vision of its practitioners. I have always thought very positively about biography and never felt that there was a necessary contradiction between the writing of an individual life and history generally. Quite the contrary in fact; a life can be construed as a sampling device – as a controlled and internally coherent batch of data, a chronologically ordered set of realities and relationships as perceived and understood by a particular actor. Biography, like the aggregated data of the historical demographer or student of voting behavior, constitutes an indispensable tool for the collective historical enterprise. •

Social scientists have long been aware of the difference between the way a social reality is perceived and construed by those living within it, and the way it is understood by individuals distant from it in space, time, or cultural assumption. For the historian, this is in some sense a distinction without ultimate significance. Common sense and the best historical practice agree that we must seek to assume both viewpoints: that is, to see the past as contemporary actors saw it, yet at the same time be prepared to impose a different meaning on the past, as experienced, while remaining aware that those past perceptions, no matter how self-deceiving or self-serving, were a *real* aspect of that particular past. The historian must be embedded in, yet abstracted from, the documents he or she studies.[1]

At a more practical level there is the problem of data and interpretation. It is easy enough to speak of attempting to approximate a particular historical reality with ever-greater precision, a great deal harder to do it. Only infrequently, for example, can a medical historian reconstruct the texture of a past practitioner's career as construed and lived. The following pages attempt to do just that. They are largely based on one atypically detailed and revealing source, the letters exchanged between a New York physician and his fiancée, later his wife. The young physician, John Sedgwick Billings, was no anonymous toiler in the therapeutic vineyards, but the well-educated son of one of America's most prominent leaders in public medicine, the polymathic John Shaw Billings.[2]

Nor was this a random time or place. New York City provided the most competitive and intense of battlefields in which to establish a medical career – while the years between the early 1890s and 1914 marked a period of dramatic transition for the medical profession. A new scientific medicine was beginning to make a place for itself in the worlds of teaching, practice, research, and public health. For the first time, most contemporaries felt, the intellectual products of the laboratory were beginning to effect fundamental change in patterns of morbidity and mortality. Like many of his contemporaries, young Billings sought to live in both the world of practice

---

1   I have developed this emphasis at somewhat greater length elsewhere. See Charles E. Rosenberg, "Woods or Trees? Ideas and Actors in the History of Science," *Isis* 79 (1988): 565–570; "Science in American Society: A Generation of Historical Debate," *Isis* 74 (1983): 356–367.

2   For a biography of the indefatigable senior Billings, see Fielding H. Garrison, *John Shaw Billings: A Memoir* (New York: G. P. Putnam's Sons, 1915). The John Sedgwick Billings letters are contained in the Hammond-Bryan-Cumming Family Papers deposited in the South Caroliniana Library at the University of South Carolina, Columbia, South Carolina. Unless otherwise specified, all letters cited in this paper are drawn from this collection. The collection includes a number of scrapbooks as well; the most useful for documenting Billings's life is Scrapbook 4, "An Autobiography by John Sedgwick Billings Prepared Principally to Cover his Education and Professional Career, 1869–1928 . . ." I should particularly like to thank Dr. Allen Stokes, Director of the South Caroliniana Library, for bringing this correspondence to my attention and for granting permission to quote from the letters. An arresting selection of the Hammond family's letters, including some between John Sedgwick Billings and Katherine Hammond, have been edited and published by Carol Bleser in *The Hammonds of Redcliffe* (New York: Oxford University Press, 1981). The great majority of the medical incidents and reflections cited below are not included in Bleser's volume, which does, however, document the personal relationship between John and Katherine.

and that of the academy. An intricate web of patronage and training, of medical practice and laboratory procedure, of personal services and nascent bureaucracy, helped shape the personal and professional options he understood and evaluated – and through which he sought success.

The Hopkins connection

After attending private schools in the District of Columbia, Billings graduated from the Johns Hopkins University with a B.A. in 1889. He then spent two years at Columbia University's College of Physicians and Surgeons before transferring to the University of Pennsylvania for his last year of medical school. He graduated in 1892, and the self-confident twenty-two-year-old soon received an appointment as assistant resident physician at the Johns Hopkins Hospital, a position he held through the fall of 1894.[3] As an undergraduate he had already begun to accumulate laboratory skills, taking summer courses in bacteriology and histology, chemistry, and pathology at the Army Medical Museum. In the spring of 1891 he had assisted A. C. Abbott in teaching a hygiene course at the Johns Hopkins Hospital, then spent the summer doing hematological research under William Osler, the hospital's eminent chief of medicine.[4] Billings was to evince a strong and continuing interest in hematology; while still a house officer, he published several articles on the blood in infectious disease.[5] Despite this atypical cultivation of skills in clinical pathology, the bulk of Billings's hospital training came in the area of what would today be called internal medicine. He was a practitioner first, a laboratory worker second.

Thus far I have outlined the typical career of a well-connected prospective member of America's late nineteenth-century medical elite, accumulating special clinical and laboratory training, publishing, making a place for himself in the hospital system. But Billings soon began to veer away from this well-understood path to prominence and success.

3 Scrapbook 4 in the Hammond-Bryan-Cumming Papers contains his letter of appointment from the Johns Hopkins Hospital. Dated December 13, 1892, it appointed him assistant resident for the period December 1, 1892, to December 1, 1893. During the summer of 1892, young Billings had served as substitute intern under Osler. The scrapbook also contains a detailed curriculum vitae that Billings prepared in 1914 for the New York City Department of Health.

4 With a father so prominent and respected, young Billings enjoyed easy access to influential superiors. Osler, for example, maintained a long-term personal interest in the young man's career. John Sedgwick Billings (hereafter JSB) to Katherine Hammond (hereafter KH or, after her marriage, KHB), October 8, 1894; JSB to KH, January 29, 1894.

5 See John S. Billings, Jr., "The Leucocytes in Croupous Pneumonia," *Bulletin of the Johns Hopkins Hospital* 5 (November 1894); 105–113; Billings, "The Leucocytes in Malarial Fever," *Bulletin of the Johns Hopkins Hospital* 5 (October 1894): 89–92.

As was so often the case in Victorian dramas of downward mobility, sex played a crucial role. While working in the Hopkins wards, Billings met an engaging young student nurse from a prominent South Carolina family – just the sort of young lady whose family origin and personal demeanor might have promised a successful administrative career in nursing. Katherine Hammond, however, was neither suited to nursing school discipline nor easily bent to authority; she found most of her fellow nurses coarse and Nurses' Training School Superintendent Isabel Hampton cold and authoritarian. Most important, she and young Billings became emotionally involved, kissing in linen closets and "walking out" together.[6] She was soon to part ways with the disapproving Miss Hampton (whom they referred to as "Miss Half-ton" or "Imperial Juno").[7] She returned home without her diploma, but not before establishing a serious relationship with young Billings. He too was less than enamored of the demanding and physically exhausting Hopkins world; a house officership meant endless cups of coffee and endless hours on call. "I am simply a bundle of nerves and exhaustion this afternoon," Billings complained in August 1893, "working steadily since 8 yesterday morning. I spent the whole of last night in the wards, working up malaria and drank quarts of coffee and smoked pounds of tobacco." His grueling routine was not to change. "Every one of the medical staff look like the devil," Billings wrote in September of 1894, "even [G. Alden] Blumer who is just back from his holiday looking fat and blooming, is beginning to get dark under the eyes & haggard. I must be losing a pound a day."[8]

The hard-working house officer was resentful, moreover, at having to minister to the coddled private patients of attending physicians, who presented the bills for the house officer's work and collected handsome fees. Nor did he appreciate serving as stand-in for his immediate clinical superior, William Henry Thayer, during the summer or on those days when the senior consultant traveled to see paying patients. "Thayer went away early yesterday morning on a $50 consultation trip," he complained on September 6, 1894. "He left the wards, private & public full of new patients and it has been a case of hustle to get them up to date, and do his work besides." Thayer's "short holidays" were always a hardship: "I am

6 On recollecting kissing, see JSB to KHB, May 21, 1905; on the need to avoid being seen in public, JSB to KH, August 8, 1893. Katherine's frequent letters home provide a detailed record of a student nurse's experience. I have cited a number of these in illustrating the social character of the late nineteenth-century hospital. Charles E. Rosenberg, *The Care of Strangers: The Rise of America's Hospital System* (New York: Basic Books, 1987), pp. 307–309.

7 On pejorative nicknames, see JSB to E[mily] Hammond, November 14, 1893, JSB to Emily Hammond, March 17, 1894.

8 JSB to KH, August 25, 1893, September 9, 1894.

expected to do as little that is decisive as possible in C [a private service] and at the same time be held responsible for anything that should have been done and was not."[9]

Billings began to reorder his personal priorities during the spring and summer of 1894. He decided to start in practice immediately so as to earn enough to support a wife. This was not the way one climbed the ladder of medical eminence. Family responsibilities had ruthlessly to be postponed. Henry Hurd, Superintendent of Hopkins Hospital, like many other administrators, always advised postdoctoral aspirants to avoid marriage. "If your time of preparation for your profession is limited," Hurd had explained a few years earlier to an applicant for specialist training, "or if like many other men you are in haste to marry I would not advise you to think of coming here."[10] Thus Osler was surprised when Billings turned down the ordinarily coveted opportunity to stay another year at the Hopkins.[11] Billings also decided not to visit the Continent for advanced training, although at this time such training was almost a necessity for an ambitious would-be academic clinician.

Getting started: The web of patronage

Billings decided to make his start in the enticing yet competitive world of New York medicine, and here John Shaw Billings's connections provided immediate help. John Sedgwick made a number of valuable contacts through his distinguished father's network of friends, clients, and colleagues.

First, Billings was able to locate a secure if modest position in the city's Department of Health; some income had to be assured while a novice physician toiled to accumulate a private practice. The New York Health Department had established an ad hoc bacteriology laboratory when the city was threatened by cholera in 1892.[12] In 1894 the Board of Health was

9 JSB to KH, September 6, 1894; August 10, 1894. "Interrupted again – this time to see a man who was fairly itching to pay some one ten dollars, but as Thayer is somewhere in the house, I have to keep my hands off." JSB to KH, August 10, 1894.
10 H. M. Hurd to R. R. Ross, October 28, 1890, Superintendent's Letterbooks, Alan Mason Chesney Archives of the Johns Hopkins Medical Institutions, Baltimore.
11 JSB to KH, July 8, 1894.
12 For background on the Board of Health in this period, see John Duffy, *A History of Public Health in New York City, 1866–1966*, vol. 2 of 2 (New York: Russell Sage Foundation, 1974); David A. Blancher, "Workshops of the Bacteriological Revolution: A History of the Laboratories of the New York City Department of Health, 1892–1912" (unpublished Ph.D. diss., City University of New York, 1979); Charles-Edward Amory Winslow, *The Life of Hermann M. Biggs, . . . Physician and Statesman of the Public Health* (Philadelphia: Lea & Febiger, 1929); Wade W. Oliver, *The Man who Lived for Tomorrow, A Biography of William Hallock Park, M.D.* (New York: E. P. Dutton, 1941).

allowed to organize a permanent "experimental station in the line of bacteriological work." A. A. Smith, an associate of John Shaw Billings and professor at Bellevue's medical school, assured his old friend that

> There will be six positions each paying a salary of $1,200 per year. I am promised one of the appointments. My idea was to appoint your son to that position which will take about four hours a day. The remainder of the day he could use as he saw fit (cultivating practice etc.) My associate Dr. Carlisle has a flat in this street which your son could share with him. In this way he could have a good living place at moderate expense for NY and be in a way to do work which would ultimately make him independent.[13]

Billings was soon appointed to one of these places. In addition, Smith promised that the young man could help him in his practice and with his library and clinical research – and possibly do some teaching at Bellevue. Billings was not altogether pleased, although the arrangement was one that would have seemed heaven-sent to most new-fledged practitioners. "Well – I know my fate," he wrote to Katherine on November 5:

> briefly it is this. To be in New York Nov. 25th, so as to start work by the 1st of Dec. To live in a narrow dark little flat with a "small, good" man – you know the kind – and to have the two worst rooms. To help another man make a literary reputation for himself – to do his night work when his regular assistant will not condescend. To teach in Bellevue – by all accounts one of the dirtiest, "smelliest," political jobs there is – next Spring, if they start a post-graduate course. Finally, to work four hours a day in a Tammany bacteriological laboratory.[14]

Young Billings needed more income than was provided by his $100-a-month salary from the Department of Health. With his father's help, he found another part-time position – this with the street-cleaning department, examining job applicants and caring for employed "White Angels" (as the city's sanitation workers were called) in their homes when they fell ill.[15] This provided another fifty dollars a month, although he could not be appointed as a full-time physician and, like any hourly laborer, had to line

---

13 Abram Alexander Smith to John Shaw Billings, October 23, 1894. Scrapbook 4, Hammond-Bryan-Cumming Papers. (Hereafter I follow JSB's custom of referring to his patron as A. A. Smith.) See also in the same scrapbook a letter from the Secretary of the New York Health Department, dated January 25, 1895, to JSB provisionally appointing him assistant bacteriologist at a salary of $1,200.

14 JSB to KH, November 5, 1894. See also JSB to KH, October 25, 1894.

15 John Shaw Billings was a friend of George Waring, Jr., New York's well-known street-cleaning commissioner. See also JSB to KH, January 12, 1895. John Shaw Billings had also expedited his son's New York State licensing so that the young man was spared the inconvenience of passing an examination before beginning practice. JSB to KH, February 22, 1894.

up each month at the stables to be paid. "I had to stand in line two mortal hours to get my money," he complained on May 6, 1898. "Garlic in front of me – and behind me – stale beer and whiskey every where – mingled with perspiration and plug tobacco."[16] Moreover, the self-important young man found the routine of examining prospective street cleaners demeaning in itself, underlining in its unpleasantness Billings's pressing financial needs.[17]

It was private practice, however, that loomed as fundamental. Like most young physicians, Billings opened an office and posted hours; but this was no more than a prudent mechanism for attracting marginal patients. His primary tactic for establishing a practice lay elsewhere: in assuming the role of assistant to an established clinician. After a decade or more of useful subordination, one might hope to inherit a patron's practice – while in the interim gradually building up one's own. Again following a familiar pattern, Billings sublet a bedroom and sitting room from Robert R. Carlisle, who served as Smith's primary assistant.[18] Billings filled in when Carlisle was unavailable, often sitting for usually tedious although occasionally stressful hours of "night duty" in the bedrooms of affluent private patients.[19] Billings's laboratory skills, atypical for physicians of the time, allowed him to play another auxiliary role: he performed blood and urine analyses and thus provided an informal clinical pathology service. He also acted as "etherizer" for surgeon friends in both hospital and home procedures.

But these varied tasks did not fill an entire work day. Time was still available in which to organize an ascent of the first rungs on the ladder to hospital eminence. As so many of his peers and predecessors were doing and had done before him, Billings sought an entering-level hospital position – which meant volunteer outpatient work. "I will not have very

---

16 JSB to KHB, May 6, 1898. In 1898 the system changed and Billings was able to submit bills for payment monthly. JSB to "Dear Lady" [Emily Hammond], July 20, 1899.

17 "I am getting slightly weary," he explained to his mother-in-law in the fall of 1897, "of the procession of rum-soaked Irishmen, garlicky Dagos, sauerkrautish Dutchmen and last but not least Oh Lord, nigger-smelling Afro-American brothers, that defile past me daily from eight to nine and six to seven." JSB to "Dearest Other Mother" [Emily Hammond], September 16, 1897.

18 The house rented unfurnished at $1,600 per year, which did not include gas or servants. Billings and Carlisle were each to get an office and bedroom and share the drawing room and bathroom. JSB to KH, November 24, 1894.

19 Billings also undertook library research at the New York Academy of Medicine for his father's friend, the prominent surgeon Frederick Dennis, as well as for A. A. Smith. JSB to KH, January 14, 1895. Such tasks were a well-accepted aspect of traditional patronage relations. William Henry Welch, for example, helped Austin Flint in preparing the fifth edition of his *Principles and Practice*. Donald Fleming, *William H. Welch and the Rise of Modern Medicine* (Baltimore: Johns Hopkins University Press, 1987, orig. ed. 1954), p. 62.

much time to devote to private practice," he explained to Katherine, "but not having any p.p. there will be no great harm done. What I must do however is to get some afternoon dispensary work – I am getting very rusty in the one thing I want to keep up – and must."[20] Here too, he could call upon his father's connections. "Lobbying again," he wrote two months later, "this continual wire-pulling and drumming up of influence makes me very weary."[21] Finally a letter from the Sister Superior at Washington's Good Samaritan Hospital to her counterpart at New York's St. Vincent's helped produce a staff position at the latter hospital's outpatient clinic.[22]

Struggling in practice

But these institutional and academic interests did not obscure Billings's primary interest, the desire to accumulate income from his private practice. His first office patient was a servant girl: "splinter *** thumb *** forceps *** $2.00. There you have it. I have a good mind to have the bill framed, and hang it on the wall." But he could hardly have lived on the handful of such cases he saw.[23] He soon found, moreover, that a solo practitioner's life could be stressful as well as discouraging, and that the demands of the profession could be dismayingly novel to a young clinician accustomed to the Johns Hopkins Hospital, where residents could "take [their] time at making a diagnosis. . . . It is different now – oh so different." This was Billings's conclusion after describing his "first dive into private practice," an emergency call to a two-year-old in convulsions, "blue in the face, [with] no pulse. . . ." The emergency left the novice practitioner a "nervous wreck."[24] But in his first decade in Manhattan, such ventures into private homes were never regular enough to establish his own practice on a secure basis. Most of Billings's private calls were made in his role as stand-in, first for A. A. Smith, and after a few years for Austin Flint, Jr., who replaced Smith as his patron.

20 JSB to KH, January 14, 1895.
21 "Especially," he continued, "when it is in vain as in this case. St. Vincents is a straight-out Roman Catholic institution and the appointment I am after is made by the Sister Superior – the Medical Board only confirm her." JSB to KH, March 31, 1895.
22 Sister Mary Laurentia, [St. Vincent's] New York, to Sister Anthony, Good Samaritan Hospital, April 26, 1895, Scrapbook 4, Hammond-Bryan-Cumming Papers.
23 JSB to KH, January 12, 1895.
24 "Nature and I brought him out of his fit. . . . I have been paying three calls a day since and am undone. . . . I have asked for a nurse. . . . The people are heavy swells, rich as the classical damp earth, and have given me a free hand. So much for luck. They were homeopaths – it remains for me to convert them." JSB to KH, January 4, 1895.

These subordinate relationships meant continual insecurity and dependence. Perhaps a physician with a different personality might have proven more successful in accumulating a stable pool of patients, but in all likelihood Billings was no more than typical in his ups and downs. Clients were few and far between, and when billed they often failed to pay. "If my patients would only pay up," he complained in 1896, "but that is the hopeless despairing cry of every D.[amn] F.[ool] of a young doctor in New York – or elsewhere."[25] His physician patrons also proved slow or grudging in compensating him for patient care and laboratory work. Billings's father warned him in the fall of 1896 that the young couple would "have to have at least $300 a month, or we will come to grief."[26] In his first years of practice, Billings rarely attained this goal. It was not until the spring of 1897 that the aspiring clinician could afford to marry his South Carolina sweetheart.

Billings soon came to realize that a stable and remunerative practice in New York was by no means guaranteed; many well-trained and well-connected practitioners were never to achieve such success. In the summer of 1895, he wrote to his fiancée that New York City was most depressing, for "no one seems to succeed who is not willing to eat a little blacking – who has (a word that I hate) push and 'hustles' for practice."[27] Carlisle, his fellow tenant and assistant to Smith, had finished his house officership ten years before and was just getting started in his own practice.[28] Billings asked rhetorically whether there was a "place here for the exact sort of good-for-nothing that I am. One must have money, must be a member of a well known N.Y. family – or must have monumental brazen nerve, cheek, impudence, assurance – whatever you may chance to call it."[29] A year and a half later, things had not changed substantially.

> Bill, my chief at the Presbyterian who has been in practice here for ten years, told me yesterday that he would have to give up in the Spring,

25 JSB to KH, March 5, 1896. "If people would only pay us what they owe us – we would be on velvet," he wrote to his wife as late as 1900. "As it is, I am hustling around for rent money today. I have it all but a little and will surely have that by to night – it is the having to hustle that makes me sick and tired." JSB to KHB, May 14, 1900.
26 JSB to KH, September 26, 1896.
27 JSB to KH, [July 22], 1895.
28 JSB to KH, December 9, 1894. Billings complained that his relationship to Smith "pays fairly well, but is almost useless as an aid to getting practice of your own." See also JSB to KH, December 11, 1894.
29 JSB to KH, May 17, 1895. Billings had been anxious all that spring as he came to realize how difficult it would be to attract private patients. "I have had no outside work now for over a week," he wrote in March, "and am growing apprehensive. . . . And we are thinking of taking a house, which will raise our expenses about 800 a year, apiece. The Governor [his father, John Shaw Billings] will be able to paper his room with my notes of hand." JSB to KH, March 6, 1895.

and go to some small town – he said he wanted to marry, and had waited three or four years, but his practice had not grown.[30]

Meanwhile, Billings lived a life of genteel poverty.

> I have no money to go anywhere or to do anything with – have had no clothes – could take no vacation on that account. . . . I go to a base-ball game once a month, and twice a month (about) have gone to cheap and nasty roof gardens, to drink some very poor beer – keeping my expenses under a dollar each time.[31]

A year later Billings could still complain about his inability to find time for a vacation to visit his fiancée: "I could not leave my half dozen patients who I see regularly – my practice. 'It's a wee thing, but it's my own.'"[32]

Economic pressures allowed few academic – or ethical – luxuries. Billings treated every pay patient he could find, even those more suited to a specialist's care; he simply could not afford to refer.[33] He solicited patients at his several dispensary clinics, even stamping his private office address and hours on appointment cards. Early in 1897, he bought a "rubber stamp with my name, address and office hours – this I will stamp on the back of all the tickets of my Dispensary patients – they say it pays to do it."[34] Billings was well aware that such means of attracting dispensary patients were ethically suspect, and in many institutions explicitly forbidden, but felt that he could not forgo the opportunity. "I hardly like that way of getting them [patients], but everything goes!"[35] Billings's work as clinical pathologist, testing bloods, feces, and urines, while it provided some income, kept him in a status subordinate to other physicians – without direct access to

---

30 "Low down J.S.B. Jr. – for even as I sympathized with him, I could not help thinking that I would get the clinic when he left." JSB to KH, December 4, 1896.

31 "My actual living expenses (bed & bread) are some eighty dollars a month in excess of my income – of which my unfortunate parent has to bear the brunt, so that naturally I do not exceed that amount by any more than I can possibly help." JSB to KH, September 3, 1895. A letter of September 15, 1895, provides more detail about Billings's genteel poverty, including his habit of turning up trousers and finding a tailor who sent bills only once a year.

32 JSB to KH, March 11, 1896.

33 "I should have called in a specialist immediately," he reflected on a case of otitis media, "but like a fool thought I could earn the money as well as he. Well – I get the money anyway." JSB to KH, February 21, 1895. See also JSB to KH, April 6, 1895.

34 JSB to KH, February 3, 1897. In later years, Billings also used prescription pads with a pharmacist's name and address printed on them (and sometimes used them in place of letter paper!).

35 JSB to KH, June 20, 1895. For examples of opposition to this practice, see, for example, Cooper Medical College, Committee on Clinics, January 22, 1889, Lane Medical Library, Stanford University; T. Grange Simons, M.D., to Trustees of the Shirras Dispensary, Shirras Dispensary Papers, Record Group 31, Charleston City Archives, Charleston, S.C.

the city's limited pool of paying patients.[36] In the spring of 1900, he wrote to his wife that he had just gone over his books for the past three years: "'On my own hook' I made $520 the first year (1897) – $684 in 1898 – and $1,020 last year."[37]

Billings remained dependent during these years on the tiring but secure part-time work for the Board of Health and the street-cleaning department. He had found the latter work particularly exhausting and unpredictable, and gave it up at the end of the century. In addition to examining healthy applicants, sometimes as many as 200 in a busy morning at the department's stables, he had to visit the sick in their often distant tenement homes; and these time-consuming duties had to be fit in among other tasks in the laboratory, the dispensary, the library, and his private practice.[38] In the summers, when the city's elite practitioners vanished *en masse* to such watering places as Newport and Bar Harbor, private practice was always unpredictable – sometimes busy, but often sparse.[39] His days were nevertheless always hectic and exhausting. "Tuesday is my busiest day," he explained to Katherine on March 2, 1897:

> I did not stop "going" today until 6:30. Down town, two sweepers, a call, early lunch, 65 patients at our clinic in the Dispensary, down to Bellevue to examine a jaundiced man's blood for A. A. Smith, and then home where I managed to finish the blood examination by dinner time.[40]

36 Billings sought to increase his medical clientele for such services but never succeeded in attracting steady referrals except from his patrons Smith and Flint. (See also JSB to KH, September 27, 1896, and October 15, 1896.) The tests were, moreover, quite detailed and presumably time-consuming. His standard form, entitled "Report of Urine Examination," listed values for nineteen different parameters ranging from sugar and urea to leucocytes. (Part of a letter of May 8, 1900, is written on a blank printed report form.) Billings was able to use the laboratory facilities at the Board of Health; establishing a commercial clinical pathology laboratory was never a real option in that decade.

37 These were his third, fourth, and fifth years in practice. JSB to KHB, April 23, 1900. "We are doing a little better all the time," he concluded, "if we had not, how could we have got on without the S.C.D. money?"

38 For the 200 applicants, see JSB to KH, April 9, 1897.

39 The comparative handful of prominent physicians who monopolized "society's" medical custom experienced no hiatus in *their* practice; "I have been rushed as usual," Austin Flint, Jr., wrote Billings from Newport, "about 30 calls a day lately and at all hours." Flint to "Dear Billings" (JSB), September 2, 1906.

40 JSB to KH, March 2, 1897. Such hectic days were no more than routine. "I have been hustling," he explained on February 8, 1897. "Just listen – Left the house at 8:25, got 5 calls to make from Rogers [a friend in surgical practice], went to the Laboratory & signed the time book, ([Walter] Bensel did my work for me today, as I did his for him yesterday), then 1 Rutgers Place, away down below the Bridge to see W.A. [White Angel] no. 1, back to Lab. then to my Hebrew Patient whom I injected and have $\frac{1}{2}$ hr's massage – and I want you to know that it was the hardest work I have done in years –

Every year brought with it mixed emotions, as Billings's income from private practice varied but never became steady and abundant. With A. A. Smith and later Austin Flint, Jr., Billings maintained his role as "associate" in the establishments of the wealthy and socially prominent, treating servants and family members alike. But no matter how competent he was as a clinician, direct access to a reliable supply of such desirable patients escaped him.

What is most revealing about young Billings's private practice, in retrospect, is the way in which he functioned in a transitional role, bridging the gap between an impending era of institutionally sited scientific medicine (with its clinical laboratories, radiology departments, purpose-built operating rooms, and the like) and a period marked by the lingering unwillingness of the prosperous and respectable to be treated in a hospital.[41] When Billings stayed overnight with an ailing Vanderbilt, or in any prolonged typhoid case or protracted labor, he was serving as the functional equivalent of a house officer; when he drew bloods and collected urine samples, then took them to the Department of Health for evaluation and reported his results, he was serving as ad hoc clinical pathology laboratory; when he administered anesthesia in a patient's home or hospital operating room, he acted as an anesthesiologist before the specialty had come into being and had become firmly situated in the hospital.[42] It was a multifaceted role that came easily to a young man with Billings's training, ambition, and financial needs, but a role that implied economic subordination and ultimate obsolescence. Nevertheless, his varied sources of income, supplemented by loans and free office space in his father's house, allowed Billings to piece out a steadily increasing if somewhat erratic income after his first few years in New York.[43]

But with marriage and the arrival of two children, costs rose as well. His

then away up Second Ave above 48th to see W.A.'s no. 2 & 3, then across town to 42nd St & North River W.A. 4 – then home to lunch at 1:30, but I found a patient here (that Mrs. Willis we met at the San Remo) and I had to examine her blood and go all over her (we will make $40 or 50 out of her) – then luncheon – then I made out my W.A. reports and took them to the Stable ... then to the Academy Library when I worked on the literature of the relative fatality of pneumonia of the upper lobes of the lungs for A. A. S.[mith] ... then down to 14th St & 2nd Ave to see a sick Sweeper who was to pay me $1.00 but was out – and finally home here at 5:45." JSB to KH, February 8, 1897.

41 As late as 1906, he was still concerned about the need to "fumigate" a private patient's bedroom so that he could "look forward to her confinement with a relatively easy mind." JSB to KHB, April 12, 1906.

42 Billings regularly charged five dollars for administering anesthesia. See JSB to KHB, April 8, 1898.

43 It should be emphasized that John always posted regular office hours, no matter what the variety and intensity of his other duties. But as will be emphasized, private practice never became an adequate source of income for his steadily increasing needs.

new wife would not live with his parents for a day longer than necessary, and the young couple soon moved into their own house.[44] Moreover, Billings had an image of an appropriate status and style of life that assumed servants, preferably white ones, and vacations at the shore.[45] He was even upset at the thought that his wife might be seen walking their baby herself in Central Park.[46] It was difficult to give up the security provided by the Department of Health.

In the heroic age of public health

New York's municipal health board enjoys an enviable place in the history of public medicine, especially in the application of bacteriology and immunology in the fight against infectious disease. Every historian familiar with the field is aware that New York City is generally credited with creating the first modern municipal bacteriological laboratory; the work and names of Hermann N. Biggs, William Hallock Park, and S. Josephine Baker are equally well known. The city's turn-of-the-century health department screened cholera cases, manufactured and distributed diphtheria antitoxin, tested cultures for tuberculosis and diphtheria, pioneered in applying the Widal test for typhoid, and battled tuberculosis with a varied program that included bacteriological diagnosis, the testing of cattle, and an aggressive community-oriented program of education and isolation.

Billings was involved in all those activities, but for many years he occupied a position in the trenches, not at the more visible command posts, in the war against infectious disease. From the lowly position of "assistant bacteriologist," realities looked rather different than they do in historical retrospect. First, the bacteriologist's workload was enormous and the level of diagnostic accuracy less than impressive. One day in 1902, for example, he examined 104 diptheria cultures by eleven in the morning; tuberculosis

44 Soon after Katherine arrived in New York, the young couple rented a house on East 53rd Street for two and a half years. JSB to Henry [Hammond], August 6, 1898. John had long made clear that he regarded "boarding" as beneath him. JSB to KH, September 29, 1896.

45 "My saying white servants was pure inadvertance," he apologized to his South Carolina−born wife. " I am perfectly content to have colored ones...." JSB to KHB, January 24, 1908.

46 In 1898, Katherine wrote to her mother that she was going to take the baby to the park herself since it was the nurse's afternoon out. "I am afraid that John does not like it very much, but it is perfectly absurd that the poor child should suffer because of a foolish prejudice. I have been living in N.Y. a year & a half − & in that time I never met anybody on the street that I knew so there is not one chance in ten thousand that I will meet anybody I know when I have the baby." KHB to Dearest Mother [Emily Hammond], [1898, undated].

slides were even more time-consuming, each one taking as much time as twenty diphtheria specimens.[47] When the Widal test was first described, the informally trained Billings soon found himself charged with mastering it and adapting it to laboratory routine. "I got a formal order today," he wrote on November 18, 1897,

> to familiarize myself with Widal's test for typhoid fever and be ready to do it as a routine thing – for the Board of Health is going to make the diagnosis free of charge, just as they do in diphtheria and tuberculosis now – that is if the test turns out to be reliable. It is simple and does not involve very much eye work – if I do that, I will give up tuberculosis, and limit myself to diphtheria and typhoid – it is the tuberculosis work that strains my eyes and gives me headaches.[48]

Desperate ailments, moreover, inspired desperate countermeasures; an epidemic of cerebrospinal meningitis in 1905, for example, demanded visible action. "'Something must be done,'" Billings reported Hermann Biggs as exclaiming. And something was done. "At Gouverneur Hospital where they have many cases, they have injected diphtheria antitoxin in the last thirteen cases – and twelve have recovered!!! Why? – don't ask me. But we are going to inject – or offer to inject – all cases reported to us."[49] The abstract criteria of scientific method had little to do with such casual procedures.

Funds were always short and staffing often inadequate. Billings had on occasion to wash walls, plane and rehang doors, and clean glassware with a 5 percent solution of carbolic acid. ("I don't know whether you remember carbolic," he complained to his fiancée, "or perhaps your hands were tough – but mine are burning and tingling as they used to when I had been snowballing, even now – an hour and a half later: why it is hard to hold a pen even.")[50] On another occasion he found the work space contaminated by carelessly handled tetanus cultures.[51] Billings was, in addition, an imperious and quarrelsome young man; he had a particularly difficult relationship with Anna Williams, an energetic and more senior bacteri-

---

47 JSB to KHB, July 9, 1902. For the comparison of diphtheria and tuberculosis diagnosis, see JSB to KH, March 3, 1897. When there was a diphtheria scare, things could become hectic indeed, as physicians awaited the reports on specimens they had turned in to the board's laboratory. One March morning in 1903, for example, Billings arrived at the laboratory to find 587 diphtheria cultures awaiting diagnosis. JSB to KHB, April 1, 1903.
48 JSB to KH, November 18, 1896.
49 JSB to KHB, February 23, 1905.
50 JSB to KH, October 16, 1896. For Billings's carpentry, see JSB to KH, October 7, 1896.
51 JSB to KH, October 1, 1896, contains a circumstantial account of this incident.

ologist, and later with S. A. Knopf, the prominent antituberculosis worker and advocate of social medicine.[52] And there was, of course, a constant need to anticipate political shifts and pressures, for the Department of Health was a microcosm ultimately controlled by politicians, ordinarily by Tammany Hall.

More dramatic than Billings's bureaucratic guerrilla warfare were his encounters with poverty in the city's tenements. As a Hopkins resident he had treated poor Baltimoreans, but he had never imagined conditions like those he found on New York's Lower East Side, or in Hell's Kitchen on the West Side.[53] Like many of his elite medical contemporaries, Billings experienced and communicated a mixture of contempt and sympathy for the working poor; even as shallow and unreflective a young man as Billings could not avoid responding to the misery and deprivation he encountered. "I had another diphtheria case in the slums assigned to me today," he wrote to his fiancée in rural South Carolina.

> It is an awful nuisance these hot days to potter around in the reeking filthy dens these people live in. If one could only help them, but it is impossible, and the sight of the weazened stunted children and the beast-like parents – why I am really depressed for at least three minutes after each visit.[54]

Two years later his sentiments had changed little. "Great Zeus, but it is hot," he complained on July 6, 1897,

> I had to go into the very heart of the district of the poorer Italians and Polish Jews this morning – and the mephitic vapors fried out of those sweltering mortals (to say nothing of garlic, weary fruit, etc) were

52 Billings complained on October 6, 1896 (JSB to KH), that the "'lady bacteriologist' thinks I am treading on her toes, taking her assistants and stopping her work." A week later, he noted that she "still fights me hard about everything. I feel like giving her a spanking with a hair brush – the good old fashioned way." JSB to KH, October 13, 1896; see also JSB to KH, October 14, 1896. A year later their mutual hostility remained undiminished. "Here *is* something nasty," Billings reported, on February 19, 1897. "Dec. 30th when I was on duty down town alone, I had 130 cultures to examine. Biggs, without telling me, had the cultures and my results, sent up to the 16th St Lab, where Dr. Williams examined them, and now sends down word that 30% of my diagnoses were wrong. She is the woman with whom I had the row last summer, and poison is not a circumstance to the way she hates me." On Knopf, see, for example, JSB to KHB, April 28, 1904; JSB to KHB, May 28, 1906. For Anna Williams's recollections, see her unpublished autobiography "A Life Time in the Laboratory," 1936, Anna Williams Papers, Schlesinger Library, Radcliffe Institute, Cambridge, Mass.
53 JSB to KH, April 7, 1897. He was often a "target for empty tomato cans and other missiles" hurled by truculent local urchins when he made tenement visits. He was grateful when such visits coincided with school hours.
54 JSB to KH, August 6, 1895.

enough to make even an Irish legislator put a $100 poll tax on every immigrant entering New York.[55]

He could also be moved by the plight of his clinical charges, especially the children. "I am tormenting myself," he reflected in the summer of 1895,

> over a little diphtheric child I am in charge of – down in the Chinese
> quarter on Mott St – one room inhabited by father, mother, grown son
> and four children. The first impluse of a civilized being is to rush to
> the window, throw it up, and sit on the sill, with head outside. . . . Well
> – no antitoxine has been given so that I could study an untreated case
> – the child is very ill, it is too late to give the antitoxine now – and do
> what I may, I can see or think of nothing else but that poor wretched
> scrawny little atom – I shall never forget it, if it dies. I went down early
> this morning, fearing to find it dead – but it was still alive . . . dimly
> wondering why *it* should have to bear all that.[56]

Although Billings shared the enthusiasm of his contemporaries, and most subsequent chroniclers, for the accomplishments of late nineteenth-century laboratory medicine, he lived and worked in the elusive world in which those laboratory findings had to be applied. Billings's reality was far more ambiguous than that recorded in the standard textbook sentences celebrating Behring's discovery of diphtheria antitoxin or Koch's identification of the tuberculosis bacillus.[57]

Even the harried and self-consciously blasé Billings felt that some of his public health work was at least dramatic, if not in a measure heroic. "Last night *was* the night, for fair," he reported on March 16, 1897.

> I got a police telegram from the President of the Department of
> Health telling me to report down town at 8 p.m. last night. Cursing &
> groaning inwardly (for I was sure it meant antitoxin work) I went
> down, and found to my astonishment, every doctor in the Board of

55 JSB to [Emily Hammond], July 6, 1897. Billings was consistently anti-Semitic and
  hostile to "colored" men and women. On Jews, see, for example, JSB to KH,
  December 10, 1896; JSB to KH, February 25, 1897; JSB to KH, April 2, 1897. On
  his racism, see his comments some years later when he anticipated attending "a
  meeting of colored physicians – as per enclosed notice. My – I hope the windows will
  be open and the room large." JSB to KH, June 2, 1905.
56 JSB to KH, September 1, 1895. One need hardly underline the attitudes toward
  clinical experimentation and "informed consent" – to employ an anachronistic term –
  illustrated in this incident.
57 I refer here primarily to the gap between an agreed-upon laboratory understanding and
  its clinical application. There are obviously a different set of epistemological questions
  as well, relating in this instance to the cognitive history of immunology and serology.
  See the pioneering study by Ludwik Fleck, *Genesis and Development of a Scientific Fact*
  (Chicago: University of Chicago Press, 1979). The original German edition was
  published in 1935.

Health (sixty odd) there and twice as many policemen – not every doctor, for Anna Williams was "excused." It seemed that a case of small-pox, coming from the lodging-houses, had been found in the New York Hospital – so the President determined to cover the whole of N.Y. city in a single night, and vaccinate all the lodgers in the lodging houses. Our corps was first, and I was 3d man – of course they began with the Bowery, and No's 39 $\frac{1}{2}$ and 41 Bowery were assigned to me. I filled my pockets with vials of vaccine, papers of needles and bundles of toothpicks, got my two big burly attendant policemen and started. Oh what a night – I told them where we were to go, and with one voice they said "That's Hell's Morgue" – nice cheerful nickname. It is a great big 5 cent lodging house – capacity 400 lodgers. I cannot describe to you the filth, and dirt and rank, reeking, penetrating foulness of the place. Only 180 men were there, and I vaccinated over 140 of them – one eighth too dead drunk to even remonstrate – another eighth fighting drunk – and one and all the veriest dregs of humanity. As those sodden, vicious, drunk-[scarred] caricatures of faces would glare at you out of their black holes, blinking at the candle, and every nerve and muscle on the alert, like some cornered wild animal – truly they were nearer beasts than men. I got through by eleven – gave my "coppers" and the clerk who carried the candle, a drink and a cigar all round, and came home to hang my clothes and overcoat out of the window – and they still had the reek of the vile den in them this morning. I had one row – the fellow struck me, and I knocked him down and the policeman arrested him – I told him I would let him go if he would be vaccinated. He came around like a lamb, and all the other men in the room (the "roost" they called it) could not come up and bare their arms quick enough. Ye Gods – there will be "Hell on the Bowery" sure enough in a weeks time – that virus of ours takes like oil of vitriol, and every Bowery Bum will have a beautiful arm on him in six or seven days.[58]

The would-be academic: Dispensary, hospital, and classroom

Throughout his busy days and years in the 1890s, Billings sought a foothold in New York's patronage-structured academic world. "You will be Mrs Professor before we are through," he wrote to Katherine on November 10, 1896, as he eyed a position for the coming year at Columbia University's College of Physicians and Surgeons, which he described as "a foot on the ladder to better things."[59] Billings began to ascend that ladder

58 JSB to KH, March 16, 1897.
59 JSB to KH, November 10, 1896.

by occupying an assortment of unpaid dispensary positions – the unavoidable first step in an elite medical career.

The quality of New York's institutional outpatient care was, Billings
felt, far below the Johns Hopkins standard. At both St. Vincent's and
Presbyterian (where he moved after serving a brief tenure at St. Vincent's),
outpatient medicine was rushed and routine – and at St. Vincent's even the
physical facilities were inadequate. "Rotten – rank – beastly – that is my
opinion of the St. Vincents dispensary: small dark dirty rooms, no system
and no therapeutics – simply a lot of mixtures called no. 1, 2, 3 &c. –
which are the only things allowed to be given."[60] Limited resources
coupled with chronic and trivial cases in enormous abundance guaranteed
that little of educational or research value would take place. The youthful
clinician described a typical afternoon's work as "admiring babies and
cheering up chronics." In a more thoughtful vein, Billings, like other
dispensary physicians, was well aware that his patients' grim personal
circumstances militated against his having any long-lasting impact on their
health. "I am worrying not a little about my dispensary work," he reflected
in mid-1895, "you see three-fourths of the cases are babies and what they
need is good food – and fresh air. Well they cannot get them, so in
consequence I have lost three cases in the last three weeks, which could
just as well have lived."[61]

By the next year, Billings found a place (with his father's help) at the far
more prestigious Presbyterian Hospital – where he hoped to "get in on the
ground floor."[62] But here too, he lamented, the outpatient service was far
from what it might and should have been.

> It makes me angry to see such a good service as we have at the
> Presbyterian wasted as it is – it could be almost as good as the one at
> the J.H.H. but – no histories are taken, examinations of heart & chest

60 JSB to KH, April 24, 1895. Billings's anti-Catholicism and Hopkins background
   combined to intensify his dislike for St. Vincent's. "I went to St. Vincents for the first
   time to day – it is a dirty hole compared to *the* hospital. The Sister Superior looked me
   over and, I think, gave me the marble heart – 'Dispensary Physician, Nit 'as they say in
   the fourt' ward." He was also unenthusiastic about subordination to a female, religious
   or not. JSB to KH, April 3, 1895.
61 The "admiring babies" phrase is from JSB to KH, August 28, 1895, and the quote
   from JSB to KH, [July 22], 1895.
62 JSB to KH, December 6, 1896. Billings senior, who served on the Board of Managers
   at the Presbyterian, was a significant factor in his son's appointment. See JSB to KHB,
   July 9, 1898. The young man displayed no small degree of arrogance when attaining
   what would have seemed a desirable appointment to most aspiring clinicians. He
   expressed annoyance, for example, at the effrontery of "a little Jack-in-office who has
   charge of the place," who "insists on my going through all the formalities." JSB to
   KH, November 14, 1896.

and so on, are not recorded – no clinical laboratory work is done – and yet they have the money and the space and the patients.[63]

The patient load was, however, far too abundant for careful evaluation of individuals; on one "heavy" afternoon, for example, Billings arrived at the outpatient clinic at 12:40, stayed until 4:00 – and treated fifty-five patients.[64]

Billings was well aware, however, that dispensary work was the necessary first step on the road to a more desirable position "on the inside" as visiting or attending physician. "I want to be on my best behaviour there [in Presbyterian's outpatient department]," he explained to his fiancée, "so as to stand a chance for a House appointment some day."[65] Such hospital status was almost synonymous with professional status. Thus, even with his hectic schedule and scorn for New York's prevailing outpatient care, Billings had no choice but to continue his dispensary work. The need to maintain and expand clinical skills, the opportunity to attract a few private patients, and the possibility of teaching small groups of fee-paying students, as well as the need to make the contacts and put in the time required to compete for an inpatient position, all conspired to make volunteer dispensary work a necessity.

The next step toward the career Billings sought was obtaining a toehold in a medical school faculty. But it was not easily accomplished. At first, he hoped to teach a postgraduate course at Bellevue; he much preferred, however, to pursue a possible connection with the far more prestigious Vanderbilt Clinic or Roosevelt Hospital.[66]

Soon, however, he found himself seeking a laboratory teaching post at Bellevue's Carnegie Laboratory ("just what I wanted – Clinical Microscopy

63 JSB to KH, November 5, 1896. For details of the Hopkins outpatient record-keeping system, see Henry M. Hurd to Adam Wright, October 23, 1890, Superintendent's Letterbooks, Alan Mason Chesney Archives of the Johns Hopkins Medical Institutions, Baltimore.

64 JSB to KH, April 6, 1897. Billings resigned from the Presbyterian dispensary in 1899. Entry for April 10, 1899. Minutes, Medical Board, Presbyterian Hospital Archives, New York.

65 For JSB's use of the "inside" phrase, see JSB to KHB, April 28, 1898. The quotation is from JSB to KH, July 28, 1896. For a discussion of medical career patterns in their relationship to the hospital in this period, see Charles E. Rosenberg, *Care of Strangers*, *passim* and esp. ch. 7, "A Marriage of Convenience: Hospitals and Medical Careers," pp. 166–189.

66 "The home of the swelled-heads & would be aristocrats of N.Y. medicine, according to the outside 2/3ds – of which Smith, Dennis, Carlisle & Bellevue generally are members. But they – the s.h's & w.b.a's – are the men I have met at our table at home, and with whom all my thoughts of N.Y. medicine have been associated. So it is not all pure snobbishness on my part, you see." JSB to KH, February 16, 1895. For a detailed and candid evaluation of the Bellevue Hospital Medical School, see JSB to KH, September 30, 1896.

with Clinical ward class teaching on the side"), only to find that his "pull" was not adequate to acquiring the hoped-for position.[67] Teaching histology or clinical pathology would, in fact, have been plausible goals given Billings's particular background, but there were few such positions and the great majority even of these were poorly paid, part-time, and much sought after. At the Carnegie Laboratory, for example, Hermann Biggs's "Cousin George" was entrenched ahead of Billings. After Cornell University established its medical school and Bellevue established a new relationship with New York University, Billings sought for months to find a secure niche in this new situation. But, as he mused, "small fry" like himself had to find shelter as best they could in these institutional storms, while even the larger predators fought to establish or maintain secure places.[68] Like many others in his position, Billings explored the possibility of securing additional income by teaching quiz classes to young men preparing for the city's competitive hospital examinations.[69]

Billings worked on scientific projects as well. Some of his time at the city's bacteriological laboratory was in fact designated "research," although in retrospect development and application might seem a more precise designation. "I have been down town this morning," he wrote to his fiancée in the fall of 1896, and had a discussion with Biggs, his superior, about the winter's work schedule:

> it will be either Rabies – Pasteur's hydrophobia cure and all that, or more probably on the use of Formalin – a most vile compound – as a gaseous disinfectant for carriages, ambulances etc. It gives off a vapor, which is supposed to kill all bacteria in a short while – So we will hang strips of paper soaked in solutions of typhoid bacilli, etc. in the closed carriage with open vessels of formalin, and then try and grow the

67 JSB to KHB, June 2, 1898. Such positions were inevitably shaped by prevailing patronage relationships. Billings felt that Hermann Biggs might have been more forthcoming in supporting him, had Billings been able to reciprocate. "I have a sneaking idea that Biggs might like me better than he does – and this in turn is solely due to the fact that I was unable to get a Librarian friend of his a position in the Astor [where Billings senior served as chief executive officer]," JSB to KHB, June 2, 1898. See also JSB to KH, October 11, 1896.

68 For the "small fry" phrase, JSB to "My Dear Mother" [Emily Hammond], May 6, 1897; for the reference to "Cousin George," JSB to "Dear Lady" [Emily Hammond], August 4, 1897. Billings was, for example, disappointed when Charles Camac was appointed to teach clinical microscopy at the new Cornell Medical School; "he certainly must have an a no. 1, harveyized steel pull, that young fellow," Billings lamented sardonically. JSB to KHB, May 8, 1898.

69 "Hitherto," he explained to Katherine on June 21, 1898, "the College of Physicians and Surgeons have gobbled them all – I mean such hospitals as the Presbyterian, St. Lukes, etc. I am to quiz them on Practice of Medicine twice a week, and Rogers on Surgery as often." JSB to KHB, June 21, 1898.

"bugs" on culture media – they should be killed – at least, that is my idea. But I will have to get up the literature first.[70]

He published articles on the blood in diphtheria, and cooperated with A. A. Smith on the blood in "Levant fever."[71] Much of his laboratory activity, as we have seen, was more routine and immediately remunerative, as he performed analyses of clinical materials for individual physicians. He also supplemented his income by abstracting articles from European medical journals for local editors.[72] He continued, in addition, to spend odd hours and evenings at the New York Academy of Medicine library, checking references and working up bibliographies for busy and socially prominent, yet would-be academic, practitioners.[73]

Billings's scholarly efforts – and presumably, his impeccable connections – brought election to membership in the prestigious Association of American Physicians in 1906. Despite this evidence of continued academic commitment, however, his career was shifting inexorably toward the security of New York City's Department of Health, where he began to spend less and less time in the bacteriological laboratory and more time in administrative tasks, such as the writing of reports and the managing of programs, as he rose in the Health Department's hierarchy. Hours at the laboratory bench could not in themselves bring economic security or organizational status.

The texture of practice

For most of Billings's first decade in New York (1894–1904), both academic striving and Department of Health routine remained in the background. The foreground was occupied by his efforts to build up a private

70 JSB to KH, September 28, 1896.
71 He kept at work writing such clinical articles for some time. See "The Significance of Absence of Nucleated Red Corpuscles in the Blood in Cases of Grave Anaemia," *New York Medical Journal* 69 (May 20, 1899): 693–695.
72 Billings also wrote articles to order for relatively modest fees. The editor of the *New York Medical Journal*, for example, offered him twenty-five dollars to write a 3,500-word article on Ehrlich's side-chain theory of immunity, and gave him two weeks to finish the assignment. Frank Foster to JSB, March 26, 1903, in Hammond-Bryan-Cumming Papers, with comments, JSB to KHB, [March 27, 1903]; JSB to KHB, March 29, 1903.
73 After a full day's work on February 6, 1897, for example, he rushed to the Academy of Medicine, where he worked "from 3 to 5:15 and looked up over twenty references." JSB to KH, February 6, 1897. He also worked on clinical research projects for such prominent physicians. "I have spent the evening" with Frederic Dennis, he reported one evening, making tables from his statistics: "these are to show how far superior he is to the world of Surgeons in general and W. S. Halstead in particular. But oh me, oh my – how figures do lie." JSB to KH, April 24, 1895.

practice. "One thing is certain," he explained to Katherine, "teaching, laboratory-work, writing and everything else have got to play second fiddle to my getting a practice – and a paying one too."[74] He maintained his own office and kept regular hours, usually at lunchtime and immediately before dinner. As late as the fall of 1907, Billings could assure his wife that "I am not going to do one single thing this winter but practice medicine – for there's where our future lies."[75]

He was busiest in the summer, when his patrons were away, joining the annual exodus of the respectable from New York. And Billings did of course attract and "hold" some private patients of his own; for this was, of course, the bottom line for any successful practitioner. Experience brought new skills. He learned how difficult it was to manage nurses in private homes and how convenient it was to have an even less well-established physician to act as his assistant.

In a number of ways, Billings sought, ironically if inevitably, to replicate aspects of his own career, but in the role of patron rather than client. He rented a room and provided breakfast to another physician, just as he had himself rented from Smith's assistant Carlisle some years before. Patterns of urban medical practice were changing rapidly in the first decade of the twentieth century as the hospital grew in importance, as specialization flourished, and as the automobile made physicians more mobile.[76] But doctoring remained intensely competitive and the prospects for financial success problematic. Even as late as 1907 and 1908, when he already occupied a responsible administrative post at the Department of Health, Billings's economic insecurity made him a resentful supplicant in his relationship with Austin Flint, Jr. "I dont seem to care for any thing but seeing patients for the sake of money – and that not so much – for Flint had to talk to me for quite five minutes last night at 11:30 to get me out of bed and off to see a new patient."[77]

74 JSB to KH, [February 7, 1895]. He was, consistently enough, tempted by the possibility of a full-time job with the Equitable Life Insurance Company, but consoled himself with the thought that it would be a dead end, without guarantee of tenure, and subject to the purges that inevitably followed management reorganizations. JSB to KH, October 28, 1896.

75 JSB to KHB, November 5, 1907. "I have a lot of work to do to day – it cannot come too fast and the Department can go hang." JSB to KHB, December 2, 1907.

76 A "wheel" (bicycle) and later an automobile allowed him to juggle a diverse and demanding schedule. "To do a practice scattered over town the way mine is," he explained in 1908, "one must have an automobile." JSB to KHB, January 4, 1908. Operating cars in this pioneer automotive era could bring significant problems. "Wheel cap dropped off twice," Billings described one drive. "Then I lost the bolt from my brake bar – and finally one of the roller bearings of the right hand front wheel ground up to powder." JSB to KHB, August 3, 1905.

77 JSB to KHB, December 6, 1907. Depressed economic conditions only sharpened Billings's resentment. "Money comes in very slowly from the bills I sent out," he wrote

In late 1907, Flint was particularly encouraging. Flint "calls me his 'partner,' " Billings exulted, "to all his patients, and tells me that all of them are willing to have me when he cannot come." He promised as well that he would give up general practice and concentrate on surgery; "I got quite busy yesterday," Billings reported in November 1907, "and was on the pump all day – and have half a dozen calls to day. If this keeps up, and I can hold all the people Flint turns over to me, we should be on easy street."[78] But Flint seemed to get "cold feet"; his decision to order a "$4,500 Packard automobile" seemed to put an end to his promised sharing of practice. "Where," Billings asked, "will he get the money to pay for it?"[79] The younger man remained a supplicant, shut off from direct access to Flint's clients such as the Astors, the Vanderbilts, and the Brundages.

Whether through a series of misfortunes or a personality ill-suited to the bedside, Billings was never to become, like Flint, a prosperous society practitioner. There was no reason for melancholy, Billings wrote his wife on December 22, 1907, "except that I am so trifling I cant make a decent living for you." It was a sentiment he had repeated again and again. "Please dont think of me as sick," he had written two years earlier, "in any way except at heart that I cannot make more money for us."[80] Nor was Billings to make his mark as a teacher and clinical investigator. The Department of Health remained a viable, if residual, option.

Settling into bureaucracy

Time, hard work, and inertia – with perhaps the help of some "elephant pull" – brought him gradual advancement at the Department of Health,

to Katherine early in 1908, "now is the time when the late panic hits the doctors." JSB to KHB, January 5, 1908. At more or less the same time, Billings undertook a new part-time job, serving as examining physician at the New York Stock Exchange. JSB to KHB, November 11, 1907; JSB to KHB, January 23, 1908. Similarly, in an instance of nepotism, John Shaw Billings, who was Director of the New York Public Library, was to appoint his son as Medical Officer of the library, at a salary of $150 per month. John Shaw Billings to JSB, March 4, 1911. JSB, Scrapbook 4, Hammond-Bryan-Cumming Papers.

78 For the partner phrase, JSB to KHB, November 21, 1907; for the giving up of general practice, JSB to KHB, January 5, 1908; JSB to KHB, November 23, 1908.

79 JSB to KHB, January 19, 1908. For further details on Flint's relationship with Billings in this period, see JSB to KHB, January 21, 1908; JSB to KHB, January 5, 1908 (for "cold feet" phrase); JSB to KHB, January 2, 1908. Internal evidence indicates that some of Flint's socially prominent families were not satisfied with Billings as primary physician. "Young Townsend Burden has typhoid and the family want Flint to take charge," Billings explained in one instance, "but I suppose I will go there twice a day. It will be a hard case because of the family." JSB to KHB, December 22, 1907.

80 JSB to KHB, July 5, 1905.

despite what was clearly a difficult and combative personality.[81] But it was a gradual, almost imperceptible commitment. In December 1897, for example, he hoped that his increasing private practice and other responsibilities would mean dropping "something else – I hope it will prove to be the Board of Health." As late as 1903, he could explain that he would soon be finished with his contributions to the Department's annual reports and could then return to his normal two-hour-a-day stint at the Department.[82] Billings was named to his first administrative post, the assistant directorship of the Diagnosis and Bacteriological Laboratory, on January 1, 1899.[83] By the summer of 1904 he bore the title of Assistant Director, Division of Bacteriology; by 1906 he had been appointed Chief of the new Division of Communicable Diseases (which grew out of the Division of Bacteriology); in 1913 the Department of Health created a Division of Infectious Diseases and appointed Billings as Chief of this enlarged bureau.[84]

As early as 1908, drift and financial need had made Billings a career administrator; he already contemplated the annual pension of $1,200 he could anticipate after six more years of service.[85] With the incorporation of Brooklyn into metropolitan New York at the end of the century and the growing commitment to fighting such Infectious ills as typhoid and tuberculosis, Billings found his Division of Infectious Diseases at the center of an increasingly well-supported municipal activity. The bureau's budget grew from $58,419 in 1907 to $435,397 in 1912.[86] And Billings's responsibilities grew in proportion; he spent long hours in producing detailed reports, writing speeches, bustling from borough to borough, and, most prominently, organizing and administering a much-admired anti-tuberculosis campaign. He also became something of an authority on

81 The phrase is from a letter describing New York's impending mayoral race in September 1897. "All nominees look alike to me, tho' I must confess that my assortment of Republican 'wires,' 'lead-pipe cinches' and 'Elephant pulls' is fresher and better than my Democratic ones." JSB to "Dearest other Mother" [Emily Hammond], September 16, 1897.
82 JSB to KHB, December 2, 1897; JSB to "Dear Lady" [Emily Hammond], February 4, 1903.
83 Scrapbook 4 in the Hammond-Bryan-Cumming Papers contains Billings's formal curriculum vitae, prepared for internal use in the Department of Health. It includes details of job responsibilities and dates of assuming administrative posts.
84 Scrapbook 4 in the Hammond-Bryan-Cumming Papers contains a New York City Department of Health Executive Order, dated May 21, 1913, establishing the Division of Infectious Diseases and detailing JSB as chief. A letter from Ernest Lederle to JSB, dated October 20, 1914, in Scrapbook 4, indicates that Billings's annual salary was set at $5,000. For background, see Duffy, *History of Public Health*, pp. 264–265; Charles F. Bolduan, *Over a Century of Health Administration in New York City*, Monograph Series no. 13 (New York: Department of Health, 1916).
85 JSB to KHB, January 12, 1908.
86 "The Division of Communicable Diseases," *Monthly Bulletin of the Department of Health of the City of New York* 2 (October, 1912): 252.

municipal health administration – an expertise seen by many of his con-
temporaries as a natural achievement for a son of John Shaw Billings.[87]
When he retired in 1917 to become Medical Adviser at the Bell Telephone
Company, he had made a respectable career in public health, a career that
he had hardly anticipated and that had existed only in embryo when he left
Baltimore and the Johns Hopkins Hospital in 1894.[88]

Conclusion

I have described a career that was unique, in the trivial sense that every
life is, but not random. Although decisions are personal, they are structured and constrained by particular configurations of perceived reality. Any
individual life is, in this sense, always a legitimate sampling device.

Billings's career illustrates a number of significant realities. One is the
transitional nature of the period in which he grew to professional maturity.
Informal patronage relations still structured medical careers. The community of academic physicians was still dependent on income from private
practice, for example; patient fees still supported the families of even the
profession's institutional leaders. Hermann Biggs and William Hallock
Park, it should be noted, Billings's internationally known superiors at New
York's Department of Health, also cultivated medical practices during those same years in which they accumulated enduring reputations as
pioneers in public health.

As we have suggested, Billings became in this transitional period a victim
of his own skills, social connections, and economic need. His ability to
provide the functional equivalent of a hospital infrastructure (in terms of
backup staffing and clinical pathology) helped to lock him into a dependent
role, one that kept him from the market access that could alone guarantee
the economic success he so anxiously sought. His subordination to well-
established patrons almost guaranteed marginality in academic medicine,
no matter what his training and intellectual abilities. Billings's situation

---

87 In 1914 the Department of Health published Billings's *Hand Book of Information
Regarding the Routine Procedure of the Bureau of Infectious Diseases*. Billings sent copies to
William Osler (then in Oxford) and pioneer American bacteriologist George
Sternberg. Not surprisingly, both took the occasion to compare Billings with his father.
Osler to JSB, November 25, 1914; Sternberg to JSB, December 4, 1914, both in
Scrapbook 4. More influential was Billings's study *The Tuberculosis Clinics and Day
Camps of the Department of Health*, Monograph Series no. 2 (New York: Department of
Health, 1912). See the editorial "Municipal Control of Tuberculosis in America,"
British Medical Journal 2 (November 16, 1912): 1407, which reviews Billings's study
and lauds New York's tuberculosis prevention efforts.
88 "The Division of Communicable Diseases," *Weekly Bulletin of the Department of Health*
(New York City), n.s. 6 (January 20, 1917).

contrasts instructively with the asymmetrical decision made by another contemporary, David Edsall. Edsall made his start in Philadelphia's medical community assisting John Musser, a prominent teacher and busy practitioner; his situation paralleled Billings's relationship to Smith and Flint. Edsall, however, soon saw the relationship as a dead end. He borrowed money, as he recalled later, to escape the trap of seeking short-term economic security in private practice.[89]

Our protagonist's efforts to find a foothold on the ladder to institutional – and especially hospital – eminence was no more than typical of his peers. The roles of clinical or laboratory assistant, quiz master, and teacher of small groups in ward and dispensary all provided access to status and some small income to particular individuals, while serving useful functions within a medical system still inadequate to the pedagogical needs of those seeking clinical and laboratory training. With the twentieth century, of course, the importance of such ad hoc arrangements declined as the standard curriculum evolved and as the internship and residency became part of that new curriculum. Billings came of age just as the nineteenth-century pattern of clinical education and academic career options was evolving into something rather different – but before new structures and institutional choices became routine. As we have seen, Billings's career illustrates as well the key role of patronage, an ancient mechanism but one that still played an enormous role in structuring career choices, even in an era that saw substantial change in the direction of a more bureaucratic and formally meritoratic system.[90]

Billings was also the victim of another sort of conflict – between his desire for the rewards of scientific status, on the one hand, and for mundane prosperity, on the other. He was genuinely attracted by both, but found it difficult to forge a career in which both could be achieved. In this sense, his ambivalence mirrored a more fundamental tension within Anglo-American medicine. Both kinds of equity were real; and it was no easy task to shape a strategy in which one could pursue economic as well as intellectual goals with hope of achieving both.[91]

89 Joseph C. Aub and Ruth K. Hapgood, *Pioneer in Modern Medicine, David Linn Edsall of Harvard* ([Boston]: Harvard Medical Alumni Association, 1970), p. 34. There are a good many other parallels between the early lives of Edsall and Billings.

90 This is not to argue that patronage has disappeared from the world of academic medicine in the course of the twentieth century. Now, however, it functions within the legitimating constraints of credentialing, peer review, and other putatively universalistic mechanisms.

91 In his first New York City years, Billings maintained a commitment to the cosmopolitan world of clinical investigation. In early 1895, for example, he boasted that "my articles have been reviewed in four German and two French journals up to date." JSB to KH, February 5, 1895. A year and a half later he could ask his fiancée to "rejoice with me ...; in a long article in the London Lancet I was quoted approvingly

This was also a period of interrelated cognitive and demographic change. And public health was a particularly significant area of growth. When Billings began to work in New York, the ability of medicine to intervene in infectious disease was minimal. Infant mortality rates remained high; for example, the death rate from pneumonia was still enormous, and typhoid and diphtheria still ravaged the city's slums. A *career* in public health or the laboratory was almost a contradiction in terms; a physician worked in these areas part-time, and especially during one's youth. Billings arrived in New York, it must be recalled, just after the seeming victory over an impending cholera epidemic precipitated and legitimated the establishment of a permanent bacteriological laboratory; and almost simultaneously with the city's initial efforts to produce and utilize diphtheria antitoxin. When he retired a generation later, things were rather different. New York's Department of Health had evolved into a large, well-funded, and increasingly bureaucratic entity. He had drifted unwillingly, unwittingly, and ambivalently into a public health career – a career that had been gradually and imperceptibly created around him. (One might argue that society too had drifted into a growing commitment to public health.)

Which, of course, leaves the personal equation. Although the dangers of retrospective psychologizing are obvious, it is tempting to make some suggestions. Billings explicitly rejected his father's example; he did not wish to become the kind of driven and demonic slave to work that he associated with his father's enormously successful yet painful life. "These great men are wedded to their work," he explained to his future wife in 1896,

> always, and their wives and children and friends are minor considerations. This is always so. . . . It is not an enviable life to me – I would not have lead my father's life for twice his name and fame – we children love him, but oh how much more we would, if he would let us – but he cannot – he is shut off from that. . . . I have always hated my father's life – hated it fiercely and vindictively, for what it deprived him of, and have often sworn to myself that never, never would I isolate myself in that way – for you have to do it.[92]

no less than three times." JSB to KH, October 4, 1896. "I go on duty with my beloved diphtheria bacilli again tomorrow," he enthused in 1895. "I have been leading a life of elegant leisure for a week – the life of the untrammeled original investigator." JSB to KH, June 6, 1895. His increasingly conflicted goals are illustrated nicely in a letter of 1907, which complains bitterly about "poor business" and reflects his economic dependence on his patron, Flint, while noting that "I had the honor yesterday of a personal call from a very distinguished German professor (Neisser) who brought me the greetings of another (Prof. Ehrlich)." JSB to KHB, November 20, 1907.

92 JSB to KH, October 22, 1896. On another occasion, the youthful Billings complained that his father wanted him "to write, write and to keep on writing – a thing that is utterly distasteful to me." JSB to KH, May 20, 1895.

In contracting a "premature" marriage, Billings had made a life decision that could not easily be reversed.

In other ways, too, he was a victim of his father's success; the younger Billings had enormous expectations and presumed a class-bound lifestyle that shackled him in another way. His Ohio-born father always knew who he was and what he had been; his son constantly sought affirmation.[93] Perhaps the young man's snobbery, immaturity, and defensiveness made it difficult for him to succeed in private practice; it certainly helped make his marriage a miserable one. "John has been selfish and thoughtless too long to change," Katherine wrote despairingly to her mother in 1904. "I hope I wont be living with him when I come to die – for I would not find even death restful if John were around looking out for his own comfort & interest."[94] At least from the historian's parochial viewpoint, however, that unhappy marriage had the virtue of producing regular absences and a stream of revealing and circumstantial letters.

In those direct and personal documents, young Billings provided a richly circumstantial account of one individual's choices among a variety of structured alternatives. His conscious awareness of those options illuminates them nicely for the historian. But his life suggests another point as well: an individual's decisions are not predictable from social location alone.

93 At the Board of Health, Billings saw himself as a "gentleman" in contradistinction to some of his administrative rivals. The laboratory staff, he explained in 1905, was discontented: they "need a firm hand. I can see nothing else than for *me* to take it in hand. They speak disrespectfully of [Walter] Cronk – and he is no gentleman – and they know it." JSB to KHB, May 16, 1905. Billings's best friend, Rupert Norton, shared many of his class attitudes. Norton's apartment mate had struck "'pay gravel'... while we poor others," the young physician reflected, "who haven't his tact must grovel down deeper. But his class of patients would never satisfy me, even if they came in crowds, ordinary second class people most of them. You know the sort I mean. I can't make that class my friends as S does. They don't interest me, and I do not care to dine with them. I may be setting myself too high, – I am sorry if I do – I do not mean to be a cad." Norton to JSB, November 12, 1896.
94 Mrs. Billings had just had a baby. "Well this is the first time John has been with me when one of the children was born – and if it was worth while to say such a thing – I would say it would be the last. I think if I had staid here when Johnny-boy was born there would never have been any more. There is much to be desired in his treatment of me at such a time." KHB to "Dearest Mother" [Emily Hammond], March 13, 1904. This bitter letter is also cited in Carol Bleser, *The Hammonds of Redcliffe*, pp. 352–353.

PART III

The past in the present:
Using medical history

11

The crisis in psychiatric legitimacy: Reflections on psychiatry, medicine, and public policy

෫ This essay was written for a meeting held in Williamsburg, Virginia, in 1973 to commemorate the bicentennial of the British North American colonies' first public hospital for the mentally ill. The celebration was invested with a certain irony, an irony that needs little explanation. The reputation of inpatient psychiatry was at a particularly low level in the early 1970s. The movement to deinstitutionalize men and women diagnosed as "mentally ill" had already begun, crystallizing generations of criticism. Clinical optimism, psychopharmacology, and a new kind of assertive liberalism had made the state hospital's custodial back wards seem an indefensible relic of a more primitive social order, and the population of America's state hospitals had already begun to decline. This was a period marked by a more general skepticism toward the medical enterprise, and in particular toward psychiatric diagnoses and the medical authority that legitimated and enforced them. To a generation wary of credentialed authority, the gap between the labeling of deviance and the diagnosis of illness had begun to narrow; the diagnosed had thus become more victim than patient, more stigmatized than understood. Social control rather than humane care was psychiatry's perceived purpose; women, the poor, and the deviant generally were seen as its chosen targets.

In the years since 1973 things have changed a great deal – and very little. Somatic views of the etiology of mental illness have become increasingly central. Deinstitutionalization has produced – or perhaps more accurately reproduced – more problems than it has solved; mental illness has not gone away and neither will psychiatry's burden of clinical responsibility. In that respect and several others, this essay describes realities which have not changed very much in the decades since it was written: the ambiguous relationship between psychiatry and the rest of medicine, the paucity of effective solutions to society's enormous accumulation of emotional pain and mental illness. These aspects of psychiatry's social legitimacy remain largely unchanged. We live in a society that demands rationalistic care provided by credentialed men and women. Even if we should find a definitive explanation – and cure – for the most grave and disabling psychoses, our culture will still provide an endless supply of depression and anxiety, of eating disorders and marital distress. Adjusting to life has never been easy and dealing with the pain of that adjustment has always been a crushing task. ❦

Attempting to define the term *psychiatry* is as difficult as it is enlightening. Psychiatry can be defined simply as a medical specialty with attendant forms of certification and accepted practice. But this is a minimal conception; in its most comprehensive meaning psychiatry is a social function, not a specialized group of physicians and their practice. The broader definition implies the response of society and its institutions to the needs of those who either see themselves as "mentally ill" or are so regarded by others, and involves all would-be healers of the mind and emotions – psychiatrists, clinical psychologists, psychiatric social workers, pediatricians, and gynecologists, as well as practitioners of the most ephemeral and opportunistic psychotherapies. The gap between the limited and the comprehensive definitions of psychiatric responsibility begins itself to suggest the dimensions of the problems faced by contemporary psychiatry – problems so grave that our very public awareness of them implies a crisis in psychiatry's social legitimacy.

While American psychiatry shares all the dilemmas faced by medicine in general, it must also confront a number of difficulties peculiar to itself. First, psychiatry has been – and is being – shaped by social values and needs and consequent decisions of social policy to a far greater degree than most other specialties in medicine. A second area of stress concerns the relationship between psychiatry and medicine in general. Discontinuities within the internal structure of the psychiatric community itself contribute to a third kind of problem. All three relationships – to society and its needs, to medicine, and among the several groups that make up psychiatry – are ambiguous and labile, yet they are rooted in history and tenaciously articulated in present attitudes and institutional arrangements. They will not easily be altered.

From its nineteenth-century beginnings as a distinct specialty, psychiatry has been shaped by decisions made outside the medical profession. The creation of asylums, for example, can hardly be interpreted as a medical decision based on a new consensus of professional opinion. Yet the establishment of such institutions created a group of physicians whose concerns centered more and more exclusively on asylum administration and on problems of human behavior. The first title of the American Psychiatric Association was the Association of Superintendents of American Institutions for the Insane. Psychiatry was very much a specialty organized in response to a specific social need rather than the logical institutional expression of an expanding body of knowledge or the crystallization of particular techniques. Within the past generation we have seen the internal institutional structure of psychiatry, and even its intellectual framework, repeatedly affected by government policy decisions. Pressing needs after the Second World War, for example, led to the use of Veterans Administration hospitals and federal funds for psychiatric training. More recently, federal commitment to something called the community mental health center has had broad implications for the internal organization and personnel of psychiatry. Similarly, recent trends toward deinstitutionalization reflect, among other things, shifts in economic and social priorities and perceptions side by side with advances in pharmacology, and a changing intellectual consensus within psychiatry.

The term *social policy* implies conscious decisions – more and more in the twentieth century those made at the levels of state and federal government. But, as we are well aware, such decisions are a consequence of more general social phenomena, such as, for example, attitudes toward aging, deviance, and ethnicity – as well as more fundamental structural changes like those involved in urbanization, industrialization, and consequent shifts in social values and ideology. I enumerate such factors not to shroud the discussion in a haze of diffuse and plausibly profound words, but because psychiatry relates to such structural factors somewhat differently than does medicine generally. For with the growth of technology and science a good many areas in clinical medicine have been provided with some understanding of pathological mechanisms and therapeutic resources which define at least some aspects of the clinical interaction between the physician and particular patients.

The discovery of insulin and its subsequent synthesis, for example, provides a relatively well-defined therapeutic framework within which emergent cases of diabetes are managed. Yet social and economic factors play a role even in this relatively distinct and treatable condition; a particular patient may be poor and isolated or perhaps a Christian Scientist, or his physician may fail to make the proper diagnosis. Each clinical entity – and medicine's technical means for dealing with it – creates a somewhat different configuration of necessity and available therapeutic options. Thus quite a different assortment of social and economic variables structures the treatment of a particular case in which renal dialysis might be needed. In this instance, of course, such factors play a greater role than they normally would in cases of diabetes, but in both these examples the technical means at hand and insight into pathology and physiology define the parameters within which clinical decisions are made.

Psychiatry can only rarely stand on such firm ground. We still debate the fundamental basis of the most common psychiatric diagnoses and their relationship to belief systems and the realities of social structure. The contrast with most somatic ills is clear enough; if there are indeed biological mechanisms underlying even the most marked psychiatric syndromes we cannot as yet define them; if there are not, we are equally unable to demonstrate their absence; if their etiology should depend on some particular interaction of constitutional endowment and environmental stress we cannot define that relationship in more than the vaguest of terms. Every aspect of psychiatry, from its most general social conditions to the level of individual interaction between physician and patient, is inevitably shaped by extramedical factors – with comparatively few defining technological boundaries.

Of course, every area within medicine is to some extent shaped by such considerations. Who is to pay for medical care, for example, and who is to regulate and certify hospitals and how are they to do it? Almost every visible twentieth-century social trend relates in some way to clinical medicine. We have seen, for example, how the management of sickle-cell anemia has begun to reflect a growing black activism; we have seen the women's movement add a novel element to debate over the surgical treatment of breast cancer. But differences over mastectomy or screening for sickle-cell anemia do not alter our views of cell physiology. These debates seem merely tactical when compared to the way in which contemporary criticisms of psychiatric theory and practice have decried their most fundamental assumptions. Methodologically oriented critics have dismissed that diffuse yet generally cumulative consensus which constitutes dynamic psychiatry as being arbitrary, insusceptible of proof, and willfully quasitheological; social activists have attacked it as the ideology of an antihuman status quo. In the past fifteen years we have seen the concept of mental illness itself assailed as an ideological construct more useful in enforcing the values of society and expressing its inability to tolerate deviance than in expressing the data of empirical observation.

As a result of such repeated criticism we have become increasingly conscious of the possible social content of psychiatric diagnoses – of the necessary tentativeness of even the most widely used diagnostic categories. We have at the same time become more conscious of the ways in which social values and structure and consequent ideological needs affect individual behavior through their shaping of role options, including those of the patient and the psychotherapist. We have, at the same time, become more conscious of the problematical quality of most cognitive therapies – not to speak of the more theoretical formulations drawn from such clinical interactions. Not surprisingly, contemporary psychiatric theory has become increasingly eclectic and hesitant. And, as we have tried to suggest, these shifts reflect not only changes in the medical and behavioral sciences, but – equally important – a changed temper in our intellectual life generally. Psychiatry could not well escape that critical mood which has questioned – among other concerns – the nature of traditional sex roles, our courts, and our prisons, and denounced three-centuries-old attitudes about the relationship between man and nature.

Yet despite such repeated criticisms, despite the fact that much of its theoretical foundations are still based on the exegesis of clinical intuitions, despite the fact that its therapeutic means are problematic and ill defined, psychiatry must still deal with the clinical burdens of a society which "produces" vast numbers of individuals whose behavior is stigmatized by that society as mental illness. It must deal as well with even greater numbers suffering emotional pain and varying degrees of incapacity – behavior and emotions which many of us have come to interpret in terms of disease process.[1] We are no more willing, many of us, to suffer the pain of depression or anxiety than that of some more readily localized and meliorable physical ailment; in our society neither stoicism nor traditional religious viewpoints seem ordinarily to provide a context of meaningfulness for such ills of the soul. Health has come to imply the absence of emotional as well as physical pain and disability, and the physician has been defined – not entirely without his participation – as the individual best suited to deal with it. Society has, in other words, shaped over the past century and a half a special role for the psychiatrist, and has provided him with a limitless abundance of clinical material – without at the same time providing him with a generally agreed-upon body of etiological and therapeutic knowledge.

Because the specialty of psychiatry has so diffuse a responsibility and possesses so little limit-defining knowledge, it is prone to border disputes; its status is critically dependent on its medical identity. Even if the formal logic and institutional appropriateness of this relationship remain problematical, its social necessity is unquestionable. Psychiatrists benefit from the status and autonomy society grants physicians – a status which may

1 We have no way of knowing or understanding the possible relationship between the reality of society's structure, values, and emotional demands, and the production of such symptoms. Thus the continuing historical and social debate as to the changing incidence and pattern of mental illness; we have, for example, no firm evidence that the incidence of felt mental illness and emotional pain is necessarily greater now than it was in the eighteenth or twelfth or fifth centuries. We have similarly no evidence to indicate that the gravely ill were treated somehow more humanely, their experience seen as simply another dimension of the human condition. Our ignorance, of course, has implied no slackening in the vigor of the debate surrounding such problems; the relationship to a growing criticism of psychiatry, to a fashionable antirationalism, illustrates with clarity the ongoing relationship between psychiatric thought and the shifting intellectual winds of the society in which the discipline of psychiatry exists.

indeed serve a therapeutic role in particular doctor–patient relationships.

Yet the relationships between contemporary medicine and contemporary psychiatry are ambiguous throughout. The problem begins with medical education itself. Few will deny that the standard medical education, which, despite a generation of reform, has been stubbornly resistant to change, is not ideally suited to the needs of those aspiring to become psychiatrists. Of course, there are the familiar justifications: the ability to differentiate genuinely functional ills from possible somatic alternatives, the assimilation of a certain detached concern. (And the expansion of drug therapy has somewhat revitalized the argument for a conventional medical education.) But these contentions have come to seem a bit shopworn. A justification heard with increasing frequency in recent years contends that traditional clinical training is an appropriate prerequisite for psychiatric practice in its inculcation of the responsibility implicit in the physician's control over life and death.[2] This claim, even if valid, is surely a marginal justification for a five-year commitment.

Another ambiguity relating to the identification of psychiatry with medicine centers on the claim of medicine to exclusive control of therapeutics. Insofar as psychiatry has voiced a similar claim, it has had a rather hollow ring; for neither available manpower nor therapeutic resources enable psychiatry to undertake realistically the exclusive care – and control – of all those defined as mentally ill. The state hospital, for example, with its formal legitimacy resting ultimately on its status as a medical institution and thus on the status and autonomy of the medical profession, illustrates dramatically the problematical nature of such identifications. It is not simply as a result of contemporary social and intellectual ferment that we entertain a crisis of what might well be called psychiatric legitimacy. The crisis also reflects the gap between the demands of medical exclusivity and the inability of psychiatry to provide either understanding or relief consistent with the pretentiousness of such demands.

And, as a matter of fact, society recognizes these realities in its unwillingness to grant holders of the medical degree exclusive control over the treatment of those who suffer emotional pain and disability. Organized psychiatry, on its part, fails to regulate effectively either its own members or other holders of medical certification who may choose to practice some form of psychotherapy.[3] Thus the unending production of would-be

---

2 Even if contemporary biochemical insights prove fruitful in bringing understanding of schizophrenia, let us say, it is not at all clear that the physician's clinical preparation constitutes an appropriate training for such new orientation.

3 Of course, general medicine has similarly failed to regulate the ethics and standards of practice of physicians, and this in many cases in which definitions of acceptable practice are more easily agreed upon. The profession has been more successful, however, in curtailing the activities of individuals who do not hold the medical degree.

psychotherapies – under both lay and medical auspices – unregulated by either the profession or the state.

Most professions are marked by sharp distinctions between the elite and the average practitioner. In the sciences and in medicine, the growing specialization and autonomy of careers oriented to basic science have only sharpened such distinctions. In psychiatry, however, the distance between elite and other practitioners is structured rather differently than in most other fields of applied science.

Historically speaking, there have been two principal styles and loci – and thus, origins – of psychiatry in the United States. One was developed out of a growing medical response to patients sufficiently ill or aged or "difficult" to require hospitalization; the other grew out of the work of physicians who treated the still-functioning though symptom-bearing patient outside of institutional settings. This distinction has existed for a century. The late nineteenth-century neurologist, with his prestigious private practice and earnest worship of European authority, practiced quite a different brand of psychiatry from that of the hospital-oriented curator of severely ill and often economically deprived hospital patients. Though it would be naive to contend that these categories have remained absolute and unchanged since the late nineteenth century, they still reflect a persistent dichotomy in psychiatric practice.

In some way, indeed, the differences are greater now than at the beginning of the century. Not only is the state hospital a locale of low status in which to practice psychiatry; it is, in general, a place where a different kind of psychiatry is practiced. In the years before the First World War, ambitious young psychiatrists still frequently served in hospital positions, partly because of a lack of other available institutional niches, partly because of the intellectual concern about the psychoses and their then-still-hoped-for elucidation through pathological and biochemical approaches. (And the state and municipal hospitals were, of course, also populated by victims of organic syndromes.) With the increasing numbers of teaching and clinical positions becoming available in university medical centers, and the parallel growth in the intellectual relevance of dynamic views, the state hospitals grew progressively less attractive to many able and well-educated young psychiatrists. In the years before the First World War, moreover, it was the spiritual – and in some cases institutional – descendants of the late nineteenth-century neurologists who provided leadership in the adoption of dynamic psychiatry and its therapeutic implications. Advocates of this orientation and their institutional successors have since the Second World War consistently achieved the highest status in the profession, written most influentially, and occupied leading positions in our most prominent medical schools.

As one consequence among many others, many of the major figures in twentieth-century American psychiatry have been students of the neuroses and personality disorders, not of the most severe and incapacitating conditions. (This is a pattern of interest which reflects the continuity between the neurologist's office and sanitarium practice of the late nineteenth century and that of the dynamically oriented psychiatrist of the mid-twentieth.) Not surprisingly then, much of our century's most influential psychiatric writing has consisted of general statements about the human condition, in the form of hypothetical etiologies of particular personality types and related modes of behavior. Such works have been as relevant to the educated community generally as to the narrower constituency of medical men and psychiatrists. Rather less attention has been paid to the great and dismayingly intractable clinical burdens of age, grave illness, and deviance which have traditionally filled our state hospitals. Such tendencies toward differentiation in practice and the preoccupations of research have only exacerbated distinctions within that group of physicians who term themselves psychiatrists; the channels of communication have functioned fitfully at best.[4]

If we see psychiatry as a function rather than as a group of appropriately certified practitioners, a number of other structural problems become apparent. One lies in the fact that physicians without formal psychiatric training habitually practice ad hoc "psychiatry." We all know pediatricians and gynecologists, for example, who casually dispense psychiatric dicta with their infant formulas or birth-control pills. This segment of what might be called psychiatric practice is little amenable to control and far removed from the work and attitudes of the elite within psychiatry.

The intellectual relationship between the several levels of practice and investigation is even more tenuous in psychiatry than in most other areas of medicine, although it is, of course, problematical to an extent in every area of applied science. The most isolated or provincial internist or general practitioner routinely employs drugs the physiological activity and chemical structure of which he understands little. But the laboratory man who ascertained the activity of a particular substance, the technicians who developed and tested it, have communicated with the practitioner through a cultural artifact. This species of communication has – with the comparatively recent exception of the psychoactive drugs – hardly existed in

---

4 And there is a further irony. Almost all twentieth-century psychiatrists have been clinicians (at least until they became administrators). Yet this identity as clinicians has not helped create a community of interest. In addition to the fact that the clinical concerns of both groups have differed, the concern with clinical situations and the elaboration of clinical intuitions created (or, perhaps more accurately, preserved) an ethos inhospitable to more positivistic standards of scientific proof – an ethos grounded in a need to find and accept explanatory formulas, almost a necessity for physicians who must actually deal with patients.

psychiatry. The psychiatric elite has in general given the state hospital physician, the pediatrician or urologist, or the general practitioner little in the way of discrete and portable artifacts. Even if one assumes a certain validity for the insights of the dynamic tradition, they are neither easily communicated nor easily utilized, though they are easily vulgarized.

The last half century, with its generally increasing public acceptance of psychiatry, has only intensified the profession's dependence on lay values and policy decisions. In no area has this been more clearly demonstrated than that of society's search for the means of dealing with deviance. Psychiatry cannot win for winning; the more confidence laypeople have placed in psychiatry and psychiatric procedures, the more importunate are the demands made upon it, and inevitably the greater the gap between expectation and performance. American psychiatry, not without the participation of certain of its own spokesmen, has become to an extent committed to finding solutions for such perceived problems as juvenile delinquency, drug addiction, criminality, and variant sexual behavior. Psychiatry has in this sense become a kind of residual legatee for the attempt to solve some of society's most intractable problems – and not without a certain logic and even idealism informing the series of attitudes and decisions which brought about this involvement.

The situation is again ambiguous. Many individuals who behave in ways perceived as antisocial do exhibit symptoms of personality disorder. It is abundantly clear as well that society's other institutions – preventive and remedial – have shown themselves consistently incapable of dealing with such individuals. Thus a measure of social commitment as well as a necessary faith in the efficacy and meaningfulness of their own clinical orientation have, in the past half century, convinced may psychiatrists that they should play some role in society's attempts to deal with such problems. (A normal component of personal ambition and pride of profession has presumably played a role as well.)

Thus the often vigorous demands for a greater role in the adjudication and treatment of the criminal offender that were made by certain forensic psychiatrists in the first half of this century. It was natural for such psychiatrists to endorse or articulate rhetorical onslaughts against the "obscurantism" of the law and lawyers – and the harsh and seemingly dysfunctional punishments meted out to criminal offenders who might be mentally irresponsible; legal ideas and institutions seemed to reflect the nature of human motivation inadequately. But a half century of such debate and a few hesitant experiments have brought few results. State and federal legislators and administrators have been unwilling generally to underwrite even the widespread experimental application of individual psychotherapeutic techniques – and it has become increasingly clear that even if they had, beneficial results could not well have been guaranteed. The demands of the psychiatric establishment that it participate in judging and treating the criminal offender seem more and more remote in intellectual history as would-be reformers increasingly concern themselves with the nature of the penal institutions and structural realities and values of the society that produces the individuals incarcerated in them. The gift of social responsibility is always dubious insofar as it implies an embittering gap between expectations and performance.

Nevertheless, some of my best friends are psychiatrists. I have several explanations for this, some more complimentary than others, but I have decided that it is principally because of our parallel marginality to the world of medicine. Psychiatrists are more likely than other medical specialists to take an interest in the history of their subdiscipline; there may even be a kind of truth in the hostile whimsy that such historical interest reflects the fact that psychiatrists practice medicine as it was practiced a century or more ago.

But insofar as this is true it should evoke sympathy rather than condemnation. All societies need physicians to deal with those conditions that cause pain and disability and are defined as illness. The mid-nineteenth-century physician could neither cure nor explain tuberculosis or typhoid, but he had to treat them nevertheless. They would not go away, nor will those grave forms of disability our society calls psychoses, or those less disabling ones that cause "only" depression and anxiety.

Indeed, the contemporary psychiatrist is in some ways in a position even more difficult than that of his mid-nineteenth-century predecessor. There are two reasons for this. One is the way in which psychiatry has, as we have argued, inherited a bewildering variety of social problems. The psychiatric profession obviously cannot make – or even plausibly formulate – policy in regard to racial discord, crime, or optimum modes of schooling, yet it bears in the minds of at least some Americans a certain burden of responsibility (in some minds, ironically, a responsibility for curing, in others for somehow causing such problems). There is a second and far more fundamental difficulty. Even if developing scientific knowledge should restructure the doctor–patient relationship in severe conditions of mental disability, as insulin has done in the treatment of diabetes and antibiotics in the treatment of pneumonia, it seems most unlikely that we will find analogous understanding for all those conditions we call neurotic or label as personality disorders.[5] They are presumably modes of adjustment and thus expressions of our emotional reality; as long as our social values venerate

5 It should be recalled that pellagra and paresis were in this century problems for the psychiatrist.

medical and manipulative solutions and fail to provide other sources of consolation, the psychiatrist (or some other designated figure) will continue to inherit a goodly share of this burden. A major justification of medical psychiatry's legitimacy lies not in its ability to diagnose, predict, and cure – nor even in its possible ethical superiority to rival schools of emotional healing – but in the very gravity and scale of the responsibility it must undertake. Psychiatry has a second claim to social legitimacy, one that upholds and justifies its continued relationship with medicine: while we await the unpredictable gestation of research to tell us more of etiology and mechanisms that may underlie mania, depression, and what is called schizophrenia, psychiatry provides the principal link between laboratory and clinical research and the social reality of these ailments.[6] Not effectiveness, but orientation, values, and responsibility are the basis of psychiatry's legitimacy.

Criticism of the theoretical frameworks used most frequently in the past half century to explain such conditions cannot obviate the implacable reality of the conditions themselves. And such explanatory frameworks have a certain legitimacy of their own, even if they are arbitrary and perhaps ultimately inadequate. Just as society needs someone to treat those it labels sick, such designated healers need an ideological framework with which to rationalize their ministrations. It is true that these formulations have, in the absence of limit-defining physiological and pathological data, provided an ideology that on the one hand supports the practitioner's role and status, and on the other incorporates general social norms and values.

The assumptions of certain psychiatrists may have seemed to endorse particular patterns of family, caste, and sex roles, and to be suspiciously consistent with the needs of an urban, rationalistic society unwilling to tolerate certain kinds of deviance. But it is not clear where this observation leaves us; for even if we change the assumptions of American psychiatry, we are unlikely to alter those social and individual factors that figure in the causation of mental dysfunction. A change of viewpoint may have an enlightening, but hardly a healing, effect. Even if one assumes that the

6 This second argument can be clarified by returning to the analogy with mid-nineteenth-century medicine. It is sometimes tempting for the historian to look with scorn upon the medical establishment of a century ago, to make its therapeutics and speculative etiologies an object of ridicule. At least the irregulars, the argument follows – the homeopaths, botanics, and eclectics who were little hindered by traditional dogma – did little to harm their patients, and they provided a cogent criticism of the contemporary medical establishment. Yet seen in perspective, the criticism of irregulars only underlines the strength of regular medicine; it was part of a world system of knowledge and of accepted techniques for its acquisition and dissemination. It was this relationship to clinical and scientific work that distinguished leaders in regular medicine, not the shortcomings of their therapeutics or their arbitrary and speculative etiologies.

macrostructure of society and the not entirely unrelated microstructure of the family play some precipitating role in the etiology of mental illness, psychiatry is hardly the most important or effective institution through which society controls and defines behavior.

It may be that different arrangements within society would perhaps reduce the number of individuals who suffer emotional discomfort. *Perhaps*, indeed. But this conviction does not help the sick today, nor does it serve as an adequate rationale for the dissolution of contemporary psychiatry – or even the dissolution of the much maligned "medical model" as a framework within which to work. Individuals will continue to suffer in varying degrees from what will continue to be defined in our rationalistic society as mental illness. And most of those unable to live with their emotional selves will either turn voluntarily or be sent to psychiatrists who offer some rationalistic mode of therapy. (Behavioral and psychopharmacological techniques fit in general into this pattern.) Neither the growth of mystical and supposedly transcendent sects nor the growth of a fashionable antirationalism promises to change this view in the near future. Most Americans simply have no other emotional and cognitive frame of reference in which to place their feelings. The religious values which provided such a framework in the past seem no longer compelling to most of us; there is no meaning, no compensation in our emotional pain. Thus the so-called medical model – for better or worse – with its implication of disease process and expectation of cure has to a certain extent replaced these older frameworks for coping with depression and anxiety.[7]

The opening of the 1970s finds psychiatry in a particularly eclectic and labile state. One of its strongest threads of continuity lies, ironically, in the very persistence of those structural dilemmas we have sought to describe. Unless all psychiatry should thaw, melt, and resolve itself into applied pharmacology there seems little possibility of these difficulties redefining themselves. Drug therapy itself, for example, represents a potential shift in traditional modes of psychiatric practice (and, by implication, theory as well). Yet even when it provides symptomatic relief and leads to new theoretical insights, psychopharmacology seems to support the criticism that psychiatry has failed to evaluate adequately the efficacy of its cognitive therapeutic procedures. Nor have those activist critics who see in psychiatry an agent of social control been reassured by current emphasis on drug therapy. Behavioral therapies only restate and reaffirm similar ambiguities,

---

7 These remarks are only marginally relevant to conditions of extreme disability, some of which have known organic causes and others of which may well be found to be dependent upon some underlying physical mechanism. Even in such severe conditions, of course, social values and expectations help shape the attitudes of others toward the sufferer and. to an extent, his conception of self.

for these newer techniques reflect not only the influence of contemporary intellectual trends but, almost simultaneously, parallel reactions to them. Drug and behavioral therapies only reformulate the persistent problems implicit in psychiatry's social location and its sensitivity to social and intellectual currents. We find ourselves in a period of unprecedented and unashamed questioning; skepticism has become our most plausible candidate for orthodoxy. And this is perhaps not too deplorable a situation.

12

Disease and social order in America: Perceptions and expectations

ᕫ᠊᠊ Written for a conference on AIDS in the mid-1980s, this essay was intended to place a contemporary crisis in historical context. Although AIDS provided an occasion, the argument reflected a longstanding prior concern. This was my effort to understand differences among the old left of the 1930s, 1940s, and 1950s, the no-longer-so-new left of the late 1960s and 1970s, and the less self-assured critical spirit of the 1980s. The older generation shared a faith in the ultimate and unambiguous benefits of science and technology in a just society; their children accepted a parallel yet opposed certainty. They regarded the presumptive benefits of scientific progress as necessarily illusory and imprisoning – and many of its fundamental conceptions as no more than arbitrary social constructions.

The history of AIDS demonstrates the inadequacy of either species of certainty. There were no one-dimensional answers. AIDS could hardly be dismissed as an exercise in stigmatizing the deviant; it obviously had a strong biological component. It was not simply a construction even if it had been constructed. Yet at the same time nothing marked the epidemic more starkly than its ability to evoke and reproduce preexisting social values and attitudes. The diversity and complexity of reactions to AIDS has underlined the need to look carefully at the elusive process through which society constructs its reponse to disease. And we know that there will be no simple and formulaic answers; in the 1990s they are neither intellectually available nor politically compelling. ᕫᕫ

During the past two decades Americans have participated in a series of debates about the appropriate social response to disease. At first glance the issues seem to differ widely. What were the appropriate responses to hyper-activity in children? Premenstrual syndrome in women? Homosexuality? Drug and alcohol addiction? Were any of these in fact diseases or simply labels for socially defined deviance? What should or could have been done about John Hinckley and other possibly insane offenders? Are diagnosis-related groups an appropriate mechanism for rationalizing the costs of inpatient health care? Does sickness come in neat and categorically distinct units? What are appropriate governmental and individual responses to AIDS? One could continue to add examples, but the point seems obvious. Despite their diversity, these controversies are bound together by several themes. One is the way that relationships between the medical profession and society are structured around interactions legitimated by the presumed existence of disease.[1] A second theme is the negotiated aspect of disease as social phenomenon. A generation of social scientists and social critics has emphasized that there is no simple and necessary relationship between disease in its biological and social dimensions. Some ills have a well-understood physical basis, others none that can be demonstrated. Meaning is not necessary, but negotiated, the argument follows; disease is con-structed, not discovered.[2]

Critics have turned the delegitimating tools of cultural relativism on medicine as they have on so many other areas in which knowledge and power are closely linked. For such scholars, Michel Foucault, not Robert Merton, has become the sociologist of choice. "I assert," a recent student of cholera – and of Foucault – argues, "that 'disease' does not exist. It is therefore illusory to think that one can 'develop beliefs' about it or 'respond' to it. What does exist is not disease but practices."[3] Medical knowledge is not value-free to such skeptics, but is at least in part a socially constructed and determined belief system, a reflection of arbitrary social arrangements, social need, and the distribution of power.

The medical profession's institutional power has long been an object of reformist concern, but during the 1960s and early 1970s medicine's conceptual foundations have come under increasing attack. This relativist point of view has sought to undermine not only the apparent objectivity of

---

1 "Presumed," because disease does not exist as a social phenomenon until it is somehow perceived as existing. This perception can have any one of many relationships to a possible biological substrate.

An earlier version of this paper appeared in *The Milbank Quarterly* 64 (1986, supplement 1): 34–55. I should like to thank Barbara Bates, Renee Fox, Stephen Kunitz, Dorothy Nelkin, Rosemary Stevens, Owsei Temkin, and the editors of *The Milbank Quarterly* supplement for their helpful comments. I am also grateful to audiences at Cornell, Harvard, Johns Hopkins, and Columbia universities, who tolerated and criticized earlier versions.

2 For a useful – if eclectic – collection of case studies reflecting this point of view, see Peter Wright and Andrew Treacher, eds., *The Problem of Medical Knowledge: Examining the Social Construction of Medicine* (Edinburgh: University of Edinburgh Press, 1982). The sociological literature of the 1960s and 1970s on the "social construction" of mental illness was particularly influential in questioning the positivist value-free conception of sickness categories.

3 François Delaporte, *Disease and Civilization: The Cholera in Paris, 1832*, tr. Arthur Goldhammer (Cambridge: MIT Press, 1986), p. 6.

particular disease entities but also, by implication, the legitimacy of the social authority wielded by the medical profession, which has traditionally articulated and administered diagnostic categories. The physician is not above social interest, but is a social actor whose mission of defining and treating disease can express and legitimate professional, class, or gender interests. This is obviously as much a political as an epistemological position. The marriage of cultural criticism and antipositivism became an influential, if never a majority, view during the past generation.

These relativist arguments are familiar and have become, in fact, a cliché among social historians and social scientists. Yet it is a point of view that seems increasingly sectarian. The weight of scholarly opinion has in the past decade shifted toward an emphasis on biological factors in the understanding of disease and human behavior. We have seen this in a growing interest in the roles of heredity and constitutional factors in disease and behavior, a growing somaticism among students of mental illness. The perceived failure of deinstitutionalization has, for example, underlined the intractability and presumed biological underpinning of the psychoses. Such views are, at least in emphasis, a rejection of once-fashionable sociological formulations that tended to dismiss the diagnosis of mental illness as an exercise in the labeling of deviance.

But no single event has had a more dramatic and illuminating impact than AIDS. It has proved an occasion for labeling, but it is not simply an exercise in labeling. Gay leaders who had for decades urged the demedicalization of homosexuality now find their community anxiously attuned to the findings of virologists and immunologists.[4] This is not to say that the social perception of AIDS and the definition of policy choices are not shaped by preexisting social attitudes; the deviant are still stigmatized, victims are still blamed. But the biomedical aspects of AIDS can hardly be ignored; it is difficult to ignore a disease with a fatality rate approaching 100 percent. AIDS has, in fact, helped create a new consensus in regard to disease, one that finds a place for both biological and social factors and emphasizes their interaction. Students of the relationships between medicine and society live in a necessarily postrelativist decade.

But as we accept our dependence on the laboratory and its findings, a number of thoughtful Americans still find it difficult to remain optimistic about society's ability to harness that knowledge; increased understanding of the natural world does not bring automatic and unalloyed benefits. We have been made too conscious of the complex and problematic relationship between medical knowledge and its application. Our decade may be

4 For an analysis of the demedicalization movement, see Ronald Bayer, *Homosexuality and American Psychiatry: The Politics of Diagnosis* (New York: Basic Books, 1981).

increasingly postrelativist, but we are still products of a generation of relativism, conscious of the costs as well as the benefits of scientific medicine, of the provisional yet indispensable quality of medical knowledge. The meaning of disease has in the recent past become more rather than less ambiguous. It is now difficult to embrace the clarifying simplicity of either extreme: the reductionist view that concerns itself with verifiable pathological process alone, or the uncompromising relativist position that chooses to ignore that same pathological process in shaping specific social responses.

Men of goodwill

This postrelativist ambivalence about medical knowledge is an uncertain position, one that would have made little sense to men of goodwill who sought to understand the social role of medicine in the 1930s and 1940s. This generation thought very differently about disease and the doctor's role. They shared an optimistic faith in science and medicine; superstition and social injustice had, and would, impede the accumulation and distribution of knowledge – but the ultimate trend was toward a more humane, healthy, and enlightened society.

No one was more prominent in that generation than the historian Henry Sigerist, a prolific author, a defender of Soviet medicine, and a self-consciously irreverent gadfly of the American medical establishment. "Disease as we conceive it today," he wrote in 1943, "is a biological process. . . . Disease is no more than the sum total of abnormal reactions of the organism or its parts to abnormal stimuli."[5] It constituted a failure of the organism to adapt to its environment; disease could, that is, be socially induced, but it was not simply a social construct. It was a real pathological phenomenon. In fact, this very lack of ambiguity underlay the role of disease as a tool of social criticism; the etiology of pellagra (a disease resulting from dietary deficiency) tells us something specific about mill villages and welfare institutions. The etiology of lice-borne typhus tells the epidemiologist something very precise about cleanliness and even the price of clothing in communities with a high incidence of the disease. The persistence of typhoid in the early twentieth century constitutes a telling critique of those communities that tolerated a contaminated water supply. Medical knowledge could serve as both tool and rationale for social intervention.

Sigerist, like almost all of his contemporaries of whatever political

5 Henry Sigerist, *Civilization and Disease* (Ithaca, N.Y.: Cornell University Press, 1943), p. 1.

persuasion, always maintained an enormous faith in the ultimately positive role of science in human affairs. "The more I study history," he concluded during the darkest days of the Second World War, "the more faith I have in the future of mankind, and the less doubt as to the ultimate result of the present conflict. The step will be taken from the competitive to the cooperative society, democratically ruled on scientific principles."[6] Science and scientific medicine were necessary aspects of the solution, not part of the problem. Such assumptions were widespread. Pioneer students of the social history of medicine, for example, tended to see as fundamental the ways in which society could stimulate, or, too frequently, impede, the autonomous and ultimately liberating development of science and medicine.[7]

Certainly scientific ideas could be misused. The Nazis' use of a racist eugenics is an obvious example; but, as Sigerist put it, eugenics was a "socio-biological experiment that deserves to be watched carefully, even if the present Nazi regime has made it subservient to a thoroughly reactionary – and unscientific – politico-racial ideology."[8] The German advocates of a racist biology were, in other words, false priests of a true religion. It seemed inconceivable to him that science would not, in the long run, stand with the forces of enlightenment and egalitarianism.

To reformers of Sigerist's generation, disease incidence was often the result of particular social arrangements, especially economic inequalities. Disease could also become part of a vicious cycle, miring families and individuals in poverty. Such ideas were widespread among advocates of what contemporaries called "social medicine," a point of view that recognized the limits of therapeutics and emphasized instead the ways in which disease reflected environmental conditions.[9] The preservation of health therefore often required the modification of social and economic relationships. Therapeutic intervention, according to this view, was not the answer. "Medical care cannot alone eradicate pellagra and rickets," as two leading authorities explained, citing particularly telling instances:

> these conditions are for the most part diseases of poverty and ignorance, and their prevention and cure lie with the economic and social

6 Sigerist, *Civilization and Disease*, p. 244.
7 See, for example, the work of Bernhard Stern, *Social Factors in Medical Progress* (New York: Columbia University Press, 1927) and *Society and Medical Progress* (Princeton, N.J.: Princeton University Press, 1941), esp. chs. 8–10; and Richard H. Shyrock, *The Development of Modern Medicine* (Philadelphia: University of Pennsylvania Press, 1936).
8 Sigerist, *Civilization and Disease*, p. 85.
9 See, for example, George Rosen, "What Is Social Medicine?" *Bulletin of the History of Medicine* 21 (1947): 674–733; René Sand, *Health and Human Progress: An Essay in Sociological Medicine* (New York: Macmillan, 1936) and *The Advance to Social Medicine* (London: Staples, 1952).

system. Health can be achieved only as a part of a high standard of living, in which good medical care is only one of a number of essential elements.

It must be emphasized that their study was not a call for radical social change but a plea for the more effective and equitable distribution of medical care. The point is, of course, that the authors could not envisage a conflict between these goals.[10] In the 1930s the fundamental problems in health care were not perceived as intrinsic to scientific medicine; instead they seemed to lie in maldistribution of the real benefits that medicine could provide. The establishment of hospitals and the provision of well-trained physicians for the poor and isolated were moral and practical necessities. And such convictions were shaped before the availability of antibiotics and the array of therapeutic and diagnostic tools that have transformed medical care in the past half-century.

Perceptions of medicine are rather different today. Despite two generations of enormous technical change, we have become aware that medical progress implies other than monetary costs. We have allowed an increasing number of men and women to live longer, yet often more incapacitated, lives. We have seen an expanded and generally more accessible medical system accused of insensitivity and physicians charged with greed and inhumanity. We have seen Sigerist's future, and in some ways it seems not to have worked. Few would-be reformers of medicine in the 1980s have been able to share his generation's confident belief in the ultimate and unambiguous benevolence of scientific medicine – no matter how impressive its technical achievements.

Yet as a social institution and body of ideas medicine has never been more central to American society. In the past half-century we have devoted an increasing proportion of our resources to medical care. Public expectations have increased proportionately, along with a widespread resentment at medicine's inability to comply with these imperial expectations. Malpractice suits are only one – indirect – index of the pervasiveness of such hopes.

Definitions of disease have come to play a particularly prominent role at the margins of medical competence – where the authority of medical practitioners and medical ideas is most obviously subject to negotiation. We

10 R. I. Lee and L. W. Jones, *The Fundamentals of Good Medical Care*, Publications of the Committee on the Costs of Medical Care, no. 22 (Chicago: University of Chicago Press, 1933), p. 15. State hospital reform in this period provides another parallel. Albert Deutsch's widely read exposés, for example, constituted a plea for the renovation and medicalization of these neglected institutions – but the therapeutic options then available inspire no great confidence today. See Deutsch, *The Shame of the States* (New York: Harcourt, Brace, 1948).

tend not to question the appropriateness of an orthopedic surgeon's role in treating a broken kneecap, although we might his or her exclusive role (until recently) in legitimating and controlling third-party payment for that treatment. A good many more of us would question the physician's role in defining behavioral deviance. Others would question the appropriateness of contemporary medical priorities in setting health care policy in regard to the very young, the chronically ill, and the very old. We are happy to have immunologists study AIDS; we disagree about the policy implications of their findings. Americans have, in fact, asked, or have been willing to allow, physicians to play a variety of gatekeeping as well as therapeutic roles. They have been rewarded with both power and resentment. Perhaps it was inevitable that disease definition would become a key battleground in the debate surrounding the prerogatives of physicians and the responsibilities of government.

Evolving conceptions of disease

Ideas about the nature of disease have been fundamental both to the internal evolution of medicine and to the profession's complex interactions with society. But even if that centrality has remained consistent over time, the specific nature of those concepts and interactions has changed; Sigerist's confident view of disease as a discrete pathological process had already substantially evolved from traditional concepts.

Perhaps the most significant difference between his ideas and those of his late eighteenth- and early nineteenth-century predecessors lay in the areas of *boundaries* and *specificity*. In 1800 sickness was still viewed in largely individual terms. True, there were well-marked ills – smallpox, for example – that experience had come to define as relatively specific, but even in such ailments, idiosyncrasy and predisposition could shape an individual's response. Most sickness was not understood in specific terms, even if its ultimate manifestations fell into accustomed patterns. Even epidemic disease was understood to result from an unbalanced state in a particular individual – an imbalance resulting from the sum of interactions between an individual's constitutional endowment and the environment; thus the conventional and persistent emphases on regimen and diet in the cause and cure of sickness. It was natural for physicians to assume connections between physical and psychological environment and sickness; they imposed no rigid boundaries between body and mind or between individual and environment.[11]

11 See Chapter 1 of this volume.

It is tempting to see such systems from a functionalist point of view, to underline the ways in which this flexible explanatory system could serve both as behavioral sanction and as a basis for legitimating the physician's social role. Physicians could provide explanations for the inexplicable, reassure those still well that reason guaranteed their continued health, and at the same time reinforce society's moral assumptions. Individuals could and often did play a role in the development of their own ailments; volition and, thus, social norms explained why the drunkard, the financial speculator, and the glutton succumbed. But volition could also be used to explain the role of crowding, poor diet, and economic exploitation. The sick man was both actor and acted upon. Like an assortment of bricks, the elements of this speculative pathology could be put together in different forms according to the builder's requirements. Freethinkers could thus see enthusiastic religion as a cause of sickness, while the more evangelical could indict irreligion. The prominent role accorded to volition implied the possibility of control.

Disease ultimately expressed itself through physiological and anatomical mechanisms; but these pathological mechanisms were activated by a unique configuration of interactions between the individual and his or her environment. Significantly, however, the form of such explanations was always material and rationalistic, no matter how strained and speculative, no matter how transparently they incorporated social norms and attitudes.

Even epidemic disease could be made to fit into the same rationalistic framework, despite the obvious fact that some general factor had to be at work. The case of cholera is particularly enlightening. The most frightening and novel of nineteenth-century European and American epidemics, cholera is the closest modern analogy of AIDS.[12] Asiatic cholera was unknown in Western Europe before 1831; it killed roughly half of those it attacked, and did so, moreover, in particularly rapid and dramatic fashion. No other pandemic had so focused popular and professional fears since plague had receded from Europe in the late seventeenth and early eighteenth centuries.

Lacking an understanding of the etiological agent, contemporaries framed a picture of cholera that sought to reduce the threat of randomness while it articulated social values and status relationships. The dirty, the gluttonous, and the poorly nourished alike were believed to be predisposed to the disease. Predisposition was, in fact, a key term in attempts to explain this and other epidemic ailments, for it served to explain the selective

12 The analogy is obviously not exact. So far as we are aware, clinically identifiable cases of AIDS have a mortality rate of nearly 100 percent – but over a clinical course that is far more extended than that of cholera.

exactions of what was at some level a general influence. Physicians played a necessary role, providing what reassurance they could in a rational, if, in retrospect, speculative, form. With no consensus regarding the pathology of the disease or the understanding of its etiology, social variables necessarily played a prominent role in fashioning a usable framework that enabled regularly trained physicians and their middle-class patients to cope with the disease.[13] All this was soon to change. By the end of the nineteenth century, disease had become a more specific, yet at the same time more expansive, concept.

During the first thirty or so years of the nineteenth century, elite physicians began to assimilate the idea – associated with the so-called Paris clinical school – that disease was a specific, ordinarily lesion-based entity that reenacted itself in every individual sufferer. Lesions discernible at postmortem could be correlated with symptoms exhibited during the patient's life. Disease could also be (and often was) construed as a disturbance of physiological function that induced an anatomical lesion over time. The study of physiology could – some of the discipline's nineteenth-century pioneers claimed – be a study of disease causation. But whether one emphasized anatomical change or physiological function, symptoms were the consequence of specific material mechanisms. Idiosyncrasy was by no means banished; the predisposition to sickness, the clinical expression of a particular ailment, and the response to therapeutics were still seen in terms of an individual's constitution and personal habits. Physicians and laypersons alike instinctively preserved a role for choice and individual responsibility in explaining the selective exactions of disease.

The cause of these newly distinct entities remained a mystery, however. Some medical thinkers even contended that the ultimate cause of disease would always remain beyond human understanding; speculation could lead only to self-delusion. Degenerative or constitutional ailments might be assumed to be implicit in the design of the human body and the aging process. Acute infectious ailments, however, could not be so easily explained.

As we are all aware, an explanation was soon forthcoming. The germ theory, first plausibly articulated in the 1870s, promised to illuminate both the transmission of infectious ills and the particularity of pathological mechanisms. Thus, the evolving model of disease should be seen as having

---

13 Etiological speculations reflected and rationalized real or potential social conflict in particular national contexts. See, for example, Charles E. Rosenberg, *The Cholera Years: The United States in 1832, 1849, and 1866* (1962; rev. ed. Chicago: University of Chicago Press, 1987); Roderick E. McGrew, *Russia and the Cholera, 1823–1832* (Madison: University of Wisconsin Press, 1965); R. J. Morris, *Cholera 1832: The Social Response to an Epidemic* (New York: Holmes and Meier, 1976); Michael Durey, *The Return of the Plague: British Society and the Cholera 1831–32* (Dublin: Gill and MacMillan, 1979).

taken two linked steps in the nineteenth century: the first emphasized the specific, somatic, and mechanistic aspect of disease, and the second provided a discrete cause for those changes. The legitimacy of the new style of conceptualizing disease entities was related closely to both the specificity and the tightness, or unity, of individual entities. Change was gradual, especially among laypersons. Well into the twentieth century, for example, the common cold was widely regarded – and feared – as the first stage of an illness culminating in tuberculosis.

The history of nineteenth-century pathology and clinical medicine seems only to confirm the explanatory value of this new way of seeing diseases. Syphilis and tuberculosis, for example, so protean as clinical phenomena, gradually came to be seen as having fundamental unities based on cause and consequent pathology. Truth lay in discerning a more real (more universal and fundamental) causal mechanism beneath the elusive and ever-changing surface of their appearance in particular individuals.[14] The intellectual tools for constructing an understanding of that underlying truth came increasingly from the insights and techniques of the laboratory.[15] A minority of early twentieth-century physicians did protest the tendency toward mechanistic reductionism in diagnosis and treatment. Their successors have continued. But such warnings could not compete with the laboratory's allure; they still cannot.[16]

Even before medicine possessed resources for treating these newly elucidated clinical phenomena, the gradual acceptance of the notion of specific disease entities by laypersons and practitioners helped reshape the physician's role – enlarging the importance of the technical, and increasing the gap between lay and professional medical knowledge. Early twentieth-century reforms in medical education and the standardization of hospitals were both, to an extent, responses to this emerging consensus. Sickness was now a discrete, material phenomenon, best understood by the tools of science and best treated by individuals who had mastered those tools.

But if medical knowledge was gradually becoming segregated in credentialed hands, laypersons were compensated with greater expectations and an increasing faith in medical ideas and medical experts. It was a kind of

14 Owsei Temkin, "The Scientific Approach to Disease: Specific Entity and Individual Sickness," in *Scientific Change: Historical Studies in the Intellectual, Social and Technical Conditions for Scientific Discovery and Technical Invention from Antiquity to the Present*, ed. A. C. Crombie (New York: Basic Books, 1963), p. 629–647.
15 For an influential, if rather categorical, statement of this point of view, see N. D. Jewson, "The Disappearance of the Sick-Man from Medical Cosmology, 1770–1870," *Sociology* 10 (1976): 224–244. See also Chapter 1 of this volume.
16 A significant antireductionist tradition has always existed among clinicians. For a recent statement of this continuing tradition, see Richard J. Baron, "An Introduction to Medical Phenomenology: I Can't Hear You While I'm Listening," *Annals of Internal Medicine* 103 (1985): 606–611.

implicit contract: society received a measure of emotional reassurance and clinical efficacy in exchange for the increased status and autonomy of medicine. Beginning in the 1880s the laboratory provided a series of dramatic insights. The discovery of the causes of cholera, tuberculosis, typhoid, and diphtheria were not esoteric events isolated in the pages of technical journals, but front-page news. And to laypersons and physicians alike, much of medicine's new explanatory power was construed in terms of specific ills and the ability to understand, diagnose, prevent, and, in a minority of cases, treat conditions previously intractable and mysterious. Even if the demographic impact of rabies immunization and diphtheria antitoxin was minor, these treatments provided striking public evidence of medicine's new powers.

The problem, of course, with this vision of disease is not that it was wrong – although in retrospect it appears incomplete and prematurely reductionist – but that it was, in fact, so powerful and seductive. No group in society was more impressed than the medical profession itself. Professional status and prestige were soon recast in these new forms. Scholarship had always been important in elite medical circles. But now that scholarship had increasingly to be expressed in the form of laboratory research or systematic clinical investigation, the library and bedside no longer defined the boundaries of professional excellence. This shift in values was also effective in helping to recast the institutional shape of the medical profession, legitimating and providing content for a proliferating specialism and an increasingly self-conscious hospital and academic elite. It is true that an appropriate role remained to be defined for the so-called basic sciences in clinic and medical school; but this is irrelevant. As we are well aware, an acute-care-, specific-disease-oriented approach came to characterize both the twentieth-century hospital and the career priorities of doctors. Insofar as the laboratory and basic science disciplines were incorporated into the hospital and academic medicine, they were most frequently bent to the purpose of elucidating and monitoring pathological mechanisms.

Disease as behavioral sanction

In the last third of the nineteenth century a related, yet potentially inconsistent, development was taking place in that contested cultural terrain where society's tendency to prescribe and proscribe behavior intersected with the prerogatives of medicine. Disease boundaries were expanded to include behavior patterns that might have been dismissed as perverse or criminal in earlier generations. Most conspicuous was the way in which deviance was increasingly, if by no means universally, being defined as the consequence of a disease process and, thus, appropriately the physician's responsibility. Toward the close of the nineteenth century, for example, neurologists widened the categories of ailments they chose to treat: phobias, anxieties, and depression could now be classed as symptoms of neurasthenia, and alcoholism, drug addiction, and homosexuality became potential diagnoses rather than culpable failures of volition.

What is particularly striking here is the way that the contemporary prestige of somatic models gradually redefined these behaviors as appropriately within the purview of medicine. The very fact that these novel but omnipresent "ills" manifested themselves exclusively in the form of behavior only emphasized the need to presume an underlying physical mechanism; without one, they could hardly be seen as acquired ailments or constitutional proclivities (the only presumed bases for genuine sickness).

The boundaries of medicine were expanding in the late nineteenth century and, to an articulate minority of self-consciously progressive physicians, that expansion constituted progress toward a more just and enlightened society. A growing secularism paralleled and lent emotional plausibility to this framing in medical terms of matters that had been previously construed as essentially moral. Science, not theology – most physicians believed – should be the arbiter of such questions.

The physician, not the priest or judge, was now viewed as the most appropriate guardian of the rights of society and the individual. The sufferer from phobias and anxieties, the victim of sexual incapacity, the man or woman consumed with desire for a socially unacceptable love object, could be seen as the product of his or her material condition rather than as an outcast. By no means all contemporaries accepted such views. But to the stigmatized themselves these hypothetical diagnoses may well have been palatable; given the choice, an individual might well prefer to regard his or her deviant behavior as the product of hereditary endowment or disease process. It might well have offered more comfort than the traditional option of seeing oneself as a reprehensible and culpable actor. The secular rationalism so prevalent in the late nineteenth century freed many Americans from a measure of personal guilt at the cost of being labeled as sick. Not until the second half of the twentieth century, however, has this come to seem a problematic bargain.[17]

17 The psychodynamic models of behavioral disorder so influential in the first half of the twentieth century shared the determinism of their somatic forerunners, although differing in etiological emphasis. Dynamic psychiatry, however, remained a minority and in some ways atypical aspect of American medicine – even when it loomed prominently in the world-view of educated laypersons. In any case, the areas of its greatest clinical responsibilities were ones that had already been claimed for medicine before 1900.

Late nineteenth-century medical practitioners became active in another area, apparently reflecting the laudable and inexorable expansion of medical responsibility. This new area was public health and, in particular, the shaping of an interventionist social agenda. These reformist and environmentally oriented policy guidelines seemed no more than appropriate responses to the findings of contemporary epidemiology. Sickness was repeatedly connected with poverty and deprivation. The conclusions seemed obvious to reformers. An enlightened society should purify its water, provide pure milk for its children, inspect its food, and clean its streets and tenements. The expansion of public medicine was connected in a score of ways with the style of self-consciously and self-righteously enlightened government we have come to associate with progressive reform. Moreover, there appeared to be no inherent conflicts among the expansion of medical authority, the clothing of that authority in the guise of scientific reductionism, the proliferation of disease entities – and the vision of a good society. In fact, this confluence of factors seemed necessary and necessarily benevolent. This optimistic and activist tradition still informed the assumptions and hopes of most advocates of social medicine in the 1930s and 1940s.

Contradictions and crisis

In the past two decades, however, this configuration of views has appeared to many social critics as neither necessary nor unambiguously benevolent. Medicine has been confronted with a multisided crisis in public expectation. Even those Americans least critical in their attitude toward the benefits of continued medical progress are concerned about the monetary cost. Others who are more skeptical, but still willing to concede the real advances of contemporary medical practice, deplore the ethical and human costs of bureaucratic, episodic, high-technology care. Again and again these concerns focus on the definition of disease.

The first widely expressed concern arose in regard to mental illness; it constituted what I have called in Chapter 11 a "crisis in psychiatric legitimacy." It might with equal justice have been termed a crisis in the cognitive and administrative management of deviance. Beginning in the early 1960s sociologists and social critics began to emphasize the arbitrariness of psychiatric categories and to contend that they were in essence labels, culturally appropriate ways of stigmatizing deviance. Psychiatric thought was in good measure a mechanism for framing, and thus controlling, deviant behavior. The force of this radical critique was augmented by a nagging truth.

Medicine had already come to play a prominent role in relation to just those areas – such as sexual deviance, addiction, and even criminality – where supposedly pathological behaviors fit least comfortably into the pathological model that has explained and legitimated conventional categories of somatic illness. Psychiatry still lacks a mechanism-specific understanding of the great majority of the syndromes it treats. A dramatic tension thus persists between psychiatry's cognitive legitimacy and its clinical responsibilities. Nor is it an accident that the specialty fits uneasily into medicine's status hierarchy. The recent expansion of interest in somatic approaches to psychiatric ills demonstrates these inconsistencies as much as it does the accumulation of new knowledge and new techniques.

A second area of disease-related conflict has resulted from the dominance of acute, interventionist models in medical-career priorities and institutions. The prestige of medicine and the personal health expectations of Americans have increasingly come to depend on the efficacy of scientific, interventionist medicine – a system of values and expectations that has been built into the economic as well as intellectual basis of American health care in the past half century. Yet it is a system that is widely perceived as having failed to provide adequate care for the old and chronically ill, or even humane death for the moribund.

Third-party, employer-based insurance has also been structured around the hospital and explicit disease entities. So have federal health insurance schemes. Disease has served as a moral and logical rationale for these bureaucratic reimbursement systems even though payments correspond to days of hospitalization, physician visits, or particular procedures. Specific disease entities have come to mediate between the conceptual world of medicine and the expectations of laypersons. Interactions between doctor and patient ordinarily take place in units defined and bureaucratically justified by the existence of real or presumed sickness. Health insurance has provided a measure of care and emotional security for millions of Americans and a steady flow of income to hospitals and hospital suppliers. But the levers controlling that cash flow can only be pressed by physicians. The language of diagnostic categories at once helps to expedite and to legitimate this special relationship among physicians, patients, and health insurers. Physicians in the mid-1980s complain of the growing influence of cost accounting and bureaucracy and their decreasing role in making care decisions. Diagnosis-related groups seem an obvious justification for such fears. Yet these diagnostic categories are product and symbol of, and condign punishment for, the rigid and unresponsive aspects of our cost-plus, disease-legitimated system of third-party payment. It is a system, moreover, in which physicians and the values of scientific medicine have played a pivotal role.

Rising costs have helped remind us that sickness as experienced comes in units of people and families – and not of discrete, codable diagnostic entities. It is significant that socially minded physicians throughout the first half of this century repeatedly cautioned that patients had families, that managing an acute episode of sickness or trauma did not exhaust the possible universe of medical care options.[18] As early as the 1920s a minority of clinicians warned that chronic and geriatric problems would become increasingly significant as the incidence of acute infectious ills declined; they warned as well that episodic, hospital-based treatment was inadequate for the optimum care of such ailments. Few contemporaries bothered to disagree, yet such concerns became, in fact, increasingly marginal to the actual work routine of many physicians – especially the specialized and often research-oriented academic elite.

A third kind of conflict grew out of the success of medicine itself in helping banish the randomness of acute infectious illness from the perceived life chances of most Americans. The great majority of our children live to adulthood. We enjoy a greater confidence in predicting our future, but at the cost of granting enormous social power to medical practitioners and institutions. It was in some ways a mutually advantageous contract – like that between the psychiatrist and the depressed or deviant patient. But even the most dramatic and undeniable achievements of medicine have their social costs.

One such cost lies in the growing problem of chronic and degenerative ills. Another lies in our cultural habit of dealing with a diversity of elusive social problems by reducing them to technical terms – holding out the promise of neat solutions. Even the most dramatic technical achievements may simply redefine problems, not solve them; or they may create new difficulties in the process of solving old ones. The neonatal intensive care unit is a case in point; so are renal dialysis and cardiac transplants. The elusive phrase *quality of life* has become increasingly familiar in the past decade. It is hardly an accident.

As the economic and emotional stakes increase, so does the likelihood of conflict. The social meanings of disease have become increasingly the subject of debate and negotiation. Matters of cost are in some ways simple enough. Questions of value can be even more elusive. Is the prevention of sickle-cell anemia through genetic counseling a blow for equal rights or an opportunity for masked genocide? Does a collective social interest require that individuals be forced to use seat belts? Does calling premenstrual syndrome a disease liberate or enslave women? Does the imposition of

---

18 See, for example, H. B. Richardson's pointedly titled *Patients Have Families* (New York: Commonwealth Fund, 1945).

mandatory maternity leave constitute justice or handicap women in the economic marketplace? Things were much simpler for the majority of reformers in Progressive-era America. The control of women's hours and conditions of labor seemed to them an unambiguous social good, and woman's role seemed ultimately and unambiguously domestic.

In still another area, dominance of the disease entity has left the profession ill-prepared to address other medical problems that are not as easily construed in such terms. This is certainly one reason for the comparative lack of interest in geriatrics, chronic care, and maternal and child health. The old and chronically ill cannot – except episodically – be seen as sufferers from discrete and meliorable ills. Neither conceptually nor actuarially do they fit comfortably into contemporary practice patterns. The monitoring of particular organs, or intervention in acute episodes, has already become the responsibility of one specialty or another; the patient constitutes a residual category. Similarly, victory over the most important and accessible causes of infant and early childhood mortality has left the profession little concerned with the "lingering" aspects of the problem, which are politically sensitive and not easily amenable to exclusively technical solutions. It is clear, for example, that the neonatal intensive care unit is not an all-sufficient answer to the problem of low weight and prematurity, but it is a more congenial and prestigious approach, and seemingly less diffuse than the economic and political measures that are its natural counterparts. Similarly, the laboratory response to AIDS has been better funded and more focused than logically parallel efforts in the sphere of education and prevention.

The status of the medical profession, like the meaning of disease, has in the past decade become more rather than less ambiguous. As the technological capabilities of medicine become ever more dramatic, as we transplant hearts and fertilize ova in vitro, we have seen the parallel growth of skepticism and even hostility among laypersons. Such ambivalence is in fact an important component of attitudes toward medicine, technology, and the bureaucracies that embody and administer medical care. At the same time, we have by no means banished disease, even if we have altered the forms in which it is most likely to become a part of our lives. We still have to construct frameworks of understanding and reassurance within which we make sense of its inevitable exactions. Scientific medicine provides a fundamental, and to many individuals well-nigh exclusive, element in shaping that understanding, even in those ailments for which no effective treatment is available.

For many Americans, the meaning of disease is the mechanism that defines it; even in cancer the meaning is often that we do not yet know the mechanism. To some, however, the meaning of cancer may transcend the mechanism and the ultimate ability of medicine to understand it. For such individuals the meaning of cancer may lie in the evils of capitalism or of unhindered technical progress, or perhaps in failures of individual will. We live in a complex and fragmented world and create a variety of frameworks for our manifold ailments. But two elements remain fundamental: one is a faith in medicine's existing or potential insights, another is personal accountability.

The desire to explain sickness and death in terms of volition – of acts done or left undone – is ancient and powerful. The threat of disease provides a compelling reason to find prospective reassurance in aspects of behavior subject to individual control. Mental illness was, for example, commonly explained in the past as a possible consequence of habit patterns gradually hardened into uncontrollable pathologies. Those who avoided even occasional lapses would have little to fear. In the nineteenth-century epidemics of cholera, as we have seen, there was much talk of predisposition. The victims' behavior or place of residence explained why they, in particular, succumbed to a general epidemic influence. With decreasing fear of acute infectious disease in the mid-twentieth century, Americans have turned increasingly to a positive concern with regimen – diet and exercise – as they seek to reduce their real or sensed risk, to redefine the mortal odds that face them. The other side of the coin is a tendency to explain the vulnerability of others in terms of their acts – overeating, alcoholism, sexual promiscuity.

Conclusion: The social construction of AIDS

It is into this world that AIDS arrived – almost as novel and frightening a stranger as cholera a century and a half ago. We were not entirely pre-pared. Antibiotics had removed much of the fear traditionally associated with acute infectious ills. Most laypersons have come to assume that such afflictions had succumbed to the laboratory's insights. Children no longer died of diphtheria; plague and cholera no longer killed masses of men and women. Tuberculosis, too, had declined, along with typhoid and other waterborne diseases. Penicillin had robbed syphilis of much of the dread that had so long surrounded it.[19] The age of great and intractable epi-

---

19 The most recent history of venereal disease in twentieth-century America emphasizes a continuity in social attitudes that rendered sexually transmitted ills resistant to eradication campaigns. See Allan M. Brandt, *No Magic Bullet: A Social History of Venereal Disease in the United States Since 1880*, expanded ed. (New York: Oxford University Press, 1985).

demics seemed to have passed, and most laypersons assumed – whether accurately or not – that medical therapeutics deserved the credit.

But AIDS is both mortal and intractable. It provokes memories of the fear that helped create cautionary and reassuring explanations for plague or cholera in earlier centuries. An ailment that combines sexual transmission with a terrifyingly high mortality, AIDS was bound to attract extraordinary social concern (in clear contrast with the more shallow and transitory social response to herpes; despite the media attention showered on herpes, it could not mobilize the same level of social concern).

The response to AIDS reminds us of the way society has always framed illness, finding reasons to exempt and reassure in its agreed-upon etiologies. But it also reminds us that biological mechanisms define and constrain social response. Ironically, this new disease reflects both elements – the biological and cultural – in particularly stark form. Only the sophisticated tools of modern virology and immunology have allowed it to be defined as a clinical entity; yet its presumed mode of transmission and extraordinary fatality levels have mobilized deeply felt social attitudes that relate only tangentially to the virologist's understanding of the syndrome. If diseases can be seen as occupying points along a spectrum – ranging from those most firmly based in a verifiable pathological mechanism to those, like hysteria or alcoholism, with no well-understood mechanism but with a highly charged social profile – then AIDS occupies a place at both ends of that spectrum.

The social response to AIDS also reminds us that we live in a fragmented society. To a substantial minority of Americans, the meaning of AIDS is reflected in, but transcends, its assumed mode of transmission. It was, that is, a deserved punishment for the sexual transgressor; the unchecked growth of deviance was a symptom of a more fundamental social disorder. "Where did these germs come from?" a writer to an urban newspaper asked in the fall of 1985. "After all this time, why did they show up now? . . . God is telling us to halt our promiscuity. God makes the germs, and he also makes the cures. He will let us find the cure when we straighten out." It is significant that this same correspondent felt compelled to add that he was not "a religious fanatic,"[20] for the great majority of Americans accept the authority of medicine and the truth of its agreed-upon knowledge. They look to the National Institutes of Health, not to the Bible, for ultimate deliverance from AIDS.

The meaning of scientific knowledge is determined by its consumers. When certain immunologists suggest that predisposition to AIDS may grow out of successive onslaughts on the immune system, it may or may not

20 Charles Realdine, letter to the editor, *Philadelphia Daily News*, October 31, 1985.

prove to be an accurate description of the natural world. But to many ordinary Americans (and perhaps a good many medical scientists as well) the meaning of such a hypothesis lies in another frame of reference. As was the case with cholera a century and a half before, the emphasis on repeated infections explains how a person with AIDS had "predisposed" him- or herself. The meaning lies in behavior uncontrolled. When an epidemiologist notes that the incidence of AIDS correlates with the number of sexual contacts, he may be speaking in terms of likelihoods; to many of his fellow Americans he is speaking of guilt and deserved punishment.

Of course, it was to have been expected that patients who contracted AIDS through blood transfusions or in utero are casually referred to in news reports as innocent or accidental victims of a nemesis both morally and epidemiologically appropriate to a rather different group. The very concept of infection is and always has been highly charged; enlightened physicians have always found it difficult to make laypersons accept their reassurances that particular epidemic ills might not be infectious. The fear of contamination far antedates the germ theory – which in some ways only provided a mechanism to justify these ancient fears in modern terms. It is hardly surprising that many remain unconvinced by authoritative medical assurances that AIDS is not (or is not very) contagious.[21]

Knowledge needs to be understood within highly specific contexts. And the specific content of that knowledge itself needs to be seen as a social variable. AIDS exposes the inadequacy of an approach to understanding and controlling disease that ends at the laboratory's door. But it also reveals the parallel inadequacy of disregarding the specific biological character of an ailment – and the status of our understanding of that character.

Our experience with AIDS emphasizes this commonsense point. As our knowledge of the syndrome changes, so do choices and perceptions. Aspects of our culture as diverse as insurance, civil rights, education, and policy toward drug addiction have all been illuminated by our increasingly circumstantial knowledge of AIDS as a biological phenomenon. Knowledge may be provisional, but its successive revisions are no less important for that. With each revision, the structure of choices for individuals and society changes. Without a serological test for exposure to AIDS, for example, there would be no debate about screening, access to insurance, and civil rights (not to mention the dilemma of millions of individuals who seek to define their own risks and predict an unpredictable future).

There are some morals here. Perhaps we cannot return to the optimistic

---

21 During the first European cholera pandemic in the early 1830s, ironically, laypersons also tended to dismiss advanced medical opinion that reassured them the disease was not contagious.

faith so general in the 1930s and 1940s; we are too much aware of the costs. But we can share the fundamental understanding of the need to study the interactions between society and medicine if we are to bring the benefits of medicine to the greatest number. We are products of what might be termed a generational dialectic. Most students of the social aspects and applications of medicine cannot easily return to the optimistic faith of the 1940s. But our very wariness, our need to place medical knowledge in a cost–benefit as well as cultural context, dictates an important agenda for social medicine. If the recognition of disease implies both a phenomenon and its social perception, it also involves policy. And that policy inevitably reflects phenomenon and perception. If an ailment is socially defined as real, and nothing is done, then that, too, is a policy decision. This *process* of interaction between phenomenon, perception, and policy is important not only to medicine but also to social science generally. The brief history of AIDS illustrates both our continuing dependence on medicine – for better or worse – and the way that disease necessarily reflects and lays bare every aspect of the culture in which it occurs.

13

What is an epidemic? AIDS in historical perspective

❧ Like the previous essay, this chapter was a product of the academic world's collective response to AIDS. More generally, however, I was intrigued by the challenge of trying to define and describe an epidemic. We have come to use the term so casually and metaphorically that I felt the logical way to think about the root meaning of *epidemic* was to see it historically, to create an ideal-typical picture of an epidemic based on repetitive patterns of past events. And in the following pages I have tried to abstract and present the narrative structure of an epidemic as historically experienced.

In some ways our generation's encounter with AIDS fits nicely into the dramaturgic pattern I suggest; in other ways recent events have evolved so rapidly that it does not. Within the space of a decade America's perception of AIDS as an acute, epidemic phenomenon has shifted subtly but inexorably: the social identity of this novel ailment has shifted into that of chronic and intractable illness, more akin to tuberculosis than cholera, leukemia than plague. In either guise, however, experience with AIDS has precisely reflected the varied realities that constitute the world's health care system as well as the social-structural and attitudinal factors that have interacted to create patterns of social response to the disease. ❧

We use the term *epidemic* in a variety of ways – most of them metaphorical, moving it further and further from its emotional roots in specific past events. Even in relation to health, we employ the word in contexts decreasingly related to its historical origins. Medical historians speak of an epidemic of tuberculosis in Europe between 1700 and 1870 and of an epidemic of rheumatic fever in the century and a quarter after 1800. In the mass media every day, we hear of "epidemics" of alcoholism, drug addiction, and automobile accidents.[1] These clichéd usages are disembodied but at

---

1 These are endemic phenomena, and a fundamental aspect of the root meaning of *epidemic* lies precisely in its contrast with such "domesticated" phenomena. The *Oxford English Dictionary* tells us that when referring to a disease, the adjective *epidemic* denotes "prevalent among a people or a community at a special time, and produced by

the same time tied to specific rhetorical and policy goals. The intent is clear enough: to clothe certain undesirable yet blandly tolerated social phenomena in the emotional urgency associated with a "real" epidemic.

Defining aspects of that millennia-old reality are, of course, fear and sudden widespread death. It is plague and cholera, yellow fever and typhus that we associate viscerally with the experience of epidemics, not alcohol and automobiles. AIDS has reminded us forcefully of that traditional understanding. But there is another defining component of epidemics that needs emphasis, and this is their episodic quality. A true epidemic is an event, not a trend. It elicits immediate and widespread response. It is highly visible and, unlike some aspects of humankind's biological history, does not proceed with imperceptible effect until retrospectively "discovered" by historians and demographers.

Thus, as a social phenomenon, an epidemic has a dramaturgic form. Epidemics start at a moment in time, proceed on a stage limited in space and duration, following a plot line of increasing and revelatory tension, move to a crisis of individual and collective character, then drift toward closure. In another of its dramaturgic aspects, an epidemic takes on the quality of pageant – mobilizing communities to act out propitiatory rituals that incorporate and reaffirm fundamental social values and modes of understanding. It is their public character and dramatic intensity – along with unity of place and time – that make epidemics as well suited to the concerns of moralists as to the research of scholars seeking an understanding of the relationship among ideology, social structure, and the construction of particular selves.

For the social scientist, epidemics constitute an extraordinarily useful sampling device – at once found objects and natural experiments capable of illuminating fundamental patterns of social value and institutional practice. Epidemics constitute a transverse section through society, reflecting in that cross-sectional perspective a particular configuration of institutional forms and cultural assumptions. Just as a playwright chooses a theme and manages plot development, so a particular society constructs its characteristic response to an epidemic.

Contemporary America's experience with AIDS has already provided materials in abundance for analysis based on such assumptions. In many

some special causes not generally present in the affected locality." Epidemics have a unity of place as well as time – and even worldwide epidemics are experienced and responded to at the local level as a series of discrete incidents.

In addition to fellow authors in *Daedalus* 118/2 (1989), in which this essay first appeared, I should like to thank Drew Gilpin Faust, Chris Feudtner, Renee Fox, Elizabeth Long, Harry Marks, and Rosemary Stevens for helpful comments on an earlier draft.

ways we have reenacted traditional patterns of response to a perceived threat. But if we are to understand our contemporary reaction to a traditional stimulus, we must distinguish between the unique and the seemingly universal, between this epidemic at this time and this place and the way in which communities have responded to episodic outbreaks of fulminating infectious disease in the past. We have become accustomed in the last half-century to thinking of ourselves as no longer subject to the incursions of such ills; death from acute infectious disease has seemed – like famine – limited to the developing world. Life-threatening infectious ills had become, almost by definition, amenable to therapeutic or prophylactic intervention. AIDS has reminded us that this sense of assurance might have been premature, the attitudinal product of a particular historical moment. AIDS has shown itself both a very traditional and a very modern sort of epidemic, evoking novel patterns of response and at the same time eliciting – and thus reminding us of – some very old ones.

Epidemic incident as dramaturgic event

The narrative of Camus's *The Plague* begins on a strikingly circumstantial note.

> When leaving his surgery on the morning of April 16, Dr. Bernard Rieux felt something soft under his foot. It was a dead rat lying in the middle of the landing. On the spur of the moment he kicked it to one side and, without giving it a further thought, continued on his way downstairs.[2]

The dead rat symbolizes and embodies the way in which epidemics seemingly begin with minor events – little noticed at the time, yet often revealing in retrospect. The rat's plague-stricken body suggests as well the way in which man is bound in a web of biological relationships not easily comprehended or controlled. From a very different point of view, it also illustrates the way in which the implacable circumstantiality of an epidemic coexists with – in fact necessarily invokes – larger frameworks of meaning. The peculiar texture of any epidemic reflects continuing interaction among incident, perception, interpretation, and response.

No matter what Camus's philosophical intentions, he chose to embed that intellectual agenda in the morally and historically resonant structure of an ongoing epidemic. And his narrative in fact follows closely the

---

2 Albert Camus, *The Plague*, trans. Stuart Gilbert (New York: Alfred A. Knopf, 1952), p. 7.

archetypical pattern of historical plague epidemics.[3] Like the acts in a conventionally structured play, the events of a classic epidemic succeed each other in predictable narrative sequence. The first of these acts, which I term progressive revelation, turns on the initial appearance and gradual recognition of the intruding disease.[4]

Act I. Progressive revelation

Like the citizens of Camus's plague-stricken Oran, most communities are slow to accept and acknowledge an epidemic. To some extent this is a failure of imagination; perhaps even more, acknowledgment would threaten interests – specific economic and institutional interests and, more generally, the emotional assurance and complacency of ordinary men and women. Merchants always fear the effect of epidemics on trade; municipal authorities fear their effect on budgets, on public order, on accustomed ways of doing things.

Only when the presence of an epidemic becomes unavoidable is there public admission of its existence. Bodies must accumulate and the sick must suffer in increasing numbers before officials acknowledge what can no longer be ignored. The pattern has repeated itself in century after century. Whether in early modern Italy, seventeenth-century London, or nineteenth-century America, whether the unwelcome visitor was plague, yellow fever, or cholera, the first stage of an epidemic acts itself out in predictable fashion. Physicians find a few "suspicious" cases and then either suppress their own anxiety or report their suspicions to authorities, who are usually unenthusiastic about publicly acknowledging the presence of so dangerous an intruder.

The stakes have always been high, for to admit the presence of an epidemic disease was to risk social dissolution. Those who were able might be expected to flee contaminated neighborhoods, while men and women

3 There is an important parallel, moreover, between the biologically determined chronology of an epidemic and its social chronology. I refer, on the one hand, to the increasingly steep curve of case incidence, the exhaustion of susceptible individuals, and the gradual decline in mortality and morbidity, and on the other, to the social pattern of gradual recognition, negotiated response, and gradual decline.
4 One might contend that there is a prior first act, or prologue, at the biological level. In the case of plague, this would have been acted out in the linked relationship among rats, fleas, and bacteria. The existence of these events prior to human awareness of them communicates the chastening moral message that humankind exists in an intricate web of biological relationships. In periods with well-developed channels of communication such as the nineteenth century, another sort of prologue takes place "offstage," as particular communities follow the gradual spread of a pandemic and anticipate its arrival.

remaining in stricken communities could be expected to avoid the sick and
the dying. And disruption of trade and communication was certain. Ever
since the fourteenth century, the institution of quarantine has provided a
feared yet politically compelling administrative option for communities
during an epidemic. Even when – as has frequently been the case –
physicians have questioned the contagiousness of a particular disease, most
laypersons have simply assumed that epidemic disease was almost by
definition transmissible from person to person and have shunned those
who might be potential sources of infection. In the United States, this
pattern was regularly acted out during epidemics of yellow fever and
cholera in the late eighteenth and early nineteenth centuries. Yet physicians
then were often skeptical about contagion.[5]

In any severe epidemic, inexorably accumulating deaths and sicknesses
have brought ultimate, if unwilling, recognition. If we were in fact writing
the story of an epidemic in conventional dramatic form, that recognition
might be an appropriate conclusion to a first act increasingly ominous in
mood.

Act II. Managing randomness

Accepting the existence of an epidemic implies – in some sense demands –
the creation of a framework within which its dismaying arbitrariness can be
managed. Collective agreement on that explanatory framework may be seen
as the inevitable second stage in any epidemic. For most previous centuries
that framework was moral and transcendent; the epidemic had to be
understood primarily in terms of man's relationship to God; consolation
was grounded in submission to the meaning implicit in that framework. In
plague-stricken London in the seventeenth century, for example, and in
New England villages afflicted with diphtheria in the eighteenth century,
most individuals construed an ongoing epidemic in just such otherworldly
terms.[6] The sudden outbreaks of mortal illness were epiphenomena, force-

---

5 On the vexing question of contagion in these ills, see E. H. Ackerknecht,
  "Anticontagionism between 1821 and 1867," *Bulletin of the History of Medicine* 22
  (1948): 562–593; J. H. Powell, *Bring Out Your Dead, The Great Plague of Yellow Fever in
  Philadelphia in 1793* (Philadelphia: University of Pennsylvania Press, 1949); Margaret
  Pelling, *Cholera, Fever and English Medicine 1825–1865* (Oxford: Oxford University
  Press, 1978); Charles E. Rosenberg, "The Cause of Cholera: Aspects of Etiological
  Thought in Nineteenth-Century America," *Bulletin of the History of Medicine* 34 (1960):
  331–354; William Coleman, *Yellow Fever in the North, The Methods of Early
  Epidemiology* (Madison: University of Wisconsin Press, 1987).
6 Ernest Caulfield, *A True History of the Terrible Epidemic Vulgarly Called the Throat
  Distemper Which Occurred in His Majesty's New England Colonies between the Years 1735
  and 1740* (New Haven, Conn.: Yale Journal of Biology and Medicine, 1939).

ful reminders of more fundamental realities. Since at least the sixteenth century, however, such spiritual assumptions have always coexisted with – and gradually yielded in emphasis to – more secular and mechanistic styles of explanation.[7]

Men and women have often expressed moral convictions as they have sought to explain and rationalize epidemics, but such values have ordinarily been articulated in terms of those mundane biological processes that ordinarily result in sickness or health. Individual and community sins could invite or prolong an epidemic – but only through the body's physiological mechanisms, not through miracles or God's direct interposition. This eclectic mixture of moral assumption and mechanistic pathology provided a style of explanation that has been fundamental to the social management of epidemics in the West for the past three centuries.

When threatened with an epidemic, most people seek rational understanding of the phenomenon in terms that promise control, often by minimizing their own sense of vulnerability. Not surprisingly, such consolatory schemes have always centered on explaining the differential susceptibility of particular individuals – what was ordinarily termed predisposition in the eighteenth and nineteenth centuries, or what might be discussed today under the rubric of risk factors. How else explain why one person or class of persons succumbed while others did not? If susceptibility was not to be seen as a random accident or as the result of constitutional idiosyncrasy alone, it had to be understood in terms of physiological mechanisms suggesting the physical – and risk-enhancing – effects of behavior, style of life, and environment. Such hypothetical schemes constituted a framework within which moral and social assumptions could be at once expressed and legitimated.

Particularly important was belief in the connection of volition, responsibility, and susceptibility. During nineteenth-century cholera epidemics, for example, alcoholism, gluttony, sexual promiscuity, and filthy personal habits were widely accepted as predisposing to the disease. Such behavior was seen as increasing susceptibility (and the likelihood of a poor outcome) even in smallpox, where contagion had been accepted for centuries.[8] It was hardly conceivable that such behaviors could be anything other than debilitating physically as well as morally; that an inveterate whiskey drinker

7 See, for example, the present author's *The Cholera Years: The United States in 1832, 1849, and 1866* (Chicago: University of Chicago Press, 1962; 2d ed., 1987), which sought to trace that growing secularism.
8 After the adoption of inoculation for smallpox in the eighteenth-century West, few physicians or laypersons doubted that this endemic and often fatal disease was transmitted from person to person. Contagion was also assumed in venereal disease. In this instance, the connection between willed behavior and the incidence of disease was obvious.

might escape cholera by avoiding water could hardly have been accepted or understood. Bad was bad, culpable culpable, in every dimension of life. Even if one conceded that an epidemic might originate in some general environmental influence such as the atmosphere, selective susceptibility still demanded explanation. Everyone in a community breathed the same contaminated air; not everyone succumbed to the epidemic. Believers in contagion could entertain parallel views; infected individuals might encounter a good many people, only some of whom became ill.

Although such etiological views may in retrospect seem occasions for the expression of a crude and class-oriented moral hegemony, the eighteenth- and nineteenth-century debates about the cause of epidemics were in actuality rather more nuanced. Epidemics did tend, for example, to be associated with place of residence and occupation as well as behavior. And the environmentalist – and thus determinist and morally exculpating – implications were there to be drawn: people who worked overlong hours and lived in tenement apartments without adequate ventilation or access to water would necessarily be less able to fight off a disease.[9] The managing of response to epidemics could serve as a vehicle for social criticism as well as a rationale for social control. The same author might casually incorporate both elements; victims were predisposed by their environment to indulgence in such habits as drinking and sexual promiscuity yet could still be held responsible for the physical consequences of such indulgence. But this assumption hardly constituted a logical inconsistency for most individuals who thought about public health. Views in this field have always been murky and conflicting, and it is hardly surprising that such ambiguity should have been expressed during the course of past epidemics.

For the poor and inarticulate, other mechanisms might be invoked to impose a certain order on an epidemic. Whether it was Jews poisoning wells, doctors seeking anatomical subjects, or the landlords and employers who forced them to live in unventilated hovels, poor people often found their own structure of blame – and meaning – in which to place an epidemic. The layperson's almost universal association of epidemic with contagious disease played a parallel role. At least a presumed knowledge of the epidemic's mode of transmission could provide a measure of understanding and thus promise control.

---

9 The environmentalist emphasis fundamental to anticontagionist views of yellow fever and cholera provided a natural rationale for critical attitudes toward inattentive local government and exploitative landlords and employers.

Act III. Negotiating public response

Recognition implies collective action. One of the defining characteristics of an epidemic is in fact the pressure it generates for decisive and visible community response. The contrast with a disease such as tuberculosis is instructive; although far more significant demographically in the nineteenth century, tuberculosis did not elicit the sense of crisis that accompanied epidemics of yellow fever and cholera. Nor did it elicit moral and political pressure for immediate and decisive measures. In the stress of an epidemic, on the other hand, failure to take action constitutes action.[10] An epidemic might in this sense be likened to a trial, with policy choices constituting the possible verdicts.

This similarity suggests another dramaturgic aspect of an epidemic: measures to interdict an epidemic constitute rituals, collective rites integrating cognitive and emotional elements. In this sense the imposition of a quarantine, let us say, or the burning of tar to clear an infected atmosphere, the gathering of people in churches for days of fasting and prayer, all play a similar role – the visible acting out of community solidarity. At the same time, these collective rituals affirm belief – whether in religion, in rationalistic pathology, or in some combination of the two – while those beliefs promise a measure of control over an intractable reality. It is hardly surprising that communities should in moments of fear and incipient social disorganization seek the reassurance of familiar frames of explanation and logically consequent policies that provide both meaning and the promise of efficacy.

Since the eighteenth century, our rituals have been of a diverse sort. We have appealed in an eclectic way to a variety of sources of authority; days of prayer and fasting might be proclaimed along with the simultaneous enactment of procedures to cleanse and disinfect. For the historian and the social scientist, of course, the content of public rituals provides insight into social values at particular times, while conflicts over priorities among them provide insight into structures of authority and belief. Thus in the 1832 cholera epidemic, inconsistencies between lay and medical views of contagion shaped policy throughout Europe and North America; laypersons almost unanimously assumed the new disease to be contagious, while medical opinion was divided. In America, to cite another attitudinal variable, hostility toward immigrants and Roman Catholics played a sig-

---

10 The action need not be efficacious by late twentieth-century standards but does imply a choice among intellectually and institutionally available options. In 1832, for example, American assumptions of inherently limited federal power meant that a truly national quarantine against the threatened importation of cholera was not a real option, while municipal and state quarantines were.

nificant role in shaping responses to the epidemic, while in England class hostility and endemic suspicion of medical men and their motives played a larger role in defining policy options.[11] Nevertheless, as I have argued elsewhere, the picture of a consistent if occasionally awkward coexistence between religious and rationalistic or mechanistic styles of thought was characteristic of mid-nineteenth-century Anglo-American society and was sharply delineated in the response to epidemic cholera.

The adoption and administration of public health measures inevitably reflect cultural attitudes. The poor and socially marginal, for example, have historically been labeled as the disproportionately likely victims of epidemic illness, and they have been traditionally the objects of public health policy. Often, indeed, good empirical evidence has supported such assumptions; experience as well as ideology has enforced the association. Such views have manifested themselves in a variety of ways. Nineteenth-century quarantines and disinfection were, for example, imposed on the poor and their possessions, not on the wealthy – on the steerage, not the cabin-class, passenger – even after the germ theory was well established. Polio provides another pertinent example. In New York's 1916 epidemic, prophylactic measures were enforced in the dirty and densely populated immigrant slums, which in the past had bred typhoid and typhus, and not in the more prosperous, less crowded, and seemingly salubrious suburbs and middle-class areas that in fact produced so many of the cases.[12]

Act IV. Subsidence and retrospection

Epidemics ordinarily end with a whimper, not a bang. Susceptible individuals flee, die, or recover, and incidence of the disease gradually declines. It is a flat and ambiguous yet inevitable sequence for a last act.

But it also provides an implicit moral structure that can be imposed as an epilogue. How had the community and its members dealt with the epidemic's challenge? Not only during its reign but, most importantly, afterward? Historians and policymakers concerned with epidemics tend to

11 See, for example, R. J. Morris, *Cholera 1832: The Social Response to an Epidemic* (New York: Holmes & Meier, 1976) and Ruth Richardson, *Death, Dissection and the Destitute* (London: Routledge & Kegan Paul, 1987), pp. 223–228.

12 New York City Department of Health, *A Monograph on the Epidemic of Poliomyelitis (Infantile Paralysis) in New York City in 1916* (New York: New York City Department of Health, 1917); Naomi Rogers, "Screen the Baby, Swat the Fly: Polio in the Northeastern United States, 1916" (Ph.D. diss., University of Pennsylvania, 1986). In the 1920s and 1930s, on the other hand, a rather different social picture was created; polio-stricken children were romanticized.

look backward and ask what "lasting impact" particular incidents have had and what "lessons" have been learned. Have the dead died in vain? Has a heedless society reverted to its accustomed ways of doing things as soon as denial became once more a plausible option? This implicit moral agenda has often accompanied – and in some cases no doubt motivated – the more self-conscious and pragmatic concern of scholars with the evolution of public health policy, let us say, or the demographic transition.[13] Epidemics have always provided occasion for retrospective moral judgment.

AIDS in historical perspective: Remembering to remember

Our experience with AIDS during the past decade has reminded us of some very traditional truths. Most strikingly, we seem not to have conquered infectious disease. Death is not associated exclusively with a particular – and advanced – age. AIDS has reminded us as well that managing death has been traditionally a central responsibility of the physician (though by no means of the physician alone). We have not, it seems, freed ourselves from the constraints and indeterminacy of living in a web of biological relationships – not all of which we can control or predict. Viruses, like bacteria, have for countless millennia shared our planet and our bodies. In some ways AIDS is a very traditional phenomenon indeed.

Nor have we revolutionized the framework within which we respond as a community to epidemic disease. In a good many ways the AIDS experience has reenacted the traditional dramaturgic structure of earlier epidemics. One, of course, is the gradual and grudging acceptance of the epidemic as reality – and the resentment expressed toward bringers of bad tidings, the physicians and activists who demand a response to this new threat.[14] Equally obvious is the way in which coping with randomness provides an occasion for reaffirming the social values of the majority, and for blaming victims. Framing and blaming are inextricably mingled; the details vary, but

13 For a recent attempt to evaluate studies of cholera's social and institutional impact, see Richard J. Evans, "Epidemics and Revolutions: Cholera in Nineteenth-Century Europe," *Past & Present* 120 (1988): 123–146.

14 One might also note the desire to specify implausibly explicit beginnings – and clothe them with moral meaning. Compare the expository and narrative function of Camus's rat with the role played by "Gaetan Dugas," the antisocial and hypersexual airline steward of Randy Shilts's recent best-seller *And the Band Played On: Politics, People, and the AIDS Epidemic* (New York: St. Martin's Press, 1987). A rodent vector obviously provides the occasion for a rather differently nuanced moral agenda. One can hardly blame a rat.

the end is similar. The peculiar mixture of biological mechanism invested with moral meaning is equally traditional.

Most Americans prefer to deal with a threat that they do not see as "meant" for them. The search for a reassuring connection of volition, behavior, and pathological consequence is as much alive today as it was in Philadelphia in 1793 and New York in 1832. Transgression implies punishment; affliction implies prior transgression. The historic circumstances and epidemiological peculiarities of AIDS have made such connections unavoidable in the public mind – and in their seemingly empirical character have obscured the social and psychological functions implicit in the apparent confirmation of those connections.

AIDS has reminded us as well of the apparently inevitable juxtaposition of suffering and death with a search for meaning that has always characterized epidemics. Meanings vary, but the need to impose them does not. Most Americans find reassurance in their accustomed faith in the laboratory and its products; they see AIDS as a time-bound artifact of that unfortunate but essentially transitional period between the discovery of this new ill and the announcement of its cure. Others, of course, see its primary meaning in the realm of morality and traditional piety. Many of us, of course, impose multiple frames of meaning on these biological events. The majority of Americans retain their faith in the laboratory but at the same time believe that AIDS points variously to truths about government, the political process, and personal morality.[15] The linked sequence of biological event and its moral management seems unavoidable.

But there is another aspect of public health history that AIDS also recalls. For the sake of convenience diseases can be divided into two categories: diseases whose prevention demands individual behavioral change, like syphilis, AIDS, and lung cancer; and diseases that can be prevented by collective policy commitments, like typhoid fever, where the aggregated knowledge and decisions of bacteriologists, civil engineers, administrators, and elected officials have protected individuals whose habits need not have changed at all.[16] AIDS reminds us of the difficulty of inducing changes in behavior and thus of the intrinsic complexity of the

15 Even scientists can, and doubtless do, understand seemingly objective statements at several levels simultaneously. "When certain immunologists suggest that predisposition to AIDS may grow out of successive onslaughts on the immune system, it may or may not prove to be an accurate description of the natural world. But to many ordinary Americans (and perhaps a good many medical scientists as well) the meaning of such a hypothesis lies in another frame of reference. . . . the emphasis on repeated infections explains how an individual had 'predisposed' him- or herself. The meaning lies in behavior uncontrolled." And suitably punished. See Chapter 12.

16 The spread of AIDS through the blood-banking and processing system represents an instance of this category of intervention – one in which the transmission of a disease can be limited or halted without inducing behavioral change in prospective victims.

decisions facing local governments and public health authorities.[17]

Contemporary sensitivity to individual rights only underlines the centrality of this dilemma, as does our novel public willingness to openly discuss sexual behavior. Despite these characteristic aspects of today's social scene, parallels with earlier health campaigns are obvious. During the first decades of this century, for example, public health workers who urged the use of condoms and prophylactic kits to prevent syphilis met some of the same kind of opposition their successors in the 1980s faced when they advocated distributing sterile needles to intravenous drug users. In both cases ultimate values came into conflict. In both cases debate turned on distinctions between "deserving" and "innocent" victims: in the case of syphilis, the presumed innocents being the wives of erring husbands and their infants; in the case of AIDS, the recipients of contaminated blood or the offspring of infected mothers.[18]

These cases remind us as well of the need for ritual, even in a fragmented modern society. It is a need that is recognized in the AIDS memorial patchwork quilt that has recently circulated throughout the United States. It is recognized, I suggest, even in the whimsically self-conscious and public distribution of condoms on college campuses and in other public spaces. It is also recognized in the calling of conferences graced by individuals representing various agencies of social authority – scientists, administrators, even the odd historian. Each ritual implies collective responsibility and communal identity. Each invokes a differentially nuanced frame of meaning: in the case of the quilt, a commitment to egalitarian compassion; in the distribution of condoms, a commitment to the potential of applied science. If science and technology allow us to control and predict, it is a realm of value worth invoking collectively.

AIDS, a modern epidemic

In a number of obvious ways, however, AIDS does not fit easily into the traditional pattern I have outlined. One, for example, is the rapidity of

17 The layperson's persistent belief in contagion through casual contact despite the reassuring words of medical authority reenacts another traditional element in the history of epidemic disease.

18 Compare Allan M. Brandt, *No Magic Bullet: A Social History of Venereal Disease in the United States since 1880, with a New Chapter on AIDS* (New York: Oxford University Press, 1987). On "syphilis of the innocent," see L. Duncan Bulkley, *Syphilis in the Innocent . . . Clinically and Historically considered, with a Plan for the Legal Control of the Disease* (New York: Bailey & Fairchild, 1894). There are a good many other parallels between AIDS and syphilis, such as the proposed criminalization of the knowing transmission of the disease. Changed attitudes toward female sexuality have, however, altered presumptions of female "innocence" and responsibility.

its geographic spread and the parallel rapidity of its identification as a unified clinical entity.[19] It might well be described as modern, and even postmodern, in its relationship to scientific medicine and institutional structures. AIDS is postmodern in the self-conscious, reflexive, and bureaucratically structured detachment with which we regard it. Countless social scientists and journalists watch us watch ourselves; that reflexive process has become a characteristic aspect of America's experience with AIDS.

More generally the epidemic has existed at several levels simultaneously, mediated by the at first uninterested, then erratically attentive media. For most Americans – insofar as this epidemic can be construed as a national phenomenon – it is a media reality, both exaggerated and diminished as it is articulated in forms suitable for mass consumption. The great majority of Americans have been spectators, *in* but not *of* the epidemic.

Another significant difference between this and earlier epidemics grows out of the novel capacities of late twentieth-century medicine. Without its intellectual tools, the epidemic would not have been understood as an epidemic; we could not easily have determined that it is a clinical entity with protean manifestations. Providing substantive cognitive change during the course of an ongoing epidemic, the laboratory and its intellectual products have played a novel role in the narrative structure of our encounter with AIDS. Without the option of serological screening, for example, the intense and multifaceted debate over the imposition of such tests could hardly have been framed. Without knowledge of an infectious agent, the options for public policy would necessarily have been defined differently.

Another modern characteristic of America's experience with AIDS mirrors the institutional complexity of our society. That structured complexity has in scores of ways shaped responses to this crisis. (Response to epidemics has, of course, always been constrained by preexisting institutional forms and prevailing values, but twentieth-century institutional structures seem categorically different – if only in scale.)

Institutional complexity implies institutional interest – and thus conflict. Certainly we have seen this in the case of AIDS. Blood banks, hospitals, the National Institutes of Health and its several components, and state and municipal departments of public health have all played particular yet necessarily linked and interactive parts. Similarly, the not always consistent interests of local and national government, and of political parties, have also helped shape the nature and pace of our society's response to AIDS.

19 The contrast with the very gradual elucidation of such protean clinical entities as syphilis, tuberculosis, and rheumatic fever is instructive. Although AIDS may seem to have appeared suddenly in the public consciousness, as a biological phenomenon it has been extremely slow in developing, certainly in comparison with other virus diseases such as measles and influenza.

Even patients and their advocates have become public activists in a generation newly conscious of individual and group rights. Perhaps least surprising is the way in which our courts have provided a mechanism for resolving the difficult policy choices posed by AIDS. As we are aware, American courts have become the residuary legatee of a variety of intractable social problems. Recently, a judge in Florida, for example, decided that a child with AIDS should not be excluded from the classroom, but would have to remain within a glass-enclosed cubicle while in attendance.[20] As in many other instances in our society, conflicting attitudes and interests find their way into courts where judges and juries must of necessity make ad hoc decisions.

Finally, Americans have created a complex and not always consistent health care system, and AIDS has been refracted through the needs, assumptions, and procedures of that system. The epidemic might be seen as a socio-assay of that system. Just as costs have been problematic in the system, so have they in the case of AIDS. AIDS has, in particular, forcefully reminded us of the difficulty of providing adequate care for the chronically ill in a system oriented disproportionately toward acute intervention – and of the complex linkages between disease categories, hospital policies, and reimbursement formulas. In this sense, AIDS might be seen as an exacerbation of a chronic pathology.[21]

The gap between isolating an infectious agent in a laboratory in Paris or Bethesda and imposing a preventive program for altering the behavior of particular people in particular places is difficult and problematic. But this is no more than characteristic; clinical application does not follow inevitably from technical consensus. AIDS provides a powerful *de facto* argument for an integrated system-oriented approach to public health and health care; neither the laboratory's contributions nor the social contexts in which that knowledge is employed can be seen in isolation.[22]

AIDS as a postmodern epidemic

The role of the media and social scientists in our contemplating ourselves is obvious enough, but AIDS can be seen as postmodern in other ways as

20 *New York Times*, August 23, 1988, p. A14.
21 Of course, AIDS has also revealed the often less-than-adequate preparation of medical personnel for dealing with fatal illness. That AIDS is infectious as well as so frequently fatal provides an exacerbating element that differentiates it from the great majority of chronic life-threatening ills.
22 The epidemic has illustrated the geographical integration of society as well; AIDS has made clear North America's relationship with other countries and continents. Our traditional habit of largely ignoring African health conditions may be a luxury we can no longer afford.

well. Perhaps most strikingly, it is a postrelativist phenomenon.[23] After a generation of epistemological – and political – questioning of the legitimacy of many disease categories, AIDS has exposed the inadequacy of any one-dimensional approach to disease, either the social constructionist or the more conventional mechanistically oriented perspective. AIDS is socially constructed (as society perceives and frames the phenomenon, blames victims, and laboriously negotiates response) yet at the same time fits nicely into a one-dimensionally reductionist and biologically based model of disease. AIDS can hardly be dismissed as an exercise in victim blaming, even if it is an occasion for it. It is no mere text, words arranged to mirror and legitimate particular social relationships and perceptions. On the other hand, we can no longer remain unaware that biopathological phenomena are framed and filtered through such agreed-on texts.

Of course, a good many Americans never succumbed to the relativist mood of the late 1960s and 1970s, while others have always regarded the social claims of medicine with skepticism, even if they did not question the legitimacy of its disease categories. Others of us have tried to steer a more tentative course. We live in a fragmented society, and not even the most myopic cultural anthropologist would find it easy to impose a neatly coherent and unified cultural vision on the diverse group of individuals who inhabit the continental United States.

Yet AIDS has reminded us that we all share at least some common fears and ways of responding to social crisis. "They fancied themselves free," as Camus wrote of the citizens of the soon-to-be-plague-stricken Oran, "and no one will ever be free so long as there are pestilences." At the end of his narrative, Camus's physician-narrator reflects, even as he listens to the cries of joy that greet the opening of the city and the official conclusion of the epidemic, "that perhaps the day would come when, for the bane and the enlightening of men, it would rouse up its rats again and send them forth to die in a happy city."[24] Plague reminds us that human beings will not so easily escape the immanence of evil and the anxiety of indeterminacy. Mortality is built into our bodies, into our modes of behavior, and into our place in the planet's ecology. Like other epidemics, AIDS has served well to remind us, finally, of these ultimate realities.

23 See Chapter 12.
24 Camus, *The Plague*, pp. 35, 278.

14

Explaining epidemics

&. This essay is intended to serve as a companion piece to Chapter 13, which sought to describe an archetypical pattern of response constituting the historical phenomenon we have come to call an epidemic. That chapter generalized about events; this generalizes about modes of explanation. It suggests that there are two fundamental styles of explanation that have been conceptually "available" since classical antiquity – materials with which to construct the reassurances demanded by an epidemic's otherwise apparently random incursions. I have chosen to label these alternative styles *contamination* and *configuration*.

There is always a danger in creating such general categories; lumpers versus splitters, hedgehogs versus foxes, vitalists versus mechanists – few individuals fall neatly into one ideal type or the other. Yet such categories remain valuable as analytical tools for the historian; and I argue in the following pages for the analytic relevance of the configuration – contamination alternatives. Although rarely articulated in pure form, these styles of explanation have served in a variety of mixtures and dilutions to provide hypothetical etiologies for successive generations of physicians and laypersons. Modern-day descendants of these styles of explanation remain viable – as we have seen in our past decade's experience with AIDS. ⟨⟨

An epidemic is almost by definition frightening; numbers of unfortunates are seized with grave illness, one after another exhibiting similarly alarming and alarmingly similar symptoms. Since classical antiquity – and in all likelihood before that – people have construed epidemics as constituting a natural category, a grouping of phenomena resting on the perceived differences between one set of phenomena and its binary opposite. Epidemic illness is not, of course, the only such aspect of humankind's experience with sickness. Acute versus chronic, traumatic as opposed to nontraumatic, epidemic as opposed to sporadic, are differentiations made almost instinctively; it is not surprising that we have Hippocratic treatises on acute diseases, on internal diseases, on epidemics, on wounds, and on fractures. Each represented a distinct kind of phenomenon, accessible in that distinctiveness to laypeople and physicians when these texts were composed more than 2,000 ago.

Perception implies explanation. Certainly this is the case during

epidemics, when fear and anxiety create an imperative need for understanding and thus reassurance. Such explanatory efforts necessarily reflect
a particular generation's cultural and intellectual assumptions, its repertoire
of available intellectual tools. Each generation in its particular cultural
setting has found somewhat different materials at hand with which to
fashion an understanding of epidemic disease. Climate, sin, disordered air
or water, bacteria – in the recent past, retroviruses – have all played roles
in those generation-specific efforts through which people have sought to
explain, and in explaining control, outbreaks of infectious disease. This is
not to suggest a democracy among hypothetical etiologies; some explanations approximate the natural world a great deal better than others (and
thus provide different real-world choices).[1] But the continuity that I seek to
emphasize relates to function, not specific content; and that function is the
unavoidable act of explanation itself.

A key building block in such efforts to provide an understanding of
epidemics has been, logically and historically, the fundamental distinction
between individual and collective illness. "When a large number of people
all catch the same disease at the same time," the Hippocratic treatise on
the *Nature of Man* observed, "the cause must be ascribed to something
common to all and which they all use.... However, when many different
diseases appear at the same time, it is plain that the regimen is responsible
in individual cases."[2] Diversity of illness reflected the inevitable diversity of
human lives; uniformity of illness implied some – time- and place-bound –
uniformity of cause.

Since most pre-nineteenth-century Western models of disease causation
were individual, based that is on the unique interaction of constitution,
lifestyle, and life course, they were of necessity different from those
rationalistic speculations that served to explain epidemics. The origin of
sporadic, endemic, and chronic ills were seen in what might be referred to
as longitudinal terms, corresponding to the individual life course.[3] On the

---

1 In our postrelativist generation, it needs to be emphasized that similarity of social
    function does not mandate equality in ontological status – or dictate policy choice.
    "Knowledge may be provisional, but it is not arbitrary.... some ideas do approximate
    nature better than others – and thus provide different options for social policy. We
    must not underestimate the role of systematic cognitive activity in the making of
    nineteenth and twentieth century society simply because we disapprove of some of its
    contemporary consequences. Knowledge does not dictate the social forms of its use
    but can create the possibility of such social use." Charles E. Rosenberg, "Medicine
    and Community in Victorian Britain," *Journal of Interdisciplinary History* 11 (1981):
    684.
2 Hippocrates, *Nature of Man*, ch. 9, in G. E. R. Lloyd, ed., *Hippocratic Writings*
    (London: Penguin, 1978), p. 266.
3 For relevant background from this point of view, see Chapters 1 and 4 of this volume,
    on traditional therapeutics and on mind and body in clinical medicine.

other hand, explanations of epidemics had necessarily to be collective and transverse (sited in a particular time and place). An ailment was the outcome of an individual's life course, the cumulative consequence of patterned interactions with his or her environment. Epidemic ills, on the contrary, had to be seen in terms of a moment in time – in cross section – and as the result of causes that would impinge on a good many individuals at once.

Before physicians had any knowledge of specific infectious agents, medical explanations of epidemic disease tended to be holistic and in-clusive: an epidemic was the consequence of a unique configuration of circumstances, a disturbance in a "normal" – health-maintaining and health-constituting – arrangement of climate, environment, and communal life.[4] A vision of health as a balanced, integrated, and value-imparting relationship between humankind and its environment constituted one major building block in traditional explanations of epidemic disease. Let me refer to this as the *configuration* view.

I would like to use the term *contamination* to refer to a second and necessarily contrasting emphasis. It is a style of explanation logically alter-native to configuration, although historically the two have often been found in relatively peaceful, if not always logical, coexistence.

Contamination often reduced itself to the idea of person-to-person contagion, of the transmission of some morbid material from one individual to another; and for many laypeople throughout history the terms *epidemic* and *contagious* were synonymous. But contamination could also imply dis-order in a more general sense: any event or agent that might subvert a health-maintaining configuration. There is a stark contrast between these alternative styles of thought. The configuration theme is holistic and em-phasizes system, interconnection, and balance, while the contamination theme foregrounds a particular disordering element. The configurational style of explanation is interactive, contextual, and often environmental; the emphasis on contamination reductionist and monocausal. Much of epidemiological thought between classical antiquity and the present can be usefully understood as a series of shifting rearrangements of these thematic building blocks. In the great majority of instances, both styles of explanation were employed in combination, with one element or another figuring more prominently.

---

4 Smallpox constituted something of an exception. Although eighteenth-century physicians did not understand the nature of the "virus" that was passed from individual to individual during inoculation (introduced in Europe and the British Isles in the 1720s), it was clear that the epidemics of this great killer were caused by a specific, reproducible "matter."

There was and is a third element as well, necessary to both or either style of explanation. This is *predisposition*. Healers and laypeople have always needed to explain the immunity of some individuals from the epidemic "influence" surrounding them. Why would so many succumb, yet others remain healthy? Predisposition flexibly bridged the logical and emotional gap between individual and collective models of disease phenomena. Differential susceptibility explained an epidemic's otherwise frighteningly arbitrary selection of victims.

In most historical instances, of course, all three elements – configuration, contamination, and predisposition – were brought to bear in creating culturally appropriate explanatory frameworks. Fourteenth-century theories of bubonic plague, for example, illustrated the persistent functional utility of such conceptions. Astrological and climatological-geographical factors are, of course, quintessentially configurational, and were used widely by contemporaries in explaining the Black Death. At the same time, fear and hatred directed toward contagion bearers, or hypothetical Jewish well poisoners, illustrate the power and persistence of contamination models. Within either formulation, of course, predisposition helped explain the plague's often arbitrary incursions.

Let me cite another example from a more recent historical period. Late eighteenth- and early nineteenth-century debates over contagionist as opposed to noncontagionist models of disease causation can be understood within the same bipolar framework. Although by no means all physicians were committed to an unqualified version of either position, many prominent individuals did express "strong" versions in the course of a half century's heated and polarizing debates over yellow fever and (to a lesser extent) cholera, the most visible and frightening of the epidemics that visited Europe and the Americas in the century before the germ theory. In the terminology I have suggested, advocates of contagionism expressed their generation's version of the contamination tradition, while anti-contagionists emphasized the configuration theme.

Yellow fever elicited a particularly sharp and forceful assortment of such contrasting views. The debate turned on the disease's portability. Physicians who pointed to local origins for yellow fever tended to see the disease as arising out of pathogenic environmental circumstances, ordinarily poor sanitation and a consequent accumulation of rotting filth that in its decomposition produced a disease-inducing atmospheric miasma. That miasma might, of course, be viewed as a contaminant, but it was those disordered environmental circumstances that engendered it. A particularly dramatic local debate took place during Philadelphia's invasion by yellow fever in 1793, when contagionists and environmentalists articulated revealingly polarized versions of epidemiological positions normally presented with more caution and less intensity.[5]

Physicians advocating contagionism emphasized the specificity of the ailment's symptoms and the seeming ability of a particular person or perhaps inanimate object to "inoculate" a larger environment. In support of this position they pointed to the "transportability" of yellow fever, which seemed always to flare up after the arrival of ships from fever-infested ports. From either the configuration or the contamination perspective, predisposition explained the selective deaths of those constitutionally at risk: the poor, the "immoral," and the frail. The seeming transportability of yellow fever remained the strongest empirical basis for contagionists. Yet it was easy enough for those emphasizing local circumstances to counter that argument – even conceding the necessity of some imported "influence" to trigger the outbreak of yellow fever. The key issue lay elsewhere. Whatever the mysterious influence that might have arrived on a yellow fever-infested ship, they emphasized, it would not infect communities that maintained civic cleanliness. Without appropriately debilitating local conditions, the "morbid material" would remain harmless.[6] Similarly, in the debates over cholera, many physicians avoided ruthlessly "simple" versions of either contagionist or anticontagionist positions, but chose to construct their etiologies selectively, emphasizing both the need for a specific inoculant and an environment in which it could reproduce itself.[7]

5 J. H. Powell's *Bring Out Your Dead. The Great Plague of Yellow Fever in Philadelphia in 1793* (Philadelphia: University of Pennsylvania Press, 1949) still remains the most readable account of this epidemic and the contemporary controversies surrounding its interpretation.

6 By mid-nineteenth century there was a clear epidemiological consensus. Yellow fever seemed undeniably transportable, even if person-to-person communication was difficult to prove. In retrospect, of course, such conclusions seem quite understandable, given our knowledge of the role played by mosquitoes in its transmission. See, for example, William Coleman, *Yellow Fever in the North. The Methods of Early Epidemiology* (Madison: University of Wisconsin Press, 1987).

7 Nineteenth-century physicians energetically debated the possibly contagious nature of cholera. In the more recent past, historians of medicine have sought to understand and interpret that debate; they have not always been consistent in their views. I have described the controversy in greater detail in *The Cholera Years. The United States in 1832, 1849, and 1866* (Chicago: University of Chicago Press, 1962; 2d ed., 1987). The locus classicus for the modern debate about the social determinants of the debate over contagionism is Erwin H. Ackerknecht, "Anticontagionism between 1821 and 1867," *Bulletin of the History of Medicine* 22 (1948), 562–593. But see these more recent criticisms: Roger Cooter, "Anticontagionism and History's Medical Record," in Peter Wright and Andrew Treacher, eds., *The Problem of Medical Knowledge. Examining the Social Construction of Medicine* (Edinburgh: Edinburgh University Press, 1982), pp. 87–108; and Margaret Pelling, *Cholera, Fever and English Medicine 1825–1865* (London: Oxford University Press, 1978). Pelling may underestimate the intensity and polarization of the debate as an international phenomenon. The debate was, I feel,

Debates over typhus fever reflected a somewhat different, less polarized, explanatory consensus. Typhus had always been associated with war and famine, with crowding, with dirt and poor ventilation (as indicated by its variety of common appellations such as camp fever, jail fever, and ship fever). A mid-nineteenth-century etiological consensus turned on the acceptance of what contemporaries termed "contingent contagion," that is, the transferability of a disease from the sick to the well, but only in certain circumscribed situations. Contingent contagion represents a conceptual building style superficially different from contagionism and anticontagionism, but one that nevertheless incorporated the same building materials. An unnatural configuration of circumstances contaminated the confined environment through metabolic changes induced in people exposed to such pathogenic conditions. The aggregate of local circumstances – inadequate ventilation and light, putrefying organic material, crowding, malnutrition – interacted to create a particularly malignant microenvironment, one that detracted from the vitality of individuals and concentrated the increasingly disordered organic exudates from both sick and well. Thus both contamination and configuration were woven together so as to fashion a plausible explanation for the occurrence of typhus epidemics in military camp, asylum, or hospital.[8]

It is fair to say that the emphasis in epidemiological thought from the eighteenth through the mid-nineteenth century was on configurational – that is, environmental, additive, and aggregate – models of health and disease. A growing awareness of the morbidity and mortality associated with industry and urban population densities constituted a compelling *de facto* argument for the holistic, configurational point of view.[9] The widely observed contrast with demonstrably healthier conditions in rural areas seemed only to document the instinctive truth of this environmental perspective.

A particularly forceful version of such thinking is illustrated dramatically and prominently by the great German pathologist Rudolf Virchow's study of an Upper Silesian typhus epidemic in 1848. Assigned to report on the epidemic, Virchow, a political radical, framed his explanation of the outbreak and suggestions for preventing recurrences in terms of an eclectic, critical, and holistic vision of society. Biting the hand imprudent enough

more polarized earlier in the nineteenth century; it was more confrontational in regard to yellow fever than to cholera, and more marked in cholera than in typhus, about which, as Pelling emphasizes, a rough and ready consensus existed.

8 For a somewhat more extended discussion, see Chapter 5 of this volume for its account of Florence Nightingale and contagion.

9 For a discussion of the eighteenth-century growth in such epidemiological environmentalism, see James C. Riley, *The Eighteenth-Century Campaign to Avoid Disease* (New York: St. Martin's Press, 1987), esp. chs. 3 and 4, pp. 54–88.

to put him to work on this survey, Virchow blamed the Prussian government itself for tolerating oppressive conditions that bred disease among the largely Polish workers beset by fever. He suggested not specific medical or therapeutic interventions, but a greater degree of political participation, improved education, and measures to raise income levels. His recommendations included separation of church and state, acceptance of Polish as an official language, road building, agricultural reform, and a shifting of the tax burden from the poor. "Medicine is a social science," Virchow contended in a much-quoted aphorism, "and politics nothing else but medicine on a large scale."[10] Health and disease could, that is, be thought of as indicators – to employ an anachronistic but useful term – reflecting the moral and material character of the society in which they occurred. The incidence of preventable disease served as an index of the way in which a society treated its least fortunate members. At mid-century, when Virchow conducted his investigation, such sentiments were widespread – if rarely expressed with his thoroughgoing ideological zeal. But this style of sociological epidemiology was soon to be confronted by the emergence of a new body of data and a new way of thinking about infectious disease.

The germ theory helped swing medical opinion toward contamination in its modern, laboratory-oriented guise, but it did not banish the configurational impulse. A continuing concern for what is often called social medicine and an interest in environmental determinants of health and disease remained alive and in continued dialogue with the new bacteriological etiology. It was hard for many physicians to give up the well-understood, almost unquestioned, and seemingly causal association between inimical states of the environment and increased incidence of infectious – and especially epidemic – disease. One of the key conceptual dilemmas for the world of medicine in the last quarter of the nineteenth century (the generation following the articulation and dissemination of the

10 For Virchow's key statements in this period, see his *Collected Essays on Public Health and Epidemiology*, Leland Rather, ed., 2 vols. ([Canton, Mass.]: Science History Publications, c. 1985), esp. I: 205–319, which reproduces the text of his report; his recommendations appear on pp. 307–319. The definition of medicine as a "social science" appears in an editorial he wrote in the fall of 1848. *Collected Essays*, I:33. For background, see Erwin H. Ackerknecht, *Rudolf Virchow. Doctor Statesman Anthropologist* (Madison: University of Wisconsin Press, 1953), pp. 15, 46. Cf. Ackerknecht, *Beiträge zur Geschichte der Medizinalreform von 1848*... (Leipzig: Johann Ambrosius Barth, 1932). Virchow's sentiments were by no means unique in tone and implication, even if atypically forceful, radical, and eloquently argued. They were clearly part of a tradition that associated exploitative – and necessarily unnatural – conditions with sickness and premature death. "The People's Misery: Mother of Diseases," was, for example, the title of an often-cited 1790 address by Johann Peter Frank, Virchow's eminent predecessor in the study of social medicine. Cf. Henry E. Sigerist, "The People's Misery: Mother of Diseases. An Address, delivered in 1790 by Johann Peter Frank," *Bulletin of the History of Medicine* 9 (1941), 81–100.

germ theory) lay in maintaining a balance between the new and old, between the role of a specific microorganism in causing a particular disease and the sick person's total environment, both internal and external. It was this particular generation's version of the much older tension between contamination and configuration.

The subsequently much-ridiculed theory of cholera's etiology advocated in this period by Max von Pettenkofer nicely illustrates this point. A founder of modern public health, Pettenkofer occupied a pioneering chair of hygiene in Munich; but he is more famous (or perhaps notorious) for one of his less successful accomplishments: his *Grundwasser* or ground-water theory of cholera. Even after Koch's discovery of the cholera organism in 1883, Pettenkofer contended that the vibrio was a necessary but not sufficient cause of the disease. It had to "mature" in subsoil water for an appropriate length of time before becoming virulent. As proof, Pettenkofer referred to records of local groundwater levels and the geological and climatological variables that altered these levels. This clearly seems an attempt to maintain the balance between contamination and configuration that was an accustomed part of his generation's epidemiological preconceptions. Pettenkofer's formulation conceded the new etiological emphasis on a specific cause, but retained an important and interactive role for the environment. Equally important, it was an eclectic and inclusive view of that environment; groundwater conditions were the outcome of a complex and interrelated set of circumstances.[11] His theory illustrates a tenacious desire to retain an older, holistic, environmentally oriented framework while incorporating a role for the specific microorganismic mechanism. He sought, that is, the intellectual benefits of a newly fashionable reductionism while avoiding its more radical implications.

Although Pettenkofer's academic prominence and intellectual ingenuity were obviously atypical, his desire to incorporate and integrate these par-

---

11 See, for example, Pettenkofer, *Zum gegenwartigen Stand der Cholerafrage* (Munich and Leipzig: R. Oldenbourg, 1887); Edgar Erskine Hume, *Max von Pettenkofer. His Theory of the Etiology of Cholera, Typhoid Fever and other Intestinal Diseases. A Review of the Arguments and Evidence* (New York: Paul B. Hoeber, Inc., 1927); Alfred S. Evans, "Pettenkofer Revisited. The Life and Contributions of Max von Pettenkofer (1818–1901)," *Yale Journal of Biology and Medicine* 46 (1973), 161–176; Alfred S. Evans, "Two Errors in Enteric Epidemiology: The Stories of Austin Flint and Max von Pettenkofer," *Reviews of Infectious Diseases* 7 (1985), 434–440; Richard J. Evans, *Death in Hamburg. Society and Politics in the Cholera Years. 1830–1910* (Oxford: Clarendon Press, 1987).

Pettenkofer's somewhat quaint niche in the history of medicine is also associated with his attempt to prove the truth of his *Grundwasser* theory by personal experiment. The Munich professor drank a beaker of fresh cholera excretions in 1892 in order to prove that such freshly excreted organisms were incapable of transmitting the disease. He survived.

ticular analytical styles was entirely typical. His medical contemporaries routinely backed away from unflinching reductionism; despite the germ theory's powerful influence, physicians sought instinctively to place these new actors in a traditional narrative, one that saw epidemic disease as the outcome of a variety of interactive factors.

Debate over tuberculosis was shifted, for example, but not revolutionized by Koch's discovery of the causative organism in 1882. Perhaps it is inappropriate to discuss tuberculosis as an epidemic, since we now see it as a chronic, endemic ailment. To physicians and public health authorities at the end of the nineteenth century, however, it was in fact an epidemic, but a uniquely omnipresent one. The very universality of the tuberculosis organism seemed in fact to argue for its dependence upon interaction with a variety of predisposing factors; more than random contact with Koch's bacillus was needed to explain the development of a full-blown case of the disease. Tuberculosis seemed so context- and constitution-dependent that clinical experience had long placed this ailment firmly at the configuration end of the explanatory spectrum. To anyone concerned with tuberculosis – especially in urban and industrial settings – this clinical truth was too obvious to be shaken by Koch's discovery of what seemed a perhaps necessary, but not sufficient, cause.

It is not surprising that tuberculosis – like infant mortality – has served as a crucial source of data in twentieth-century policy debate. Both have been used as indicators of social health or malaise, with both serving as evidence for inclusive, holistic, and multicausal approaches to public health. Since the late nineteenth century, when observers first noted a decline in tuberculosis mortality, up through the work of more recent critics such as René Dubos and Thomas McKeown, that decline – in the absence of effective therapeutics – has constituted evidence for modern versions of configurationism in a twentieth century increasingly dominated by a narrowly biopathological understanding of infectious disease.[12]

A relationship to public policy is clear as well; the configurationist view has tended to be most strongly represented in public health and in specialties such as pediatrics and occupational medicine where contextualized views of clinical realities continued to be important. But it was not only in the area of social medicine and public health that this anti-

---

12 See, for example, Arthur Newsholme, *The Prevention of Tuberculosis* (New York: E. P. Dutton, 1908); René and Jean Dubos, *The White Plague, Tuberculosis, Man, and Society* (New Brunswick, N. J.: Rutgers University Press, 1987; orig. published in 1952); Thomas McKeown, *The Role of Medicine. Dream, Mirage or Nemesis?* ([Princeton, N. J.]: Princeton University Press, 1979); F. B. Smith, *The Retreat of Tuberculosis. 1850–1950* (London: Croom Helm, 1988); Linda Bryder, *Below the Magic Mountain. A Social History of Tuberculosis in Twentieth-Century Britain* (Oxford: Clarendon Press, 1988).

reductionist style retained a twentieth-century vitality. Self-consciously oppositional movements such as constitutional medicine, psychosomatic medicine, and the related emphasis on stress can all be seen as constituting efforts to restore elements of the configurationist perspective.[13] Connected with related interests in the roles of class, gender, and race in the shaping of disease incidence, these antireductionist positions have constituted a vigorous minority voice throughout a twentieth century dominated by the inexorably increasing status of mechanism-oriented perspectives. These general positions, one reductionist, the other holistic and inclusive, have – in other words – asserted and reasserted themselves in differing guises in different times and places.

The microhistory of AIDS

And that process is very much alive. Our still-brief experience with AIDS has already demonstrated the continued relevance of these explanatory styles. Much of the short history of our encounter with the disease can be seen as a negotiation between contamination and configuration, between the laboratory and the clinic, the virologist and the public health worker. And as we are well aware, predisposition has remained central throughout these debates.

On the American scene, the role of predisposition was the first aspect of AIDS to impinge on the public consciousness in the early 1980s; it occupied a similarly prominent place in the epidemiologist's fieldwork. For the first time a large proportion of America's population became familiar with the epidemiologist's technical use of the term *risk*. But as we are well aware, the line between risk and blame is a thin one. It is an obvious and continuing – but highly functional – ambiguity. *Risk* seems a concept originating in the world of value-free science; but that technical identity, and the status connected with it, make the concept's implicit moral content only more plausible. It does not explicitly blame victims, but points to correlations between behavior and subsequent pathology – between sin and punishment.

The history of AIDS has also illustrated another enlightening sequence. This is a shift in the course of the 1980s from the comparative prominence accorded the epidemiologist's global and multicausal – configurational – strategies to the laboratory worker's necessarily technical and reductionist –

13 See, for example, the revealingly titled *Beyond the Germ Theory. The Roles of Deprivation and Stress in Health and Disease* (New York: Health Education Council, 1954). Edited by Iago Galdston, it was based on a conference sponsored by the New York Academy of Medicine.

contaminationist – orientation. Without the knowledge of a specific causal agent and in a period of confusion and even panic, epidemiologists played a prominent role. In the first months after AIDS was identified as a discrete clinical phenomenon, epidemiologists explored a variety of ecological and environmental variables. But the epidemiologist's conclusions are often treated as contingent and provisional, descriptive not definitive – the most adequate explanation society enjoys until the laboratory's higher truth provides a more satisfying closure.

And in the case of AIDS this was to take place with remarkable speed. The discovery of the HIV retrovirus quickly changed the balance of emphasis within society's understanding of AIDS.[14] The contaminationist style of thought with its implicitly reductionist and narrowly technical vision grew more prominent, and the social context in which the disease proliferated – or failed to – began to seem less immediately relevant (and in any case far less amenable to solution).

Our experience with AIDS has illuminated a reality that was in danger of being obscured during the first three-quarters of the twentieth century – when inclusive and holistic models of disease causation remained at the periphery of medical status and concern. Put simply, a monolithic version of neither position remains intellectually adequate. Without the laboratory scientist, we would have no understanding of the mechanism underlying the protean manifestations of AIDS and thus no blueprint for rationalizing preventive measures. On the other hand, a knowledge of the mechanism – as we have seen – does not constitute a policy, or even a guarantee of effective modes of prevention. AIDS reflects in its etiology as well as in its clinical course an environment-sensitive, interactive quality that reveals the need for understanding the human, organizational, and cultural contexts in which AIDS has either thrived or failed to gain a foothold.

The more we have come to understand the disease as both a biological and social phenomenon, the more we understand that our interaction with it reflects a complex and multidimensional reality – and an international and multicultural one at that. First, the history of AIDS demonstrates the arbitrariness of our habitual distinction between culture and biology. When a believer travels to Mecca, for example, that act of volition reflects a particular cultural history. Yet at the same time that believer is a biological entity whose decision may contribute to the pathological history of cholera and typhoid. We need, that is, an ethnography as well as an ecology to explain the network of interactions underlying the appearance, diminution,

14 For a valuable analysis from a parallel point of view, see Gerald M. Oppenheimer, "In the Eye of the Storm: The Epidemiological Construction of AIDS," in Elizabeth Fee and Daniel M. Fox, eds., *AIDS. The Burdens of History* (Berkeley: University of California Press, 1988), pp. 267–300.

or recrudescence of particular infectious ills. To give a concrete example, it is difficult to deal with AIDS in places like the South Bronx without an understanding of the behavior of drug users and the social-structural realities that make such communities what they are. Without history and political economy, in other words, we can have neither a meaningful ethnology nor a meaningful ecology. And certainly we cannot have an effective epidemiology.

In thinking about infectious disease, contemporary epidemiologists make a conventional distinction between agent, host, and environment. And in some sense, that distinction parallels the categories of contamination, predisposition, and configuration. But it cannot, of course, be more than analogy; late twentieth-century ways of thinking would hardly have been available to the writers of the Hippocratic treatises. History has changed the terms of each style of analysis and invested each with a particular, historically differentiated content. *Environment* means something quite different from what it did in the eras of Galen, Thomas Sydenham, or even Louis Pasteur. And so does disease.

But there remain, I think, two important morals to be drawn from the parallels between traditional and contemporary versions of these alternative emphases. One is the way in which the configuration and contamination models – even in their late twentieth-century guises – mirror and imply policy choice. They are not only ways of thinking about a specific disease or diseases, but ways of thinking about the world and sets of directions for acting in it. The other is the way in which these perspectives represent emphases, not answers – elements in a complex discourse about humankind, fate, and social organization that is never answered, but only reconfigured by each new generation.

15

Framing disease: Illness, society, and history

෫෯ This chapter too addresses the elusive problem of the ways in which society has understood, defined, and responded to disease. It was written originally to serve as the introduction to a volume made up of case studies in the framing of particular ills, ranging from coronary thrombosis to anorexia, from rheumatic fever to silicosis. I tried to categorize the kinds of factors – intellectual, attitudinal, professional, and public-policy – that enter into the complex negotiations through which society agrees to accept as legitimate the particular ills that have come to populate our nosological tables. ෯෫

Medicine, an often-quoted Hippocratic teaching explains, "consists in three things – the disease, the patient, and the physician." When I teach an introductory course in the history of medicine, I always begin with disease. There has never been a time when people have not suffered from sickness, and the physician's specialized social role has developed in response to it. Even when they assume the guise of priests or shamans, doctors are by definition individuals presumed to have special knowledge or skills that allow them to treat people experiencing pain or incapacity, unable to work or fulfill family or other social obligations.[1]

But "disease" is an elusive entity. It is not simply a less than optimum physiological state. The reality is obviously a good deal more complex: disease is at once a biological event, a generation-specific repertoire of verbal constructs reflecting medicine's intellectual and institutional history, an occasion for and potential legitimation of public policy, an aspect of social role and individual – intrapsychic – identity, a sanction for cultural values, and a structuring element in doctor–patient interactions. In some ways disease does not exist until we have agreed that it does, by perceiving, naming, and responding to it.[2]

1 Portions of this essay have been repeated or adapted from the author's "Disease in History: Frames and Framers," *Milbank Quarterly* 67 (1989, Supplement 1): 1–15, and are reprinted with permission.
2 Disease can and must also be seen as a taxonomy, with individual ailments arranged in some order-imparting structure.

Disease must be construed in one of its primary aspects as a biological event little modified by the particular context in which it occurs. As such it exists in animals, who presumably do not socially construct their ailments and negotiate attitudinal responses to sufferers, but who do experience pain and impairment of function. And one can cite instances of human disease that existed in a purely biological sense (certain inborn errors of metabolism, for example) before their existence was disclosed by an increasingly knowledgeable biomedical community. Nevertheless, it is fair to say that in our culture a disease does not exist as a social phenomenon until we agree that it does – until it is named.[3]

And that naming process has during the past century become increasingly central to social as well as medical thought (assuming the two can in some useful ways be distinguished). Many physicians and laypersons have chosen, for example, to label certain behaviors as disease even when a somatic basis remains unclear, and possibly nonexistent: one can cite the instances of alcoholism, homosexuality, chronic fatigue syndrome, and "hyperactivity." More generally, access to health care is structured around the legitimacy built into agreed-upon diagnoses. Therapeutics too is organized around diagnostic decisions. Disease concepts imply, constrain, and legitimate individual behaviors and public policy.

Much has been written during the past two decades about the social construction of illness. But in an important sense this is no more than a tautology, a specialized restatement of the truism that men and women construct themselves culturally. Every aspect of an individual's identity is constructed – and thus also is disease. Although the social constructionist position has lost something of its novelty during the past decade, it has forcefully reminded us that medical thought and practice are rarely free of cultural constraint, even in matters seemingly technical. Explaining sickness is too significant – socially and emotionally – for it to be a value-free enterprise. It is no accident that several generations of anthropologists have assiduously concerned themselves with disease concepts in non-Western cultures; for agreed-upon etiologies at once incorporate and sanction a society's fundamental ways of organizing its world. Medicine in the contemporary West is by no means divorced from such affinities.

Some of these social constraints reflect and incorporate values, attitudes, and status relationships in the larger culture (of which physicians, like their patients, are part). But medicine, like the scientific disciplines to which it has been so closely linked in the past century, is itself a social system. Even

---

3 In the sense I have been trying to suggest, an inborn error of metabolism unknown to a generation's clinicians was not, in fact, a disease but rather an analogy in the realm of pathology to the tree falling in the forest with no ear to hear it.

the technical aspects of medicine seemingly little subject to the demands of cultural assumption (such as attitudes concerning class, race, and gender) are shaped in part by the shared intellectual worlds and institutional structures of particular communities and subcommunities of scientists and physicians. Differences in specialty, in institutional setting, and in academic training, for example, can all play a role in the process through which physicians formulate and agree upon definitions of disease – both in terms of concept formation and ultimate application in practice. In this sense, the term *social history of medicine* is as tautological as *the social construction of disease*. Every aspect of medicine's history is necessarily "social" – that acted out in laboratory or library as well as at the bedside.

In the following pages I have, in fact, avoided the term *social construction*. I felt that it has tended to overemphasize functionalist ends and the degree of arbitrariness inherent in the negotiations that result in accepted disease pictures. The social constructivist argument has focused, in addition, on a handful of culturally resonant diagnoses – hysteria, chlorosis, neurasthenia, and homosexuality, for example – in which a biopathological mechanism is either unproven or unprovable. It invokes, moreover, a particular style of cultural criticism and a particular period in time: the late 1960s through the mid-1980s and a vision of knowledge and its purveyors as ordinarily unwitting rationalizers and legitimators of an oppressive social order.[4] For all these reasons, I have chosen to use the less programmatically charged metaphor of the frame rather than the construct to describe the fashioning of explanatory and classificatory schemes for particular diseases.[5] Biology, significantly, often shapes the variety of choices available to societies in framing conceptual and institutional responses to disease; tuberculosis and cholera, for example, offer different pictures to frame for a society's would-be framers.[6]

During the past two decades, social scientists, historians, and physicians

---

4 The emergence of AIDS and the intractability of certain psychiatric conditions made visible by the deinstitutionalization movement have both played an important role in calling attention to the need to factor in biopathological mechanisms in understanding the particular social negotiations that frame particular diseases. Physicians and social scientists concerned with such issues necessarily inhabit what might be called a postrelativist moment; neither biological reductionism nor an exclusive social constructivism no longer constitute viable intellectual positions. See also Chapter 12 of this volume, *passim*.

5 There is, of course, an abundant sociological literature in this area, particularly in relation to psychiatric diagnoses. The work of Erving Goffman has been particularly associated with this emphasis. He also used the frame metaphor in his well-known *Frame Analysis: An Essay on the Organization of Experience* (Cambridge: Harvard University Press, 1974), though in a somewhat different context.

6 Their very different etiologies, moreover, imply different relationships to relevant ecological and environmental factors.

have shown a growing interest in disease and its history. The attention paid to social-constructivist views of disease is only one aspect of a multifaceted concern. Scholarly interest in the history of disease has reflected and incorporated a number of separate, and not always consistent, trends. One is the emphasis among professional historians on social history and the experience of ordinary men and women. Pregnancy and childbirth, for example, like epidemic disease, have in recent years become an accepted part of the standard historical canon.

A second focus of interest in disease centers on public health policy and a linked concern with explanation of the demographic change associated with the late nineteenth and early twentieth centuries. How much credit should go to specific medical interventions for the decline in morbidity and the lengthening of life spans, and how much to changed economic and social circumstances?[7] The policy implications are apparent: what proportion of society's limited resources should be allotted to therapeutic intervention, and what proportion to prevention and to social meliorism generally?

A third trend is the rebirth in the past generation of what might be called a new materialism in the form of an ecological vision of history in which disease plays a key role – as, for example, in the Spanish conquest of Central and South America.[8] A fourth has been the reciprocal influence of demography among a quantitatively oriented generation of historians and of history among a growing number of demographers. For both disciplines,

7 The name of Thomas McKeown has been closely associated with revitalizing this century-old debate. McKeown and R. G. Record, "Reasons for the Decline in Mortality in England and Wales during the Nineteenth Century," *Population Studies* 16 (1962): 94–122; McKeown, *The Modern Rise of Population* (London: Edward Arnold, 1976); McKeown, *The Role of Medicine. Dream, Mirage, or Nemesis* (London: Nuffield Provincial Hospitals Trust, 1976); Simon Szretter, "The Importance of Social Intervention in Britain's Mortality Decline c. 1850–1914: A Re-interpretation of the Role of Public Health," *Social History of Medicine* 1 (1988): 1–37; Leonard Wilson, "The Historical Decline of Tuberculosis in Europe and America: Its Causes and Significance," *Journal of the History of Medicine* 45 (1990): 366–396. McKeown's emphasis on the elusive variables that determine tuberculosis incidence has inevitably made for controversy, but has served to focus historical and demographic attention on ecological variables generally. An example is the intellectually and politically related revival of interest in the history of occupational health. See, for example, David Rosner and Gerald Markowitz, eds., *Dying for Work. Worker's Safety and Health in Twentieth-Century America* (Bloomington: Indiana University Press, 1987); Alan Derickson, *Workers' Health, Workers' Democracy. The Western Miners' Struggle, 1891–1925* (Ithaca, N.Y.: Cornell University Press, 1988).

8 Among the most influential works in this area have been A. W. Crosby, Jr., *The Columbian Exchange. Biological and Cultural Consequences of 1492* (Westport, Conn.: Greenwood Press, 1972); Crosby, *Ecological Imperialism. The Biological Expansion of Europe, 900–1900* (Cambridge: Cambridge University Press, 1986); William H. McNeill, *Plagues and Peoples* (Garden City, N.Y.: Anchor Press/Doubleday, 1976).

the study of individual disease incidence provides a viable tactic for ascertaining the mechanisms underlying change in morbidity and mortality. Typhoid rates, for example, can tell us something rather more precise about municipal sanitation and public health administration than the aggregate annual mortality figures to which outbreaks of this waterborne disease may have contributed.

A final, and perhaps the most widely influential, focus of scholarly interest in disease has been on the way disease definitions and hypothetical etiologies can serve as tools of social control, as labels for deviance, and as rationale for the legitimation of status relationships. Logically – and historically – such views have in the past generation often been associated with a relativist emphasis on the social construction of disease.[9] Such interpretations are one aspect of a more general scholarly interest in the relations among knowledge, the professions, and social power. The more critically inclined among such would-be sociologists of knowledge have seen physicians as articulators and agents of a broader hegemonic enterprise, with the "medicalization" of society one aspect of a controlling and legitimating ideological system.

What are often lost sight of in each of these emphases are, first, the process of disease definition, and second, the consequences of those definitions in the lives of individuals, in the making and discussion of public policy, and in the structuring of medical care. We have, in general, failed to focus on the connection between biological event, its perception by patient and practitioner, and the collective effort to make cognitive and policy sense out of those perceptions. Yet, this process of recognition and rationalization is a significant problem in itself, one that transcends any single generation's effort to shape satisfactory conceptual frames for those biological phenomena it regards as of special concern.

Where an underlying pathophysiologic basis for a putative disease remains problematic, as in alcoholism for example, we have another sort of frame-making, but one that nevertheless reflects in its style the plausibility and prestige of an unambiguously somatic model of disease. The social

9 See, among numerous examples, Karl Figlio, "Chlorosis and Chronic Disease in 19th Century Britain: The Social Constitution of Somatic Illness in a Capitalist Society," *Social History* 3 (1978): 167–97; P. Wright and A. Treacher, eds., *The Problem of Medical Knowledge* (Edinburgh: Edinburgh University Press, 1982); Elaine Showalter, *The Female Malady. Women, Madness, and English Culture, 1830–1980* (New York: Pantheon, 1985). A recent growth of interest in "imperial" medicine reflects an interest both in the ideological and demographic aspects of disease. See, for example, Roy MacLeod and Milton Lewis, eds., *Disease, Medicine, and Empire. Perspectives on Western Medicine and the Experience of European Expansion* (London: Routledge, 1988); Philip D. Curtin, *Death by Migration. Europe's Encounter with the Tropical World in the Nineteenth Century* (Cambridge: Cambridge University Press, 1989); David Arnold, ed., *Imperial Medicine and Indigenous Societies* (Manchester: Manchester University Press, 1988).

legitimacy and intellectual plausibility of any disease must turn, that is, on the existence of some characteristic mechanism.[10] This reductionist tendency has been logically and historically tied to another characteristic of our thinking about disease, and that is its specificity. In our culture, its existence as *specific* entity is a fundamental aspect of the intellectual and moral legitimacy of disease. If it is not specific, it is not a disease and a sufferer not entitled to the sympathy, and in recent decades often the insurance reimbursement, connected with an agreed-upon diagnosis. Clinicians and policymakers have long been aware of the limitations of such reductionist styles of conceptualizing disease, but have done little to moderate its increasing prevalence.

Framing disease

Disease begins with perceived and often physically manifest symptoms. And medicine's historical origins lie in the sufferer's attempt to find restored health and an explanation for his or her misfortune. That search for healing counsel has constituted the historical basis for the physician's social role. And an essential aspect of the healer's role has developed around the practitioner's ability to put a name to the patient's pain and discomfort. Even a bad prognosis can be better than no prognosis at all; even a dangerous disease, if it is made familiar and understandable, can be emotionally more manageable than a mysterious and unpredictable one. It is certainly so from the physician's point of view. Diagnosis and prognosis, the intellectual and social framing of disease, has always been central to the doctor–patient relationship.

The process of framing inevitably includes an explanatory component: how and why did a person come to suffer from a particular ailment? Physicians have since classical antiquity always found intellectual materials at hand with which to explain those phenomena they have been asked to treat, imposing some speculative mechanism or another on an otherwise opaque body. The study of any entity or symptom cluster through time indicates the truth of this particular truism.

Physicians have always been dependent on time-bound intellectual tools in seeking to find, demonstrate, and legitimate patterns in the bewildering universe of clinical phenomena they encounter in their everyday practice. In classical antiquity, the metaphor of cooking provided a familiar source for a metaphorical understanding of the body's metabolism, the aggregate

10 This characteristic helps explain the ambiguous status of psychiatry in medicine, as well as the enthusiasm which has greeted recent somatic explanations of behavior and behavior pathology.

functions of which determined the physiological balance that constituted health or disease. At the end of the twentieth century, hypothetical auto-immune mechanisms, for example, or the delayed and subtle effects of virus infections often serve to explain diffuse, chronic symptoms. For a physician in the late eighteenth and early nineteenth centuries, as we have suggested, humoral models of balance were particularly important, and were used to rationalize such therapeutic measures as bleeding, purging, and the lavish use of diuretics. With the emergence of pathological anatomy in the early nineteenth century, hypothetical frameworks for disease were increasingly fashioned in terms of specific lesions or characteristic functional changes that would, if not modified, produce lesions over time. Fermentation had already provided an experiential basis for metaphors explaining epidemic disease, suggesting the ways in which a small quantity of infectious material might contaminate and bring about pathological change in a much larger substrate (as in the atmosphere, water supply – or a succession of human bodies). The germ theory created another kind of framework that could be used to impose a more firmly based taxonomic order on elusive configurations of clinical symptoms and postmortem appearances. It seemed that it would be only a matter of time before physicians understood all those mysterious ills that had puzzled their professional predecessors for millennia; the relevant pathogenic micro-organisms need only be found and their physiological and biochemical effects understood. This was an era, as is well known, in which energetic physicians "discovered" microorganisms responsible for almost every ill known to mankind.

The major point seems obvious. In crafting explanatory frameworks the physician employs a sort of modular construction, utilizing those intellectual building elements available to his or her particular place and generation. But the resulting conceptions of disease and its hypothetical origin are not simply abstract knowledge, the stuff of textbooks and academic debates. They inevitably play a role in doctor–patient interactions. Disease concepts always mediate that relationship. In earlier centuries lay and medical views of disease overlapped to an extent, and that shared knowledge served to structure and mediate interactions between doctors, patients, and families. Today knowledge is increasingly specialized and segregated, and laypersons are more likely to accept medical judgments on faith. Diagnostic procedures and agreed-upon disease categories are thus all the more important. They guide both the physician's treatment and the patient's expectations.[11]

---

[11] Contemporary patient advocacy groups can be construed as in part a response to this asymmetrical distribution of knowledge – and thus power.

Disease as frame

Once crystallized in the form of specific entities and seen as existing in particular individuals, disease serves as a structuring factor in social situations, as a social actor and mediator. This is an ancient truth. It would hardly have surprised a leper in the twelfth century, or a plague victim in the fourteenth. Nor, in another way, would it have surprised a "sexual invert" at the end of the nineteenth century.

These instances remind us of a number of important facts. One is the role played by laypersons as well as physicians in shaping the total experience of sickness. Another is that the act of diagnosis is a key event in the experience of illness. Logically related to this point is the way in which each disease is invested with a unique configuration of social characteristics – and thus triggers disease-specific responses. Once articulated and accepted, disease entities become "actors" in a complex network of social negotiations. Such negotiations have had a long and continuous history. The nineteenth century may have changed the style and intellectual content of individual diagnoses, but it did not initiate the social centrality of disease concepts and the emotional significance of diagnoses once made.

The expansion of diagnostic categories in the late nineteenth century created a new set of putative clinical entities that seemed controversial at first, and served as one variable in defining the feelings of particular individuals about themselves, and of society about those individuals. Inevitably, these often-conflicted social negotiations turned on matters of value and responsibility as well as epistemological and ontological status. Was the alcoholic a victim of sickness or of willful immorality? And if sickness, what was its somatic basis? And if such mechanism could not be demonstrated, could it simply be assumed? Was the individual sexually attracted by members of the same sex simply a depraved person who chose to commit unspeakable acts, or a personality type whose behavior was in all likelihood the consequence of hereditary endowment?

Such dilemmas are not simply an incident in the intellectual history of medicine, but an important – and revealing – aspect of changing social values more generally, and as well, of course, a factor in the lives of particular men and women. This style of social negotiation is very much alive today as physicians and society debate issues of risk and lifestyle, and as government and experts assess deviance and evaluate modes of social intervention. The historian can hardly decide whether the creation of such diagnoses was positive or negative, constraining or liberating, for particular individuals; but the creation of homosexuality as a medical diagnosis, for example, certainly altered the variety of options available to individuals for *framing themselves*, their behavior, and its nature and meaning. It offered the possibility, for better or worse, of construing the same behaviors in a new way and of shaping a novel role for the physician in relation to that behavior.

But this is not only true of such morally and ideologically charged diagnoses. A late twentieth-century diagnosis of heart disease becomes, to cite a commonplace example, an important aspect of an individual's life, to be integrated in ways appropriate to personality and social circumstance. Diet and exercise, anxiety, denial and avoidance, or depression can all constitute aspects of that integration. Once diagnosed as epileptic, to cite another example, in centuries before our own – or as a sufferer from cancer or schizophrenia in our generation – an individual becomes in part that diagnosis. Chronic or "constitutional" illness plays in this sense a more fundamental social role (both in economic and intrapsychic terms) than the dramatic but episodic epidemics of infectious disease that have played so prominent a role in the historian's perception of medicine; we have paid too much attention to plague and cholera, too little to "dropsies" and consumption.

From the patient's perspective, diagnostic events are never static. They always imply consequences for the future and often reflect upon the past. They constitute a structuring element in an ongoing narrative, an individual's particular trajectory of health or sickness, recovery or death. We are always becoming, always managing ourselves, and the content of a physician's diagnosis provides clues and structures expectations. Retrospectively, it makes us construe past habits and incidents in terms of their possible relationship to present disease.

The technical elucidation of somatic disease pictures has steadily added to – and refined – our existing vocabulary of disease entities. The nineteenth century saw a host of such developments. The discovery of leukemia as a distinctive clinical entity, for example, created a new and suddenly altered identity for those individuals the microscope disclosed as incipient victims. Before that diagnostic option became available they might have felt debilitating symptoms, but symptoms to which they could not put a name. With that diagnosis, the patient became an actor in a suddenly altered narrative. Every new diagnostic tool has the potential for creating similar consequences, even in individuals who had felt no symptoms of illness. Mammography, for example, can suggest the presence of carcinoma in women entirely symptom-free. Once that radiological suggestion is confirmed, an individual's life is irrevocably changed.[12] A rather different

---

12 With today's sophisticated laboratory medicine and screening of populations at risk we have created an assortment of pre- or proto-disease states – bearing with them a difficult variety of personal and policy decisions. Is the middle-aged male with a high cholesterol level a sufferer from disease? What are his personal responsibilities, and those of society to him?

scenario is acted out in diseases less ominous. Our knowledge of the existence, epidemiological characteristics, and clinical course of chicken pox, for example, constitutes an important social resource. A fevered child suddenly covered with angry eruptions could be extremely alarming to its parents had they not had prior knowledge of that clinical entity called chicken pox and its generally benign and predictable course.

Communities as well as individuals and their families necessarily respond to the articulation and acceptance of explicit disease entities and to an understanding of their biopathological character. Perceptions of disease are context-specific, yet context-determining as well. For example, when in the mid-nineteenth century typhoid and cholera were discovered to be discrete clinical entities, spread most frequently through the water supply, policy choices were not only reframed in practical engineering terms, but in political and moral ones as well. Vaccination, to cite another example, provided a novel set of choices for philanthropists and government policy-makers as well as individual physicians. Concepts of disease, their causation, and possible prevention always exist in social as well as intellectual space.

Individuality of disease

Disease is irrevocably a social actor. It becomes, that is, a factor in a structured configuration of social interactions.[13] But the boundaries within which it can play such social roles are often shaped by the ailment's biological identity. Thus chronic and acute disease present very different social realities, both to the individual, his or her family, and society. In a traditional society, for example, one either died of or recovered from plague or cholera. Chronic kidney disease or tuberculosis, on the other hand, might present long-term welfare problems for a community and economic and personal dilemmas for particular families. Especially in the case of chronic disease, tuberculosis or mental illness, for example, institutional programs and policies mediate the complex relationship among patients, families, medical staff, and administrators.

Our understanding of the biological character of particular ills define public health policies as well as therapeutic options. Acute ills obviously

---

13 It might be objected that the actor metaphor is inappropriate, implying volition and autonomy; only people can be actors in the strict sense. From this perspective, and remaining within the dramaturgic sphere, disease might be more accurately considered a script – specifying future behaviors. I prefer the actor metaphor because of its emphasis on the way in which disease concepts serve in some sense as independent factors, constraining the options of human actors in social situations.

provide a very different challenge to physicians, governments, and medical institutions than do chronic ones. But even acute infections vary in their modes of transmission, for example, and thus in their specific social identity. Attitudes toward sexuality and the need to change individual behavior, for example, constrain efforts to halt the spread of syphilis.[14] To cite another sort of instance, waterborne ailments like typhoid and cholera could be interdicted by the skills of bacteriologist and civil engineer and the decisions of local government – with minimal need to alter individual habits.[15]

Negotiating disease

The negotiations surrounding the definition of and response to disease are complex and multilayered. There are cognitive and disciplinary elements, institutional and public policy responses, as well as the adjustments of particular individuals and their families. And relating at all these levels is the doctor–patient relationship.

In some cases, the negotiations surrounding the definition of disease are literally – and didactically – acted out. When a court evaluates a plea of not guilty by reason of insanity, for example, or when a workmen's compensation board decides whether a particular illness is a consequence of work experience, society acts out that negotiation. In the former case, the courtroom proceedings become a proxy for a debate among competing professional ways of seeing the world, professional training, and conflicting social roles. Recent debates about brown lung and asbestosis provide another example of socially negotiated situations in which interested participants interact to produce logically arbitrary but socially viable, if often provisional, solutions. In such cases, the agreement upon a definition of disease can provide the basis for mediated compromise and a pattern of consequent administrative actions, just as conflict could turn on a failure to reach consensus in regard to the existence, origin, or clinical course of a particular ailment. Disease can be seen as a dependent variable in such a negotiated situation; yet once agreed upon it becomes an actor in that social setting, providing legitimation as well as direction in social decision-making.[16]

14 See, for example, Allan M. Brandt, *No Magic Bullet. A Social History of Venereal Disease in the United States since 1880* (New York: Oxford University Press, 1985).
15 The physician's diagnostic situation can reflect another sort of biological reality, the endemic incidence of disease in a particular society. The distribution of sickness constitutes a background against which and in terms of which the physician evaluates the comparative plausibility of diagnostic options.
16 This is not to suggest that the need to arrive at decisions in particular cases serves to end conflict in parallel instances.

In a more general sense, disease categories serve to rationalize, mediate, and legitimate relationships between individuals and institutions in a bureaucratic society. This is nicely exemplified in third-party payment schemes, where the inchoate and in some sense incommensurable experience of individuals is transformed into the neatly ordered categories of a diagnostic table – and thus becomes suitable for bureaucratic use. In this sense a nosological table is a kind of Rosetta stone providing a basis for translation between the two very different yet structurally interdependent realms. Diagnoses are in a literal sense machine-readable; human beings are not so easily construed.

Disease as social diagnosis

For centuries, disease, both specific and generic, has played another role as well; it has helped frame debates about society and social policy. Since at least biblical times the incidence of disease has served as index and monitory comment on society. Physicians and social commentators have used the difference between "normal" and extraordinary levels of sickness as an implicit indictment of pathogenic environmental circumstances. A perceived gap between what is and what ought to be, between the real and the ideal, has often constituted a powerful rationale for social action. The meaning of a particular policy stance to contemporaries might well be thought of as the outcome or aggregate of what is and what ought to be; the actual is always measured against the presumably attainable ideal. Late eighteenth- and early nineteenth-century military surgeons worried, for example, about the alarming incidence of camp and hospital disease; the frequency of death and disabling sickness in a youthful male population underlined the need for reform in existing camp and barrack arrangements. Social critics in Europe's new industrial cities pointed to the incidence of fevers and infant deaths among tenement dwellers as evidence of the need for environmental reform; the instructive and unquestioned disparity between morbidity and mortality statistics in rural as opposed to urban populations constituted a compelling case for public health reform.[17] Between the mid-eighteenth century and the present it has always played this role in the discussion of public health and social environment. One

17 See also William Coleman, *Death is a Social Disease: Public Health and Political Economy in Early Industrial France* (Madison: University of Wisconsin Press, 1982); John M. Eyler, *Victorian Social Medicine: The Ideas and Methods of William Farr* (Baltimore: Johns Hopkins University Press, 1979); Erwin H. Ackerknecht, *Rudolf Virchow, Doctor, Statesman, Anthropologist* (Madison: University of Wisconsin Press, 1965); James C. Riley, *The Eighteenth-Century Campaign to Avoid Disease* (New York: St. Martin's Press, 1987).

could easily cite scores of parallel instances. In this sense, disease became an occasion and agenda for an ongoing discourse concerning the relationship among state policy, medical responsibility, and individual culpability. It is difficult indeed to think of any significant area of social debate and tension – among issues such as those of race, gender, class, and industrialization – in which hypothetical disease etiologies have not served to project and rationalize widely held values and attitudes. It is a debate that has hardly ceased, as the recent outbreak of AIDS has so forcefully demonstrated.

Unity and diversity

In a much-quoted essay of 1963, the medical historian Owsei Temkin traced the history of "The Scientific Approach to Disease: Specific Entity and Individual Sickness." He organized his analysis of disease concepts around two distinct yet interrelated orientations. One of these he termed the *ontological* view of disease: the notion that diseases existed as discrete entities with a predictable and characteristic course (and possibly cause) outside of their manifestation in the body of any particular patient. The other was what he termed *physiological* – a view that saw disease as necessarily individual. Common sense and several centuries of accumulated knowledge tell us that these ways of thinking about disease are separable primarily for analytical purposes; it seems apparent that we do and perhaps must think about diseases as entities apart from their manifestation in particular persons.[18] At the same time, as we are well aware, disease as a clinical phenomenon exists only in particular bodies and family settings.

Temkin's distinction parallels another emphasized perhaps most prominently in recent years by Arthur Kleinman, that between illness as experienced by the patient and disease as understood by the world of medicine.[19]

---

18 Temkin himself is careful to note that he employs the terms *physiological* and *ontological* "for brevity's sake." "The Scientific Approach to Disease: Specific Entity and Individual Sickness," in A. C. Crombie, ed., *Scientific Change: Historical Studies in the Intellectual, Social and Technical Conditions for Scientific Discovery and Technical Invention from Antiquity to the Present* (New York: Basic Books, 1963), pp. 629–647, reprinted in Temkin, *The Double Face of Janus and other Essays in the History of Medicine* (Baltimore: Johns Hopkins University Press, 1977), pp. 441–455. From the present author's point of view, what Temkin refers to as the "scientific" approach should also be seen as the bureaucratic approach – one that lends itself to the functional requirements of large administrative structures.

19 For recent expositions, see Arthur Kleinman, *The Illness Narratives. Suffering, Healing, and the Human Condition* (New York: Basic Books, 1988); Kleinman, *Rethinking Psychiatry. From Cultural Category to Personal Experience* (New York: Free Press, 1988); Howard M. Spiro, *Doctors, Patients, and Placebos* (New Haven, Conn.: Yale University Press, 1986); Howard Brody, *Stories of Sickness* (New Haven, Conn.: Yale University Press, 1987).

Both deal with the fundamental distinction between the general and the specific, the personal and the collective. In a sense, of course, these distinctions – ontological as opposed to physiological, disease as contrasted with illness, biological event as opposed to socially negotiated construction – are defensible primarily for analytical and critical purposes. In reality, we are describing and trying to understand an interactive system, one in which the formal understanding of disease entities interacts with their manifestations in the lives of particular individuals. At every interface, that between patient and physician, between physician and family, between medical institutions and medical practitioners, disease concepts mediate and structure relationships.

Although we have begun to study the history of disease and have cultivated a growing appreciation of the potential significance of such studies, much remains to be done. As I have tried to argue, the study of disease constitutes a multidimensional sampling device for the scholar concerned with the relation between social thought and social structure. Although it has been a traditional concern of physicians, antiquarians, and moralists, the study of disease is still a comparatively novel one for social scientists. It remains more an agenda for future research than a repository of rich scholarly accomplishment. We need to know more about the individual experience of disease in time and place, the influence of culture on definitions of disease and of disease in the creation of culture, and the role of the state in defining and responding to disease. We need to understand the organization of the medical profession and institutional medical care as in part a response to particular patterns of disease incidence and attitudes toward particular ills. This list could easily be extended, but its implicit burden is clear enough. Disease constitutes a fundamental substantive problem and analytical tool – not only in the history of medicine, but in the social sciences generally.

16

Looking backward, thinking forward: The roots of hospital crisis

&❧ In the 1980s, the words *hospital* and *crisis* seemed almost inseparable. Growing economic pressures in the health care system made an enormous variety of Americans sensitive to the medical problems of the here and now – and anxious about prospects for the future. This chapter was originally written for a symposium on the future of the American hospital, designed to illuminate the options facing America's health care professionals, planners, and consumers. As an historian among a varied assortment of academic physicians and social scientists assembled for the occasion, I sought to make a case for continuity – and by implication, the relevance of history in understanding the present and preparing for the future.

There is a problem, of course. By emphasizing the historical roots of contemporary problems one inevitably runs the danger of fatalism; choice seems increasingly limited by past constraints and expectations. But change is inevitable – in part because of the particular shape of underlying constraints and expectations – and an understanding of such deep-seated structuring factors is a precondition to the reasoned consideration of present choices. Most important, I sought to emphasize two sets of factors that seemed to me insufficiently articulated in many contemporary discussions of health care policy. One is the power of social attitudes – especially in relation to health, welfare, and science. A second is the way in which the hospital's history reflected the medical profession's particular history. Intellectual aspirations and career options shaped the decisions of individual physicians – and thus cumulatively shaped the hospital.

In an essay written some years earlier – not reprinted in this volume – I had discussed America's hospital history under the rubric "Inward Vision, Outward Glance," a title chosen so as to underline the way in which institutional and professional needs had interacted – absent central and self-conscious planning and control – over time to create the late twentieth-century American hospital. Lack of planning is a form of planning, as we have gradually and painfully discovered. ❧

American hospitals have always disappointed. Each generation during the past century has deplored some aspect of this seemingly necessary institution. In the late nineteenth century, critics were indignant at the use – and apparent abuse – of free hospital services by men and women able to pay private physicians for care. They were concerned as well about the difficulty of imposing cleanliness, economy, and order on an intractable institution.[1] At the beginning of the present century, a concerned minority of progressive reformers assailed the hospital's forbidding impersonality and bureaucratic rigidity, while other critics (and sometimes the same ones) decried its failure to attain the standards of efficiency and productivity that prevailed in the business world. In the 1920s and 1930s, planners urged that hospitals be made accessible to all Americans regardless of class or place of residence.[2]

After the Second World War, an expanding economy brought a solution to the problem of inadequate facilities; more seemed inevitably better and a suddenly generous federal government began to support the hospital enterprise in a variety of ways.[3] By the 1960s, a new generation of critics had begun to bewail this very expansion of hospital beds and services; it had created, they charged, an institution dominated by bureaucracy and capital-intensive technology and controlled by career-driven physicians and socially insensitive administrators.

Since the mid-1970s, economic problems have seemed most pressing. Third-party payers, both private and public, have sought to cap runaway costs, while profit-making hospital corporations have sought to take advantage of a seemingly risk-free niche in the American economy. Hospital planners, administrators, and a good many physicians have fallen victim to an outbreak of acute Chicken Little syndrome, wringing their hands as they wait for some actuarial sky to fall. Probably no generation has undertaken a broader and more stressful examination of hospital services.

An institution that has never been more necessary has never seemed more problematic. Today, voluntary hospitals discuss their market share and place in what is now called "the health care industry." Their administrators negotiate with health maintenance organizations and other whole-

1 These generalizations and many of those following are drawn from the author's *The Care of Strangers: The Rise of America's Hospital System* (New York: Basic Books, 1987).
2 The most detailed and influential compendium of such health care concerns was the publications of the Committee on the Costs of Medical Care. Between 1928 and 1933, The University of Chicago Press published twenty-six monographs commissioned by the Committee, a massive summary volume, and a number of minor publications.
3 The Hill-Burton Act of 1946, providing subsidies for local hospital construction, marked a significant shift toward a growing federal health care role. See also Rosemary Stevens, *American Medicine and the Public Interest* (New Haven, Conn.: Yale University Press, 1971), pp. 509–513.

sale customers, while casting about for "profit centers" in the form of outpatient surgery units, sports medicine, and eating disorder clinics. Hospital managers measure earnings against the cost of capital and, in many regions, look over their shoulders at competition from profit-making competitors – as both nonprofits and for-profits begin to look more and more alike. The situation seems unprecedented; to many in the health care professions it is as offensive as it is uncomfortable.

All of this is very much in the here and now; conditions so novel and unsettling minimize concern for the past. "What are the hospitals' *real* problems," a questioner asked me at a seminar some months ago, "aside from emotions and history?" But both history and emotions are fused reality; attitudes and historically determined interests are as "real," and can be as constraining, as any other marketplace variable. What individuals assume, value, and anticipate are structuring – and, in fact, structural – elements in defining the boundaries within which economic and professional motives operate.

And although many of the key elements in today's medical care system seem to have come into being during the past quarter-century, they have been built upon well-established foundations. As early as the 1920s, indeed, the fundamental aspects of our contemporary hospital system were already in place. Even then, most Americans expected a great deal of these impressive institutions and such enthusiastic anticipations were already tied to a vision of the hospital as scientific and therapeutically efficacious. No longer was it merely a refuge for the poor alone, as it had been since its origins in the eighteenth century and throughout the nineteenth.[4] By the same time, an intense and intimate relationship between the hospital and medical profession had also come into being. The ambiguous and contradictory image of the hospital as social service institution, on the one hand, and, on the other, as purveyor of technically defined and legitimated services was already well established. This confusion was paralleled and exacerbated by the voluntary hospital's place in an ill-defined terrain between the public and private sectors.

There have certainly been major changes in health care and for hospitals since the Second World War, among them, the emerging role of the federal government, the expansion of third-party payment, and the enormous and capital-intensive growth of technical capacity. But all of these elements of change were assimilated into a system already rigid and

---

4 Mental illness provided the only consistent exception to this generalization. Private asylums were able attract a middle- and upper-class clientele from among families who would never have considered hospital treatment for a family member with a normal – that is, less troublesome and less stigmatizing – ailment.

precisely articulated, strengthening, rather than challenging, the fundamental aspects of that system.

The hospital medicalized

By 1920, the hospital and the medical profession had negotiated an
intricate symbiosis. It began with education and staffing and was by no
means a novel relationship. The hospital had always been important to the
training and status of a small group of elite urban practitioners. Ambitious
and well-connected medical students had always sought training on the
wards; senior physicians expected to teach on those same wards; hospital
trustees had always assumed that their staffing needs would be met by the
volunteer labor of local practitioners. Though the hospital had in this sense
long been important to elite medical careers, it was not until the twentieth
century that it became central in the education and certification of every
regularly licensed physician in an increasingly bureaucratic and tightly
ordered medical profession.

The hospital had also become important to the delivery of medical care.
During the first century of American independence, none but the urban
poor would ordinarily have been hospital patients; in the 1920s, however,
Americans of every class and almost every locality might be treated in a
hospital bed. Although the great majority of the sick were still treated at
home in the 1920s, life-threatening ills and surgery were firmly associated
with the hospital and its professional staff, its laboratories, and its antiseptic
operating room. The hospital had already become a fundamental and
quality-defining element in American medical care.

Both the legitimacy and the allure of the hospital turned on the perception of its healing promise and the necessarily technical basis for such
therapeutic expectations. Disease was a discrete and specific condition; the
task of hospital medicine was to intervene in its course. Those physicians
who practiced the most visible and visibly efficacious of such techniques
enjoyed particularly high status. Surgery fit neatly into this pattern of
prestige and expectation, as did the management of both acute infectious
ills and life-threatening episodes in the course of a chronic disease.

Yet, as was apparent to students of medical care by the 1920s and 1930s,
the crusade against infectious diseases seemed to have already borne fruit.
Cholera and smallpox had vanished from the average physician's practice;
typhoid and diphtheria were no longer major problems, and even the
incidence of tuberculosis, the greatest killer of the previous century, was
rapidly declining. With this decrease in communicable disease and the
rapid aging of the American population, the burden of medical care shifted

increasingly to "constitutional" and degenerative ills, geriatrics, and mental illness. Perceptive students of medical policy were already contending that an older population implied the need for expanded chronic and long-term care.[5]

But the hospital of the 1920s and 1930s had already become a relatively inflexible, acute-care-oriented institution. Contemporaries concerned with public health and social medicine were well aware of what they regarded as a one-sided – and disproportionately costly – emphasis on acute beds at the expense of chronic care facilities. And this was only one of a variety of criticisms leveled at the hospital's social role.

As early as the first decade of the present century, a diverse array of reformers had called for a recasting of hospital resources. One familiar criticism urged the need for more convalescent and extended care beds. Another asked for increased outreach – treating the patient as a member of a particular family and community, and not simply as a diagnosis.[6] Public health nursing blossomed during this period; and it too was characterized by an emphasis on the costs and rigidity of inpatient hospital services and the need for flexible outpatient care and the prevention of disease through education.[7] Public health workers also saw a need for more aggressive approaches to the shaping of individual regimen; diet, cleanliness, and even eugenical counseling needed to be brought to the ordinary family. Other advocates of health care reform called for an expansion of outpatient clinics and dispensaries and for increased investment in the new profession of medical social service; the hospital had to be seen as one aspect of a co-ordinated and community-oriented medical care system – not as a socially unaware, procedure-oriented repair shop. Patients were still people – and family members – when they were being treated in a hospital's wards and rooms; and they were still its patients after they left a hospital's beds.

But such reformist arguments had little impact. Outreach was tainted with the aura of charity medicine and in some of its aspects seemed to threaten the private practitioner's still often-shaky economic prospects. In the 1920s, for example, organized medicine opposed government support for both venereal disease and maternal and child health clinics. High status

---

5 See, for example, Ernst P. Boas and Nicholas Michelson, *The Challenge of Chronic Diseases* (New York: The MacMillan Company, 1929); Boas, *The Unseen Plague: Chronic Disease* (New York: J. J. Augustin, 1940); Mary C. Jarrett, *Chronic Illness in New York City*, 2 vols. (New York: Columbia University Press for the Welfare Council of New York City, 1933).

6 This paragraph is based on the discussion in Rosenberg, *Care of Strangers*, ch. 13, "The New-Model Hospital and its Critics," pp. 310–360.

7 For the most recent history of public health nursing, see Karen Buhler-Wilkerson, "False Dawn: The Rise and Decline of Public Health Nursing, 1900–30" (unpublished Ph.D. diss., University of Pennsylvania, 1984).

within clinical and hospital medicine was routinely awarded to those who intervened most dramatically and in clearly mechanistic terms; surgeons enjoyed such prestige, as did fledgling cardiologists – and, of course, the more prominent consultants in what we would now call internal medicine. Psychiatrists and outpatient physicians seemed more marginal to the medical enterprise.[8]

Consistently enough, staff and house-officer positions at chronic disease facilities were hard to fill; such institutions were depressing, the capacities of medicine in them minimal, and the "victories" of therapeutics few and fleeting. Managing long-term illness offered little to the most prestigious hospitals or to the great majority of ambitious young men. The older patient was, of course, often seen by highly trained, prestigious, and flourishing specialists – surgeons and cardiologists, for example, confident in their technical skills and hardly enthusiastic about the prospect of referring clients to another specialist. It is not surprising that geriatrics should have languished for most of the twentieth century.

Within the hospital of the 1920s, technical resources had become increasingly important – both as symbol and in substance. A gleaming antiseptic operating room and laboratories for clinical pathology and radiology served to justify an increasing concentration of personnel and capital resources. Even though nursing might have been equally significant in the actual delivery of hospital care, it failed to rouse the enthusiasm of hospital publicists – or of prospective donors. The hopes of laypeople and the new-found confidence of physicians turned on the promise of medicine's new diagnostic and therapeutic tools. The techniques that had banished so many infectious ills promised to be the most appropriate for dealing with degenerative disease as well.

Technology had also been integrated in a practical way into the hospital's day-to-day routine. At the turn of the century only antiseptic surgery had been an important aspect of hospital therapeutics; by the 1920s, both diagnosis and treatment had become increasingly technical, less and less easily practiced in the patient's home. Surgery had expanded dramatically, and clinical pathology, radiological diagnosis and therapeutics, and even the beginnings of electrocardiography were gradually – if as yet inconsistently – being incorporated into the average patient's hospital experience.[9]

8 It is not surprising that medical career choices reflected – and still reflect – such intraprofessional status relationships. But this is not simply a sociological truism, it is a political reality, a constraint that helps define policy choices within both specific hospitals and the health care system generally.

9 Certain diagnostic *tools* – the laryngoscope, ophthalmoscope, otoscope – had become a part of regular practice by the last quarter of the nineteenth century. These were not of course limited to hospital use, but were associated with specialty practice, which was in its turn associated disproportionately with hospitals.

This was an economic as well as medical evolution. At the beginning of the twentieth century, laboratory costs had seemed enormous for hard-pressed hospital budgets, but with the increase in numbers of private patients came the gradual realization that technical procedures could pay for themselves, as well as upgrade the hospital's image and improve the quality of care offered to its patients. The discovery that separate charges could be imposed for the use of an operating room, for laboratory tests, and for the work of pathologists, anesthesiologists, and radiologists meant that investment in technology could pay for itself (and, if carefully managed, could become a source of profit).

It was not surprising, then, that psychiatry, public health, and outpatient medicine should have occupied relatively low positions in medicine's status hierarchy in the decades between the wars. They represented, in their various ways, parts of the medical enterprise that seemed the least promising, the softest, and the most inconsistent with the reductionist, technical, and often impressively efficacious style of practice that had become associated with the medical profession. For all these reasons, the general hospital had become a more explicitly *medical* institution, while the meaning and legitimacy of that medicalization was construed – by both laypersons and physicians – in technical terms. Hospitals had become the appropriate place for practicing the most efficacious and prestigious medicine; such had hardly been the case a half century earlier.

But if the hospital had become "medicalized" by the 1920s, it must be emphasized that the medical profession had by the same time become hospitalized. Bedside training now began in the medical student's undergraduate years and continued through a compulsory internship – and for the more ambitious, through a residency as well. The house officers' intense, shared experience was an important element in the *esprit de corps* and self-image of physicians, regardless of where they were ultimately to practice. Specialists and consultants, of course, practiced in a hospital setting, while admitting privileges were important to the majority of general practitioners no matter how small or large their local community. All medical functions – including teaching, research, and specialty training at university hospitals – were structured into a care-based staffing system. Though many medical school faculty and attending physicians pursued clinical investigation in the 1920s, almost none boasted appointments explicitly designated and funded as research positions. The habit of confounding care, teaching, and research had its beginnings long before the advent of government research grants and fellowship programs. The status hierarchy in which teaching hospitals and their associated clinical facilities stood at the apex of influence – and philanthropic funding – had already been established.

The voluntary hospital: Public and private, neither and both

American voluntary hospitals have never been private except in the narrowest legal sense. Until the recent past, the great majority of America's important and influential hospitals were either explicitly municipal or not-for-profit institutions operating for the common good. Such hospitals paid no taxes, were immune from civil suits, and received a variety of subsidies from state and local governments. Their governing boards assumed that they acted as stewards of society's resources, which were to be expended in pursuit of the general welfare. A for-profit sector has existed ever since nineteenth-century surgeons rented houses in which to treat private patients, but until recent years it has never played a significant role in the provision of medical care.[10] Both the hospital's healing function and the presumably selfless and necessarily benevolent nature of that defining purpose have always guaranteed that hospitals would be clothed with the public interest. Their mission constituted a "sacred trust" that differentiated the hospital corporation's activities from those of an ordinary marketplace actor.

Consistently enough, cities and states have supported voluntary hospitals since the founding of Pennsylvania Hospital in 1751.[11] Even explicitly religious institutions have been the beneficiaries of public subsidies. In the realm of ideology, however, Americans have historically held fast to one consistent distinction among hospitals, but it was not the distinction between public and private that a lawyer might have understood and defended. It was a traditional differentiation between almshouse and hospital, between municipal – or county – and voluntary institution, between welfare and technical functions, and between the "unworthy" and "worthy" poor.

The eighteenth- and early nineteenth-century almshouse was an undifferentiated receptacle for the "dependent," as the conventional phraseology termed those unable or unwilling to work. Almshouse inmates

---

10 Private sanitoria for the care of mental illness, alcoholism, drug addiction, and tuberculosis have had a long history as well, but one little studied by historians. And in many small towns, of course, hospitals owned by individual physicians provided the only inpatient facilities into the 1920s and 1930s. In other communities, so-called industrial hospitals, operated by mining, railroading, or lumbering corporations, played a similar role.

11 On the history of the Quaker-sponsored Pennsylvania Hospital, see William H. Williams, *America's First Hospital: The Pennsylvania Hospital 1751–1841* (Wayne, Pa.: Haverford House, 1976); Thomas G. Morton, assisted by Frank Woodbury, *The History of the Pennsylvania Hospital 1751–1895* (Philadelphia: Times Printing House, 1895).

included the mentally and physically handicapped, the aged, the infant, and the sick. In larger cities, medical care and medical personnel soon became important in local almshouses, for many of those inhabiting almshouse beds were, in fact, the sick and the chronically ill aged – even if they had been admitted as "indigent." The categories "sick" as opposed to "indigent," "worthy" as opposed to "unworthy," dissolve under closer inspection: Were the chronically ill in the almshouse sick people deserving sympathy or indigent paupers unwilling to support themselves and thus deserving contempt or censure? To ask the question is to underline the arbitrariness of these labels.

But the tenacious belief in a fundamental distinction between the culpably dependent and the guiltless victim of random sickness was important to nineteenth-century Americans. It served not only to justify a frugal regimen at almshouse facilities, but also as a major argument to justify the founding of our pioneer nineteenth-century hospitals.[12]

The contentions of hospital advocates in the nineteenth century seemed reasonable and equitable. It was unfair to subject the honest working man or woman to demeaning contacts within the almshouse's stigmatizing walls. A hospital open only to the remediable sick could be presented as a very different sort of institution, one in which no factor other than sickness itself determined eligibility for admission. It was consistent that admission policies at most such voluntary hospitals categorically excluded the presumed victims of their own misdeeds, such as syphilitics, alcoholics, and unmarried mothers.[13]

The provision of medical care outside an almshouse setting was a necessary path to reform. So long as acutely ill patients were treated in the almshouse, the dominance of chronic and geriatric ailments would make the institution unattractive to elite physicians concerned with the hospital's potential teaching role. So long as laypeople were aware that admission to a municipal hospital was determined exclusively by dependence, they would regard the institution with fear and hostility. To be treated in New York's Bellevue, Chicago's Cook County, or the Philadelphia General Hospital

---

12 One thinks, for example, of hospitals as diverse as the Massachusetts General, Hartford, and New York's Episcopal, Mount Sinai, and Presbyterian. Even some municipal hospitals, such as the Boston City (opened 1864), were established in the hope of creating an explicitly *medical* institution – one in which the sick would not be stigmatized while receiving care.

13 Most nineteenth-century hospitals also excluded the chronically ill, on the assumption that limited resources should be devoted to those who might be cured and returned to the work force. This necessarily consigned the often worthy poor to the almshouse in their declining years. It was a moral inconsistency that disturbed some nineteenth-century hospital advocates who urged that private institutions find a place for the care of such unfortunates.

was to admit a culpable lack of options. Moreover, the frugal tradition of "less eligibility" meant that the municipal hospital's internal standards of diet and amenities would routinely be maintained at a minimum level. No one, after all, was to be encouraged to prefer public alms to even the most meager wages earned by their own efforts.

No respectable Americans were more aware of grim municipal hospital conditions than the physicians who practiced in them. It is no accident that staff physicians at such institutions were leaders in calling for the severing of hospital from welfare services. They sought to make the municipal hospital exclusively a healing institution, subject to the claims and judgments of medical science and no longer hostage to political expediency and to the crushing and irremediable burden of poverty and incapacity. Key to the logic of such reform pleas was an often-expressed faith in medicine's healing capacity, and the egalitarian corollary that every individual had a right of access to such undeniably therapeutic resources. This technological entitlement implied an increasing gap between the hospital's welfare and curative functions. It was consistent, moreover, with intellectual trends in the medical profession and the parallel lay attitudes that granted the highest status to those aspects of medicine that promised cure in a categorical and visibly technical form. Insofar as human sickness could be defined in technical – and, in practice, episodic – terms, medical care made a strong appeal for public sympathy and support. Yet much of public medical care was in fact devoted to the chronic and multidimensional miseries of families and individuals; it was difficult to subsume such grim realities to the most prestigious aspects of the hospital system.[14] The social worker or would-be improver of maternal diets has always fared poorly in comparison with the surgeon.

The pressure for increased access to hospital facilities implicit in a growing faith in medical capacities had a number of consequences in the 1920s and 1930s. One was a widely shared concern with the fact that the most technologically advanced medicine seemed available only to the very poor and very rich. The hospital ward and its subsidized beds were still marked by the stigmatizing aura of charity, while the private room with its capacity to protect individual sensibilities was limited to a small percentage

14 Average lengths of stay decreased substantially at the end of the nineteenth and beginning of the twentieth century. The increase in surgery seems to have been one factor, the careful avoidance of chronic cases another. The residue of old age and chronic illness remained the responsibility of county and municipal facilities. Not surprisingly, average length-of-stay and death rates remained higher at such institutions than those prevailing at their voluntary contemporaries. See also Chapter 9 of this volume and Harry F. Dowling, *City Hospitals: The Undercare of the Underprivileged* (Cambridge, Mass.: Harvard University Press, 1982).

of Americans. One solution, of course, was the construction of "semi-private" wings or buildings intended to serve the needs of middle-class men and women. The assumed prerogatives of class and the equally unquestioned public mission of the not-for-profit hospital made such solutions plausible. But beneath these experiments in hospital care for middle-income Americans lay a powerful conviction: if the hospital and its technical skills provided the best hope for cure, then every American should have access to these resources.

The emergence of third-party payers

The Great Depression raised the stakes in the 1930s; new solutions had to be found, tactics that would preserve both the hospital's fiscal integrity and the middle-class patient's access to the institution. The creation of Blue Cross and Blue Shield was one outcome of this configuration of need, interest, and assumption.[15] These prepaid insurance schemes also reflected the peculiar status of the hospital as clothed with the public interest and somehow above the marketplace. Faith in medicine's technical capacities – as centered in the hospital – guaranteed that these prepayment mechanisms would occupy the generally unquestioned place of quasi-public agencies, but would be little constrained by public supervision.

These assumptions, coupled with bureaucratic necessity, led the Blue Cross and Blue Shield to adopt administrative strategies that reified and exacerbated the reign of acute, reductionist models in health care. No disease was legitimate unless it could be coded in a nosological scheme. The schematic logic that divided medical care interactions into the specifically diagnosable and thus legitimately reimbursable, as opposed to the preventive or chronic, paralleled in another sphere the distinction between worthy and unworthy poor, between the voluntary and almshouse hospital. It reflected as well existing professional priorities that put acute individual care at center stage and placed preventive and chronic care on the periphery.

At the same time, of course, this particular mechanism entrenched all those interests that benefited from it, including hospitals, the doctors who practiced in them, and every participant in the "health industry." Nevertheless, physicians maintained a key role in the generally expanding system. For if the labeling of a discrete ailment legitimated the expenditure of dollars, it remained solely within the power of physicians to affix those

15 For a lucid brief discussion of these events, see Paul Starr, *The Social Transformation of American Medicine* (New York: Basic Books, 1982), pp. 290–334.

labels and thus channel and legitimate reimbursement.[16] The emergence of Medicare and Medicaid in the mid-1960s did not challenge the ideological assumptions or interests embedded in preexisting prepayment schemes; they simply added a deep new pocket to subsidize an existing system.

It is hardly surprising that powerful interests should have found this a comfortable environment: a controlled context in which cost-plus procurement replaced normal, and sometimes chastening, market transactions. Third-party payment has in general reflected the interest of providers but has never been perceived in this potentially critical and antagonistic way by most Americans; the convenient and deeply rooted blurring of distinctions between the public and private sectors, between the technical and the egalitarian, helped disarm such skepticism. It is paralleled by the way in which programs that largely benefit middle-class constituencies, such as Medicare and tax deductions for home mortgage interest, have been perceived as rights, while those designed to help the less fortunate, such as Medicaid and rent subsidies, are seen as welfare and thus demeaning. In a fundamental way, these examples parallel the attitudes expressed in an older set of polarities that distinguished between almshouse and hospital, public and private, and welfare maintenance and scientific healing.

Cultural values, medical expectations, and hospital growth

The American hospital is an American institution. As such, it partakes of and reflects more general aspects of American cultural values. It has also been seen as particularly praiseworthy, the product of a local, and in more recent years national, commitment to community in the highly valued – and value-legitimating – form of advanced technology. Throughout their history, Americans have esteemed countries and communities able to mobilize advanced technology as a social resource; such societies have seemed more admirable, more moral, somehow higher on the scale of worthiness.[17]

Thus boosterism provided one motivation for the rapid spread of hos-

16 This is not to suggest that all physicians had uniform interests or occupied the same niches; but the system supported, in different ways, academicians and general practitioners, big-city specialists and small-town surgeons. It was a formula that muted the potential diversity of interest among such medical men, so long as the system kept expanding.

17 One need only be reminded of nineteenth-century Western assumptions that the steamboat, the telegraph, the power loom, and the repeating rifle were naturally associated with the moral and social superiority of Christianity. A less developed technology was presumed to be the inevitable counterpart of "lesser" religions and their far-from-admirable moral order.

pitals during the years between the late 1880s and 1910; community pride began to demand that every middle-sized town support one of these public amenities. Such sentiments found natural allies in local practitioners who urged the founding of hospitals and volunteered to staff them. No forward-looking physician wanted to practice less than the best possible medicine, or lose his prosperous patients to consultants in larger communities with better facilities. X-ray equipment and facilities for aseptic surgery were perceived as fundamental needs by 1910, even if some communities could not muster the resources to build and maintain the hospital in which such costly facilities seemed naturally to dwell.[18]

Communities wanted hospitals not only because they provided trained nurses and twenty-four-hour care, but because they seemed to incorporate and represent the most scientific and technically advanced form of the healing art. These were decades during which most prosperous and educated Americans were fascinated both by the regalia and the rhetoric of science, even if the content remained open to debate. This was a period during which the art of warfare became military science, and when domestic science, library science, and political science all came into being. In retrospect, it seems obvious that the impact of the laboratory on medicine's therapeutic capacities still lay largely in the future; but Americans had been enormously impressed by a seeming transformation in medical knowledge during the years between 1880 and the 1920s. Newspapers and magazines were quick to report the discovery that many of humankind's greatest killers were caused by specific microorganisms. They were equally enthusiastic in reporting that some of these ills could be averted through preventive "inoculations" or, in other instances, cured by the injection of substances discovered and manufactured in the laboratory. The public health worker's ability to evaluate water quality, to diagnose ailments, and to disclose healthy carriers of disease through the use of serological tests or bacteriological screening seemed enormously encouraging.

Physicians as well as laypeople accepted the promise of these new techniques with comparatively few reservations. Most ignored or were unaware of the fact that medicine still possessed few tools for intervening decisively in the course of an infectious disease once the illness had been contracted. Some physicians in the first decades of the twentieth century did worry that traditional clinical skills and human interactions would be ignored in an uncritical obeisance to the laboratory and its enticing new tools. But they represented a minority position. The elite in American

18 Physicians also benefited from the saving of time implied by the concentration of seriously ill or postoperative patients in a community hospital and the availability of trained nurses. Without such facilities a busy practitioner would have had to make frequent home visits and arrange for patients' nursing care.

medicine were increasingly converts to this new dispensation, not so much in the role of full-time researchers or laboratory scientists, but as specialists and purveyors of the laboratory's products in diagnosis and treatment. It is no accident that private philanthropy turned with a novel, and increasing, generosity to the medical profession and medical institutions, that state legislatures proved themselves increasingly willing to support state university medical schools, and that municipalities sought to upgrade their health facilities. In each case, the reform rationale turned on the vision and promise of medicine as applied science.

These attitudes about medicine were coupled with an older American faith in technology, with the ordinarily unstated but deeply felt conviction that if something could be done, it should be done. And the healing of sickness provided an emotionally resonant and seemingly disinterested goal to justify the mobilization of social resources. This complex of assumptions about science and its necessary application constituted a compelling argument for the proliferation of hospitals and progressive upgrading of the technology that had come to provide their fundamental rationale.

To the extent that the provision of institutional health care could be uncoupled from its welfare heritage and defined in technical terms, it could mobilize powerful attitudinal support. Every human being was entitled to life and health, and if technology could provide or safeguard those equities, it should be made to do so. It is not surprising that the need to improve the numbers and quality of hospitals in America's more deprived and isolated areas was a major concern of medical policy analysts, foundation advisors, and thoughtful physicians generally in the 1920s.

Health and healing had come to play an important role in a secular society, a society that was at the same time increasingly ill-equipped to deal with acute illness and death outside an institutional context. Funds to implement these assumptions became increasingly available after the Second World War. At the same time, technology grew rapidly in complexity and cost, increasing budgetary pressures and adding substance to arguments for expanding and renovating hospital facilities. Thus occurred the intersection of material and attitudinal factors that provided the legitimacy and guaranteed the inevitability of escalating hospital expenditures; it was demeaning to place a price on a person's life or on his or her freedom from pain and incapacity. So long as the calculation could be seen in terms of a procedure or practice that might or might not be performed, the decision-making gradient would clearly be inclined in the direction of making that procedure available. And more and more of such procedures became real options in the decades after 1950; renal dialysis and coronary bypass surgery are only two such examples among a host of others. Quibbling over mundane dollars seemed inappropriate in the face of

transcendent goals. The bottom line was that there was no bottom line –
and costs climbed dramatically in a highly bureaucratic and capital-intensive
enterprise.

In this sense, it would not be inappropriate to compare hospital costs
with defense expenditures. In both cases money is spent in pursuit of a
transcendent goal, in the one case "security," in the other "health." In
both cases, cost-cutting could be equated with penny-pinching, an unworthy aim, given the gravity of the social goals involved.

In both areas material interests obviously play a role; hospitals, doctors,
and medical suppliers, like defense contractors and the military, have
interests expressed in and through the political process. But ideas are
significant as well: it is impossible to understand our defense budget
without factoring in the power of ideology; it is impossible to understand
the nature and style of America's health care expenditures without an
understanding of the ideological allure of scientific medicine and the
promise of healing. Both the Massachusetts General Hospital and General
Dynamics Corporation operate in the marketplace, but they are not bound
by market discipline; and both also mock the presumed distinction between
public and private that places them both in the category of private enterprise.

Ordering a disordered institution

Like many other institutions, the hospital of the 1920s had become a self-
consciously rational and efficient institution. It was no accident that the
efficiency movement helped shape the rhetoric and, to a lesser extent, the
practice of hospital administrators, just as it had factory and public school
administrators. At the same time, the hospital still bore the marks of its
humanitarian and paternalist origins. (Religious hospitals in particular still
reflected community values in a variety of ways.) Hospital workers were
paid less than their similarly skilled peers, and compensated with a presumed paternalist security. House officers and student nurses still bartered
their time for credentials and experience.

Nevertheless, the great majority of hospitals sought to follow the much-
admired pattern of other large enterprises: the army, the corporation,
the factory. The most efficient use of limited funds implied the careful
evaluation of expenditures; exhaustive record-keeping, it was contended,
guaranteed more consistent and higher-quality medical care as well as
the possibility of monitoring and controlling costs. Few contemporaries
anticipated circumstances in which conflict might arise between bureaucratic efficiency and the quality of care ultimately experienced by individual
patients.

In any case, it is clear that key aspects of the hospital's internal order had been transformed by the 1920s; the hospital was a very different institution from its mid-nineteenth-century predecessor. One such aspect was the professionalization of administration, another, and perhaps even more important, was the professionalization of nursing.

Nothing was – and is – more significant than nursing in shaping a hospital's internal life.[19] And the day-to-day routine of patient care in large and medium-sized hospitals of the 1920s was controlled by a staff composed largely of student nurses, supervised by a cadre of more experienced training school graduates. (In small hospitals, a trained nurse might serve simultaneously as superintendent and chief nurse.) A decisive gap had been opened between the patient as object of care and the nurse as would-be professional, allied in some necessary, if ordinarily subservient, way with the staff physicians who oversaw and legitimated the provision of that care. In earlier periods hospital nurses had been recruited from among recovered patients or from the community's servant class. They were not expected to identify with physicians or to see themselves as professional in their training or prerogatives. In the first decades of the twentieth century, nurse administrators were well aware of their less-than-secure professional identity and, lacking a prestigious and laboratory-oriented body of knowledge, dedicated themselves all the more tenaciously to the ideals of order and efficiency.

Hospital administrators, too, had come a long way from their nineteenth-century origins. Prudence, morality, and a bit of business experience described the qualities desired in a mid-nineteenth-century hospital superintendent. Trustees neither assumed nor expected any specific experience in the man entrusted with the day-to-day administration of their institution.[20] By the 1920s, however, the situation was rather different. Given the superintendent's expanded and diversified duties, most authorities agreed that experience and vocational commitment were a necessity for the job, especially in large institutions. There was some disagreement as to whether medical or lay superintendents might be more appropriate, but "professionalism" was assumed. A hospital superintendents' association was organized in 1899, and textbooks and specialized journals had already become available for the would-be hospital chief executive.[21]

The place of the medical profession in the hospital of the 1920s was

---

19 For an important recent study, see Susan M. Reverby, *Ordered to Care: The Dilemma of American Nursing, 1850–1945* (Cambridge: Cambridge University Press, 1987).

20 I use "man" advisedly, inasmuch as large urban hospitals engaged only males as superintendents. A few smaller hospitals for women and children, the Boston Lying-in Hospital, for example, did hire women as "matrons," but such instances were atypical.

21 See Rosenberg, *Care of Strangers*, ch. 11, "A Careful Oversight: Reshaping Authority," pp. 262–285.

more prominent as well as more formal than it had been in previous generations. The hospital had become more explicity and self-consciously a technical institution; medical knowledge appeared increasingly effective and decreasingly accessible to lay understanding. It seemed both natural and appropriate that medical practitioners and medical judgments should play a commanding role in hospital governance. Physicians determined admissions policies and, often, capital expenditures as well. These areas of decision-making had been tenaciously contested in the previous century – when even individual admissions might be questioned by lay trustees or superintendents.[22]

Matters were quite different by the 1920s. Whether an institution was headed by a trained physician or not, its chief executive was bound to defer to the opinion of his or her medical staff. Such deference was particularly unavoidable in those hospitals dependent on private patient fees for substantial portions of their annual income. An administrator could hardly ignore the needs and opinions of physicians whose referrals filled private rooms. The faith in scientific medicine that helped encourage the new-found willingness of respectable Americans to enter hospitals motivated a more general lay deference in any area that could be construed as technical. Hospital decision-making was increasingly responsive to physicians and medical knowledge.

Meanwhile, every stage of the physician's career was becoming embedded in the hospital – in the large teaching hospitals most prominently, but to a degree in every institution. The needs of certification and teaching helped define the role and duties of house officers, and wedded individual hospitals to a national network of certifying agencies. Accreditation made the individual hospital and its traditionally autonomous governing board subject to external bureaucratic control. Less concretely, but perhaps even more important, the individual hospital was subordinate to the dictates of an internationally agreed-upon body of medical knowledge. Such knowledge had a variety of implications – from the way in which surgical and radiological facilities should be built and maintained to appropriate doctor – patient ratios.[23] The hospital was well along in its shift from a paternal-

22 Early in the nineteenth century *all* admissions had to be approved individually by lay boards; the situation shifted gradually in the course of the century as the prestige of medical judgments increased and trustees moved gradually away from day-to-day hospital oversight.

23 The prestige of scientific medicine also legitimated hospital accreditation and the acceptance of bedside undergraduate teaching, internship, and residency programs. For a useful account of these developments, see Stevens, *American Medicine and the Public Interest*, and for the best recent account of scientific medicine and academic reform, see Kenneth M. Ludmerer, *Learning to Heal: The Development of American Medical Education* (New York: Basic Books, 1985).

istic institution controlled by local laypersons and reflecting traditional ideas of stewardship, to a professionally dominated and bureaucratically ordered institution responsive to national and even international standards and constraints.

The hospital had also entered, if somewhat more tentatively, the impersonal world of market transactions. In some ways, as suggested earlier, the hospital in the 1920s still bore the marks of its origins in a very different sort of society. The barter of services for credentials, of work for status, and of lower wages for paternalistic security still played an important role, but cash transactions were becoming increasingly important. A few physicians were paid in dollars, especially by those institutions too small or undesirable to attract volunteer labor in the form of interns and residents. Even more important was the growing role of fee-for-service practice within the hospital. Both the promise and vulnerability of the hospital rested on its ability to attract and care for paying patients. This in itself constituted a major change from earlier periods. But it reflected another reality as well: the emergence of the hospital as an important aspect of care for the wealthy and middle-class, as well as for the poor. The changing expectations and practice patterns that had helped bring about this change would play a key role in maintaining the centrality of the hospital through the lean years of the Depression and into the increasingly obese years that were to follow.

Decentralization of control, centralization of reality

As early as the turn of the century, would-be hospital reformers sought to address the institution's individualistic and seemingly anarchic nature. It was thought that regional planning and the imposition of agreed-upon standards might result in more efficient use of social resources. Philadelphia and New York, for example, sponsored organizations (both still in existence) aimed at achieving these ends.[24] But as contemporaries agreed, their effectiveness was limited. Rivalry for prestige, and competition for government and philanthropic support and for a limited supply of private patients overwhelmed the impulse toward rationalization and the subordination of institutional egos. In big cities, especially, the shared commitment to scientific medicine implied that no institution would willingly provide "second-rate" facilities to its patients; ethnic, regional, and individual loyalties guaranteed that a functional, explicit, and necessarily hierarchical division of labor would not easily be accepted.

24 I refer to the United Hospital Fund in New York and the Delaware Valley Hospital Council in Philadelphia.

That there was little effective planning does not mean that there were no policies. The strength of social expectations, needs, and attitudes, and the power of medical knowledge and the institutional requirements of medical careers, imposed similar developmental patterns on hospitals of widely diverse origin. (A number of these parallels have been discussed earlier.) But at the same time, of course, hospitals had diverged by the 1920s so as to differ in ways that have come to seem both natural and familiar a half-century later. At the top of the hospital hierarchy were America's most prestigious and influential teaching hospitals – for example, Presbyterian in New York, Massachusetts General in Boston, and Barnes in St. Louis – many of them already dynamic elements in growing "medical centers" as they assimilated or attracted smaller and more specialized institutions. Ranked somewhat below them in status were the more prestigious municipal and voluntary hospitals in the nation's largest cities. Finally, there were the so-called community hospitals, institutions defined by their local sponsorship, patient population, and involvement fundamentally in the delivery of care, rather than in the teaching of a new generation of physicians or the accumulation of research findings. It does not require a great leap of imagination to recognize the late twentieth-century future in the already vigorous hospital establishment that served Americans in the 1920s.

Structured crisis: The 1980s

The perceived hospital crisis of the 1980s had its roots in the years immediately following the Second World War. Science had never seemed more relevant, while the long pent-up economy provided resources for hospital expansion. The Hill-Burton Act (1946) granted funds for hospital construction, while the National Institutes of Health supported research and training (and, indirectly, hospital teaching and staffing). Employee-connected third-party payment expanded as well, providing a reliable, predictable, and expanding stream of revenue for previously hard-pressed institutional budgets. With the passage of Medicare and Medicaid in the 1960s, the system was complete. Health care seemed to be in the national interest and few congressmen could, or wished to, oppose so benevolent a source of jobs, contracts, and services to constituents.[25] Similarly, corporations and unions negotiated health insurance into contracts, and passed the costs along to consumers. Despite its initial opposition to third-party pay-

---

25 The class-free aspect of Medicare was to have an extremely important political impact. By using age rather than need as a criterion for eligibility, the program was able to build powerful support, while seeming to sever itself from the taint of welfare medicine.

ment schemes and federal involvement in reimbursement, organized medicine soon adjusted to this new world of guaranteed income, while hospitals expanded in the reassuring context of predictable negotiated rates.

At first, the expanding health care system seemed to be one in which everyone benefited and no one paid excessively. Certainly there remained a diversity of interest among corporations and their employees, physicians and hospitals, hospital administrators and hospital workers, the young and the old, and the employed and the unemployed, but with a steadily increasing revenue stream, potential antagonisms remained largely latent. The hospital functioned as a seemingly politically neutral and socially desirable conduit through which equities flowed to ever more generously supported constituencies. The sick received prepaid inpatient and some outpatient care; physicians, a generous income; hospital administrators, a secure and profitable salary; suppliers, enthusiastic and free-spending customers. Even nurses and workers could band together to demand salaries approaching those available in the private sector. By 1965, the system was ideally positioned for a generation of expansion.

And, for a time, it seemed that many of the older dilemmas of medical care had been bypassed. The poor could, it seemed, be treated in less stigmatizing circumstances, while the working man and woman and the middle-class family benefited from a medicine whose quality would not be constrained by cost. The technical resources of the system both structured and legitimated reimbursement. Briefly, at least, it seemed that private hospitals could and would take over the burden of poverty and dependency that traditionally had been the responsibility of municipal and (a minority of) large, urban voluntary hospitals. The egalitarian implications of a shared faith in technology made traditional distinctions between welfare and private medicine seem less and less defensible; technological entitlement became a force in itself, legitimating increasing hospital-based expenditures.

But in some fundamental ways the hospital system had changed less than the scale of its funding and the diagnostic and therapeutic tools at its disposal. The priorities and characteristics already built into American medicine a half-century earlier were in some ways only intensified by these newly abundant sources of support. The distribution of funds to existing institutions without a parallel increase in central control guaranteed that existing perceptions, structures, and priorities would determine the spending of these funds. Medical emphasis on acute care and interventionist therapeutics, for example, would hardly be questioned – nor would the status system and career patterns within the profession. The traditional conflation of education, care, and research functions continued, allowing both government and the health care system to defer difficult political and intellectual choices.

The hierarchical and increasingly academic and specialized character of late twentieth-century medicine has been accepted as necessary, even indispensable, but has created problems of priorities and personnel. No one wants to impede research or dilute the focus of the most intensely trained subspecialist; but how does one keep the prestige of such activities and individuals from skewing the provision of care? The formal egalitarianism of medical training and prerogative is belied by a far more complex and diverse reality of demands and contexts of care. Laypersons were and are part of this equation as well: they have come to expect – in fact, demand – technical solutions for problems that may have no ultimate technical resolution. We want both care and cure, humane nursing and high technology; it is only recently that it has become clear that there may be conflict structured into these expectations. Technological change brings unanticipated costs and consequences, in medicine just as in agriculture and industry.

In the 1980s, the proliferation of support for medical care has come to seem a metastatic growth, and the hospital, in particular, a brontosaurus browsing among rapidly drying swamps. It is becoming apparent that the hospital system's structure and dynamics have helped create the perception of disorder and crisis. The growth of a for-profit sector and the attempt through prospective payment systems (based on Diagnosis-Related Groups) and other reimbursement mechanisms to control expenditures are in their differing ways symptoms of the same disease. Profit-making enterprises have responded to a cost-plus environment; Medicare's DRGs are based on a literalist acceptance, a kind of *reductio ad absurdum*, of the mechanistic views of disease central both to medicine's intellectual history and to the institutional growth of hospitals and third-party payment.

Perhaps the crisis in hospital finance will stimulate some general reflections. Although that crisis seemed, in the mid-1980s, to turn on questions of financing, public dissatisfaction with hospitals implicates other aspects of health care as well. The shocked reaction to rapid private-sector growth shared by many laypersons as well as physicians and health care administrators reflects in part the deeply felt assumption that the hospital was, and is, clothed with a social mission that transcends its place as marketplace actor. It seems somehow wrong to many Americans that managers and stockholders should benefit from healing the sick.[26]

Contemporary debate has clarified a number of other issues as well. We

26 None of this is to deny that a good deal of such indignation reflects the special interests of particular institutions and individuals, who themselves benefit.

have been reminded, for example, that class and social location help
determine the nature and quality of care an individual receives, no matter
what the potentially relevant technical options. It has also become clear that
widespread acceptance of third-party payment and the assumed universal
entitlement to advanced medical care has created rigidities of its own: on
the one hand, the sense of entitlement to insurance coverage; on the other,
the growing awareness that some individuals are inadequately covered, and
others not covered at all, in a fragmented prepayment system. It has
become harder and harder to ignore the fact that some individuals have no
stable employment while others are at risk of losing that employment, and,
as a result, the health insurance that has in the past forty years come to
seem a natural right. Like reformers at the turn of the century, we have
been reminded that the modern hospital can be a dysfunctionally narrow
institution, oriented too exclusively to the episodic and the technical, as
defined and legitimated by the care of acute ills. Care must be understood
as something more than a residual category, that which is left after technical procedures have been exhausted or proved irrelevant.

While the hospital's productive capacities have been maximized, its
"product" remains problematic. The growth of faith in technology that
legitimated the need to provide quality medical care has had unforeseen
and not always desirable outcomes. We need to disaggregate the functions
of teaching, care, and research and make choices among them. We have
been reminded of some primitive truths: that technology does not always
solve problems, but may only redefine old ones or create new ones,
and that there may be conflicts between the collective interest and the
maximization of personal equities (whether those equities are garnered in
the form of dollars, status, or prestige).

The hospital can no longer conduct itself as a passive actor in a complex
medical system, serving as a trough for the distribution of social and
economic nutrients. Hospitals have interests that are not necessarily the
same as those of any particular individual or group of individuals who earn
their living in them. Our very awareness that we are experiencing a hospital
crisis, the formulation and aggressive advocacy of widely differing diagnoses and prescriptions, are all aspects of a dissatisfaction that is itself a
prerequisite to change.

For generations the hospital has seemed a necessary and inevitable, thus
laudable and legitimate, institution. Perhaps the most important truth that
has emerged in the past decade is the conviction that hospitals are not
inevitable institutional reflections of available technical capacity. Technology provides options; it does not choose among them. The American
hospital is historical and contingent; its boundaries are not necessary
but negotiated. Our contemporary sense of crisis is one aspect of an

increasingly self-conscious process through which hospitals are in fact renegotiating accustomed boundaries. But such negotiations are never easy. Boundaries reflect accustomed privileges and habits of thought. They are not redrawn without a struggle.

Index

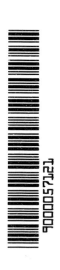